NATUROPATHY
A
CURE TO CANCER

Naturopathy
A
Cure to Cancer

Dr. Sadhna Dubey

Published by
ARAVALI BOOKS INTERNATIONAL
W-30, Okhla, Industrial Area, Phase-II
New Delhi-110020

First published 1997

© Aravali Books International 1997

All rights reserved. No part of this book may be reprinted or reproduced or utilised in any form or by any electronic, mechanical or other means, now known or hereafter invented, including photocopying and recording, or in any information storage or retrieval system, without permission in writing from the publisher.

Due care has been taken with regard to copyright matters. However, if anyone's copyright has been inadvertently infringed the author hereby offers sincere apologies. If the matter is brought to her notice, suitable acknowledgement will be made in future editions.

—Dr. Sadhna Dubey

ISBN 81-86880-30-5

Price : Rs. 625/- US$65

Designed, Typeset & Printed at New Printindia Pvt. Ltd.
8/4B, Sahibabad Industrial Area Site IV
Sahibabad, Ghaziabad India

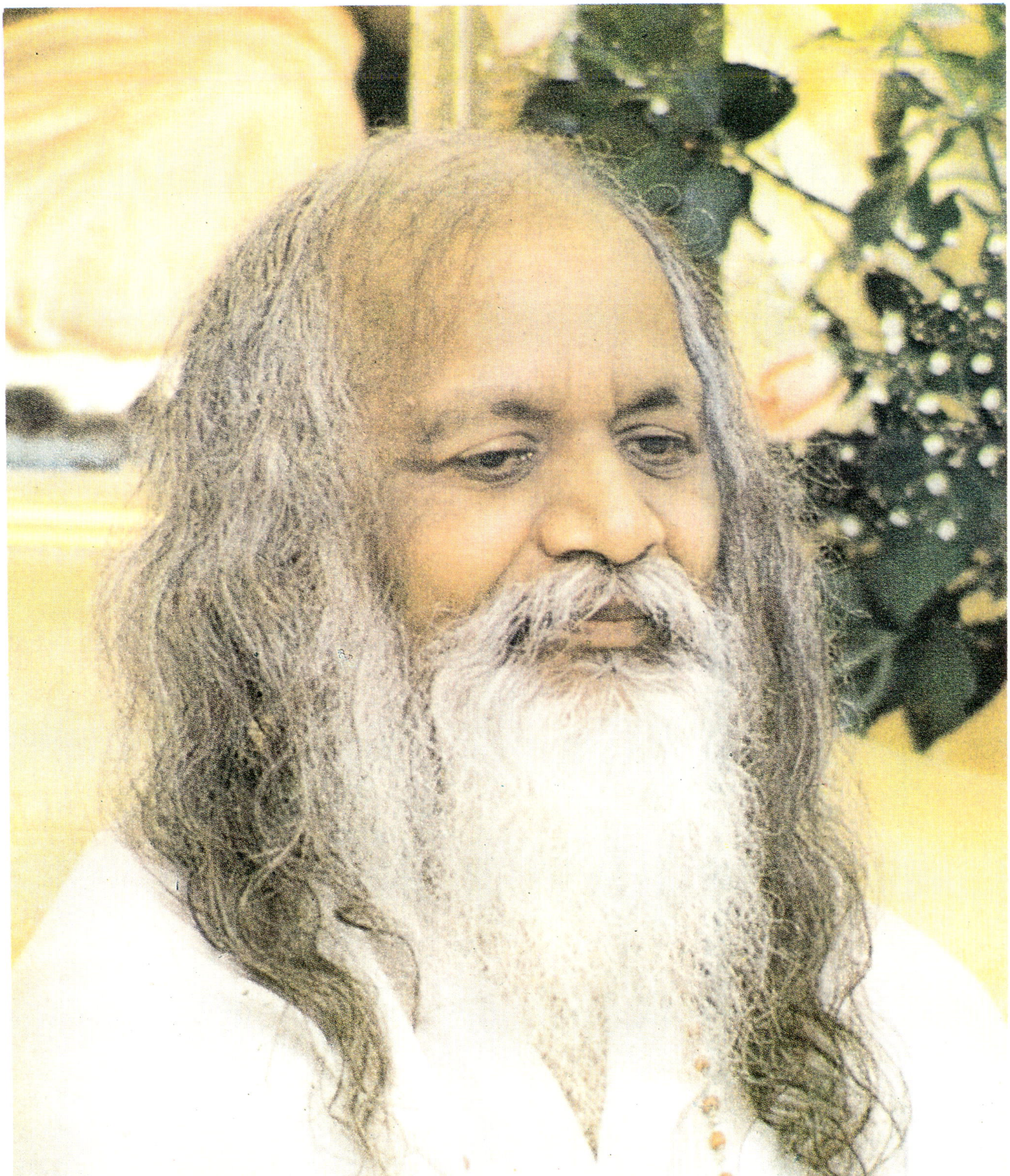

His Holiness

MAHARISHI MAHESH YOGI

Founder of the Transcendental Meditation
and TM-Sidhi Programme and the World Government
of the Age of Enlightenment

With a Full Heart and

Inspiration This Book is

Dedicated To

His Holiness Maharshi Mahesh Yogi Ji

Foreword

Cancer is as old as humanity. Its reference is given in Sushrut Bagbhta and Charak Samhita as *karta arbud.* Just as in modern medicine, a single causative factor for cancer has not been mentioned in Ayurveda. Rather most of the factors responsible for cancer have been described. The most important factor is life-style. Following wrong routine (like going to bed late, waking up late, not eating on time, etc.), bad eating habits, eating deeply fried food constantly, chemically preserved food and incompatible food over a long time could give rise to cancer of the digestive tract.

Tobacco is an important factor in causing lung cancer, cancer of the throat, larynx and pharynx. Polluted environment is also known to be causing cancer.

In modern times the incidence of cancer has gone up alarmingly. The fast pace of life, rapid industrialization creating pollution of the atmosphere, excessive use of chemical fertilizers and insecticides and over-use of chemical preservatives are the main causes.

Diagnosis of cancer in modern times has been quite satisfactory. Treatment by surgery, chemotherapy, radiotherapy, etc., has been saving lives and giving patients a new lease and better quality of life.

But almost all faculties agree that improvement in the immune status is definitely required for success in the management of cancer.

Naturopathy, which has its roots in Ayurveda, the most ancient system of health care, is known for its knowledge and practical application to improve immunity in patients.

Dr. Sadhna Dubey's book *Naturopathy: A Cure to Cancer* has dealt with this subject in great detail. All the modalities of Naturopathy treatment and yoga and pranayama aim at one thing, i.e., restoration of balance.

Modern science is now looking into the area of perfect balance, the unified field of all laws of nature, to be Samhita of Veda which is nothing but your own "self"—Pure Consciousness. So the role of Yoga and Pranayama in experiencing this state of balance is undisputed, and its effectiveness in the management of cancer is immense.

Cancer is preventable. If cancer is detected early the prognosis is good. Living a good life-style alone can keep cancer away by raising the immunity of the body. Dr. Dubey's book in this regard using Naturopathy is commendable and she has explored a new area of thrust in the management of cancer through Naturopathy. I am sure many will benefit from this book.

Brihaspati Dev Triguna

What they Say About the Book

The book *Naturopathy: A Cure to Cancer* by Dr. Sadhna Dubey makes interesting reading. The emphasis on natural methods of healing, and its importance in improving the general well-being and subsequent resistance to disease, although obvious, has not been generally appreciated. Not only that, this may even help in prevention and cure of diseases that afflict man. The book brings out this aspect in clear and easy-to-read style.

That terminal cancer can be cured by nature cure methods as described may seem a tall order—the illustration of a few cases is not convincing evidence. However, its role in preventing cancer deserves consideration. This, combined with some of the allopathic procedures, would certainly improve results.

The chapter on Naturopathic Methods of Treatment through the ages is comprehensive, and helps one to understand how Naturopathy improves the resistance of the body to fight disease. The principles and philosophy of nature cure as enumerated make sense. In this regard Section III of this manuscript deserves serious thought and is well written.

Section II describes different forms of cancer. In its treatment emphasis is on improving the resistance of the entire body to fight the local manifestations of the disease. The importance of alleviation, various psychological factors and stress by yogic exercises and meditation are well brought out. The importance of correct diet is rightly emphasized, the extensive research on diet being a causative factor in cancer, is an ongoing research; it cannot be contested, and appears plausible. In this context, the present work by using Indian herbs presents the right perspective.

By reading this book one realizes that a healthy life and relief of psychological stress by yogic meditation, a vegetarian and balanced diet which include various herbs and leafy vegetables found in nature, exercises by yogic asanas—all these would go a long way in prevention and cure of disease, including some forms of cancer.

I find this book is timely, and should be of great benefit to everyone concerned with healthy living. The book is well written, painstakingly researched and easy to comprehend. I would recommend it to all, including the medical and scientific faculty.

—*Dr. Ranbir S. Gupta*

We are pleased to certify that Ms. Sadhna Dubey was the youngest ever student to obtain a doctorate in Naturopathy. Not only did she accomplish this at the tender age of 24, but also earned a gold medal for obtaining the highest marks in her class.

Sadhna was a remarkable student in many ways. She went well beyond the normal course requirements by following up the treatment of chronic cases even after she finished her course, and by investigation of old, historical texts in Sanskrit.

Her dedication and diligence was so remarkable that late Shri Hira Lal Ji, the founder of our institute, associated with her in all his research on the Naturopathic cure for cancer.

Sadhna has the unique distinction of being the only Naturopath in the country with the largest collection of case studies in Naturopathy, especially those relating to cancer.

We wish her all success.

—*Dr. N.S. Adhikari*
Secretary General
(Naturopathy Institute)

I am very happy that Miss Sadhna Dubey has taken the trouble to write this elaborate treatise. I find it has in all 20 chapters and covers the field of naturopathy very effectively. She has also tried to correlate it to the dreaded disease of cancer. Her efforts are laudable indeed and deserve all praise. I am sure her readers will be much better informed about cancer and Naturopathy after they have read her book. In this day and age when there is so much emphasis on antibiotics, chemo and radiotherapy, Ms. Dubey's approach to the subject makes for a refreshing change.

I wish her all success.

—*Dr. Geeta Singh*
Senior Research Officer (AIIMS)

There is world-wide recognition of the importance of safeguarding and building upon indigenous knowledge system as a means to enhance sustainable development. The utility and practicability of building upon and integrating the distinctive knowledge and skill resources held by indigenous people world-wide is now well recognized. This is particularly true of traditional medicine and health care systems. The highly specialized technocentric and institutionalized approach to medicine as has evolved in the West is impracticable in isolated regions and rural areas where the majority of people reside in developing countries. Yet, as the Indian experience clearly demonstrates, the priority assigned by India to the Western medical/health system has undermined the knowledge of traditional health care systems accumulated over many centuries even though the Western world of pharmacology relies considerably on derivatives of indigenous Indian plant genetic resources for drug formulations. This in turn has (i) contributed to sub-optimal management of local health by reducing the potential for genuine local control and participation in prevention and cure, and (ii) high cost of health care which the vast majority of the Indian population now cannot afford and whose principal beneficiaries are pharmaceutical companies. The need for preserving and building on indigenous knowledge of health care systems is clearly warranted. China has made quantum jumps in this direction and today the traditional medical regime in China is almost as important as the modern health care system. In India this revolution is yet to occur. In this context, Ms. Sadhna Dubey's *Naturopathy: A Cure to Cancer* is an important contribution towards preserving and promoting indigenous health care system in India, particularly in the context of cancer.

The book provides an articulate analysis of Naturopathy in general and its preventive and curative qualities in particular. The author has provided support to the hypothesis that there is an interface between Western and traditional approach towards detection, prevention and cure of cancer. For example, it demonstrates how the able modern technology of cancer detection and its management can be effectively combined with traditional knowledge of Yoga and food attributes to benefit both preventive and curative aspects of cancer. Recent research on anti-cancer properties of certain vegetables and cereals lends support to the traditional knowledge on this issue as elaborated in the sections in the book dealing with fresh foods and nature diet. The evidence of curative and preventive power of naturopathy *vis-a-vis* cancer is provided in the case studies documented in the publication.

The practitioners of both Western and traditional health care as well as the layman stand to benefit from Ms. Sadhna Dubey's work. Community health workers are particularly encouraged to read Ms. Sadhna Dubey's work.

—*Vijay G. Pande*
Regional Director (IRDC)

Preface

Cancer is one of the most dreaded diseases of the modern world affecting people of all ages and both sexes. According to one of the World Health Organization's Reports one out of every ten persons who die of serious diseases, is a cancer patient. Unfortunately, in spite of worldwide research, no definite cause and cure for cancer has yet been found. Even worse is the fact that cancer in its early stages cannot normally be detected. Even though it originates in a specific part of the body its effects are felt all over the body. Modern medical science, through surgery and chemotherapy, however, continues to treat only the part of the body in which cancer has been detected and not the whole body.

Naturopathy believes that despite the concentration of cancer in a particular part of the body, its treatment must encompass the whole body because the disease originates and spreads due to the presence and assimilation of high amount of toxins which contaminate the entire body. Therefore, the first step towards the treatment of cancer should be the purification of the whole body.

In the present book almost all the latest research on the etiology of cancer has been taken into account. It discusses the naturopathic treatment of cancer, which comprises (i) the elimination of toxins and (ii) neutralization of cancer cells.

Modern medical science has also not taken the psychological factors causing and aggravating cancer into account. From the study of thousands of cancer patients, it has been observed that there are certain factors which always generate toxins in the body. Therefore, Naturopathy first emphasises on the release of the psychological stresses generating toxins in the body, followed by the Panch Karma treatment, Yogic exercises, proper food and Meditation. Naturopathic treatment cleanses the body of its toxins and thereby provide immediate relief to the patient.

The treatment of cancer through Naturopathy is not based on mere theoretical assumptions, but on its practical application. In the section on the Naturopathic Perspective on Cancer, a few case studies have been cited in which Naturopathy has proved very effective. Naturopathy primarily emphasizes preventive medicine and points to a very simple and natural way of leading a healthy life. Nature has given us life and the best possible mechanisms to promote and preserve it. Naturopathy is like the lap of mother nature, which provides the best possible support, protection and relief to all persons who aspire for it. Whenever we neglect the laws of nature, we invite self-ruin.

Cancer is a result of the ignorance of the laws of nature, coupled with the neglect of minor ailments. The cause of cancer is not in our body, but in our mind, habits, life-style and a flagrant disregard of nature's laws.

This book provides not only a unique and simple way of leading a healthy life with longevity, but also methods of prevention of cancer and other dreadful diseases. In writing this book, I have not neglected the modern diagnostic techniques for the detection of cancer, but my emphasis has been on the prevention of cancer and curing it in its early stage. In section IV of the book different forms of cancer originating in various parts of the body, their symptoms and naturopathic treatment have been discussed. Similarly, the Appendix deals with yogasanas which can cure cancer.

Naturopathy is not only a drugless therapy, but also a way of disease-free healthy living and, in case of disease, taking recourse to the immense gifts of nature, which like a mother is the best source of relief. The present book shows the most simple and natural way of self-treatment.

Many persons have helped and inspired me in writing this book. I remember Late Shri Hiralalji, of the Nature Cure and Yoga Health Care Centre, New Delhi, with the greatest gratitude, who initiated me into the wonder world of Naturopathy. I thank Dr. Shyam Agrawal, Chairman National Cancer Foundation, who opened vast vistas of modern science research in the field of cancer for me.

LORD KRISHNA says, "Know that work proceeds from the Supreme. I am the Pattern for man to follow; know that I have done all arts already; nought remains for me to gain by action, yet I work for ever unweariedly, and this whole universe would perish if I did not work my work".

Dr. Sadhna Dubey

Contents

Introduction

The science of Naturopathy has existed from time immemorial. Its origin dates back to the emergence of homo sapiens on this planet when early man cured himself of all ailments by eating herbs and regulating his diet.

Through the ages, man has harnessed the forces of nature not only for the development of civilization, but also for keeping his mind and body healthy. This worked wonderfully well as long as they were used in their pure, unadulterated states like, for example, fresh herbs, free flowing hot water springs, natural magnets, etc. But unfortunately, with the emergence of the artificially produced "drugs" of modern medicine, several of the infallible techniques of nature cure were thrown into the backwaters of history, only to be lost in the mists of time.

Fortunately, over the last few years the wheel of medicine has turned a full circle and, once again interest in natural methods of healing has revived all over the globe because modern medicine is sometimes found to do more harm than good and is often unsuccessful in curing chronic ailments and skin diseases.

It is a true but little known fact that Naturopathy can cure virtually every disease and ailment that afflicts mankind. Even the so-called "terminal" illnesses can be cured by Naturopathy. Of all the terminal illnesses that afflict mankind, cancer is one of the most dreaded. This book is perhaps the first known attempt which describes the manner in which cancer can be both prevented and completely eradicated from the body by the general healing processes of nature cure. It includes empirical research evidence as well as case studies of people who have completely recovered from the advanced stages of cancer by naturopathic treatment.

This book is the result of years of painstaking research which involved the culling out of information about several long forgotten techniques of nature cure from old manuscripts and the writings of naturopaths of the seventeenth and eighteenth centuries. All the different methods of naturopathic treatment that have been practised the world over, from ancient times until today have been described in this book.

The ancient Indian disciplines of yoga and meditation have been practised through the centuries for keeping the mind and body healthy and ailment-free. There is a plethora of research all over the world which has proved beyond doubt that the curative processes of these disciplines encompass every facet of the body and mind. Unfortunately, these findings are widely dispensed and no known attempt has been made to document their correlation with hard-to-cure diseases like cancer.

This book is perhaps the only one of its kind which contains detailed descriptions of each of the yoga and asanas (physical postures) and pranayama (breathing exercises) which can be used to treat and cure cancer.

This book is basically intended to serve as a comprehensive textbook, not only for students of Naturopathy, but also for those who wish to study the debilitating effects of cancer and how it can be cured through natural methods. The book, therefore, contains four sections as follows:

Part I : A compilation of the naturopathic methods of treatment through the ages, across the world.

Part II : An overview of cancer and its debilitating effects.

Part III : The role of Naturopathy in preventing and curing cancer.

Part IV : Different forms of cancer and their naturopathic treatment.

This book is perhaps the only existing publication which contains extensive data on naturopathy, cancer and cancer-specific yoga asanas. Every effort has been made to use as little medical jargon as possible, without detracting from a complete explanation of all the relevant concepts. Thus, both lay-persons as well as doctors will be able to comprehend the procedures and analysis described in this book.

To Whom It May Concern

Conventionally the wisdom of ancient ayurveda has been associated with the sages; the saints of India who developed and passed on this science from one generation to another, gifted men of vision and compassion.

Because of their vision and larger-than-life perspective on even the minutest of things, Naturopathy became a necessary base of this science.

In the ancient epic "MAHABHARATA", only the chosen one - Arjun, the epitome of human capabilities was the recipient of the message of "GITA" — the eternal song of wisdom. And he was younger than most of the renowned voices. Thus, wisdom is not the monopoly of age alone, it seeks a vibrant mindset. A dynamic seeker of knowledge, who refuses to accept any limitations. Sadhna Dubey, perhaps the youngest Naturopath in the country, belongs to the select breed of people, who know no barriers, no limitations.

And that is why she has chosen the seemingly incurable, the dreaded disease of cancer as the subject of her specialization.

Belonging to an illustrious family of saintly Brahmins of northern India Sadhna Dubey has investigated the secrets of naturopathy which have been hidden in our ancient knowledge. Her whole family is seeded deeply in the Aryan traditions of knowledge, specially in the sciences of Jyotish (Astrology), Ayurveda and cosmic gemology.

Sadhna's exposure to these disciplines has enabled her to develop greater insights into the mysteries of life and its forces. Needless to say, Sadhna has used her conventional background of formal education as a stepping stone to comprehend the higher noble and difficult areas of Ayurvedic and naturopathic learning.

Since the age of 12 years Sadhna has observed the application of natural herbs by the most respected names in the field of Naturopathy. Research, analysis, and synthesis have been the basic elements of her learning. Observation is the laboratory where Sadhna's mind has developed keen insights into the solutions of Naturopathy.

In the book Sadhna has attempted to bring together the various courses, the disciplines of Naturopathy as applied into the curing of cancer. The book is full of documentary evidence of the effectiveness of these treatments.

This book is a knowledge bank for all those who believe in the healing power of nature. It is probably one of its kind that encapsulates widely distributed pieces of knowledge. Sadhna's work has gained widespread recognition and there are many individuals who have benefited by her knowledge. Their testimonials are included in this book. This is just the beginning of her search for permanent solutions and not temporary checks and controls. Here is the case of a young dynamic mind paying tribute to the power of life through Naturopathy. She received her formal education in Delhi and has been working in the field of Naturopathy for more than a decade.

Dr. K.K. Pandey
Chief of Surgical Oncology
Rajiv Gandhi Cancer Institute &
Research Centre

Part I

Naturopathy – A Cure to Cancer

CHAPTER I

An Introduction To Nature Cure

Nature cure is a term that covers all methods of treating diseases which aim at cooperating with the natural forces and the body's defence mechanisms. It is a distinct system of healing based upon its own philosophy of life, health and illness. It is not a rag-bag of fads and notions, as is popularly supposed, nor is it a scheme of returning to life in the wild. Nature cure may be defined as an art, a science, a philosophy, and a practice which follows definite physical, chemical, biological, mental and spiritual laws for the restoration and maintenance of health and the correction of bodily disorders without the use of poisonous drugs. Naturopathy, nature cure, the new science of healing, drugless healing and healing from within may be treated as synonymous.

Naturopathy is a system of medicine to diagnose, treat and prescribe through the use of diet, air, light, water, heat and all other kinds of natural methods and modalities. Nature therapies exist for most diseases, pains, injuries, deformities and psychological conditions.

Nature therapy includes mechano-therapy, articular manipulation, corrective and orthopedic gymnastics, neurotherapy, psychotherapy, hydrotherapy and mineral baths, electrotherapy, thermotherapy, heliotherapy, phototherapy, chromotherapy, vibrotherapy, thalmotherapy, artificial dilation and other means of the stimulation of the nervous system through the body's orifices and diet. The latter includes the use of foods such as bio-chemical tissue-building products and cell-salts which are found in the normal body, and the use of vegetable oils, dehydrates and pulverized fruits, flowers, seeds, barks, herbs, roots and vegetables which are uncompounded and used in their natural state.

Nature cure is not just a therapy or system of healing. It is a complete way of life which is in tune with the internal vital life-giving forces or elements comprising the human entity, on the physical, mental and spiritual planes of being. It is this supreme force or power acting in and through every atom, molecule and cell in the body, which is the true healer, the "Vis Medicatrix Natura" which always endeavours to heal, to repair and to restore to perfection. All that the physician can do is guide the patient, so that healing can take place naturally, from within his own body.

In general, naturopathy investigates, scientifically, all the methods and procedures which are related to the correction of ills and the maintenance of sound health. It uses definite means and methods of alleviation of bodily disorders, both physical and mental. It is the practical realization and application of all that is good and sensible in all the systems of therapeutics.

Naturopathy prohibits the use of poisonous drugs, serums, invasive surgery, X-rays and radiation for therapeutic purposes.

The nature cure way of life involves educating people in self-control and the right habits of living, thereby preventing disease by following the laws of nature. It improves constitutional health by using the life force within us to effect cures and create internal defences against ill-health and disease. It is a way of life in tune with the internal vital life-giving forces or elements which comprise the human entity on the physical, mental and spiritual planes of being. It is this supreme force, acting in and through every atom, molecule and cell in the body which is the true healer.

There are three aspects of nature cure: *First*, as a natural process which uses the natural forces of air, sunlight, water and food. *Secondly*, as a philosophy of natural living which incorporates healing and the joy of life. *Thirdly*, as a practical science of restoring health with the aid of a qualified naturopathic practitioner.

Nature as the Healer

Nature cure means healing from within. It is Nature that heals and cures--the naturopathic physician merely lends intelligent assistance and interprets nature's laws for the patient. "Medicus Curat Natura Sanat" ("The doctor treats; but it is Nature that heals") is the foremost tenet of naturopathy.

The body is a remarkable and unique mechanism in the world. It can withstand danger from within because of its power to correct itself and restore its own balance. No machine made by the hand of man can do this. No machine can repair its own broken parts, but the body does this through the air it breathes, the water it drinks and the food it eats.

All healing comes from within the body itself. That is to say, there are self-curative forces inherent in the body, constantly working towards health and healing. The self-curative power of the body is commonly seen in case of a cut or a broken bone. Its self-curative power in the case of other ailments is less commonly realized. In the ultimate analysis, no cure is achieved except through the natural process, the means adopted to promote and expedite this process notwithstanding.

It is the bodily condition that makes disease possible; it is not the disease that creates the primary condition in the body. Ill-health or disease is basically a failure in or the perversion of the normal physiological condition of the material constitution or the functional integrity of the living organism. We cannot heal it with any remedy--it is the vital force within us which heals. We need but aid it.

Nature cures all kinds of diseases except where surgical intervention becomes essential or the body is damaged beyond repair. It is rightly said that there is no such thing as an incurable disease but there may be incurable patients. Usually patients who are medical rejects try naturopathy and expect miracles.

Nature cure treatments ensure that requisite amount of our own vital forces are generated, for it is only the proper stimulation of the vital force within us that can cure us. Any form of treatment can only help the curative powers of the human system to operate more intensely than they have hitherto been doing.

How Naturopathy Works

The purpose of naturopathic treatment is to restore health by assisting nature, the greatest doctor of all.

Some of the ways in which this is accomplished are:

- By purging the body of wastes, poisons and foreign substances, or by assisting nature if she has commenced her own processes of cleansing and regeneration.
- By stimulating the organs of purification and elimination to improve their functioning
- By restoring normal blood supply and proper innervation to the diseased and disordered organs and tissues.
- By freeing the nerves, the blood vessels and the lymphatic system from undue pressures and obstructions.
- By relieving nervous and muscular tension and toning up the nervous system.
- By balancing the glandular activities, thus augmenting the vital energy.
- By supplying the body with the cell-salts that it lacks. These are tissue remedies which restore the disturbed body chemistry and normalize its functions, increase it strength and enrich and purify the blood, thereby immunizing the body to diseases and the breeding of germs.
- By reducing and removing the roots of infection and freeing the body of their effects.
- By correcting abnormalities of the tissues, organs, muscles, joints, bones and skin such as swellings, strains, tensions, displacements, injuries, curvatures, over and under-development, tumours, growths, obstructions in passages, abnormalities in temperature and moisture, inflammation, discharges, sores, ulcers, eruptions, etc.
- By making necessary adjustments in the mental and emotional life of the patients, and changes in their personal habits and mode of living.
- By advising on hygiene, sanitation, the prevention of disease and how to live in accordance with nature's laws of health. The methods that it prescribes are fasting, eliminative measures, mono-diet, curative and rational dietetics, hydrotherapy, constitution building measures, and the adoption of other subsidiary healing agents like manipulation, massage, curative exercises, sunlight, etc.

Axioms of Nature Cure

Two leading axioms of nature cure are, *Unity of Disease* and *Unity of Cure*. These are briefly explained below.

Unity of Disease. There is only one cause of disease which manifests itself in various forms and with different degrees of severity. Barring trauma (injury) and surroundings uncongenial to life, the primary cause of all diseases is the violation of the laws of nature. Violation of nature's laws in thinking, breathing, eating, drinking, dressing, working and resting, as well as in normal social and sexual conduct results in both the primary and the secondary manifestations of disease. Whatever be the malady, remember that disease is a single unit. It is the result of transgression--conscious or unconscious.

All diseases are in reality Nature's self-purifying efforts. "Give me fever and I can cure every disease" said Hippocrates who formulated the fundamental laws of nature cure over two thousand years ago. Dr. Henry Linderahr, one of the best known exponents of the nature cure movement, said, "Every acute disease is the result of a cleansing and healing effort of nature. If you suppress an acute condition by drugs or by any other means, you are simply laying the foundation for chronic diseases. By making a general application of this law, we can deduce that all diseases, from a simple cold to skin eruptions, diarrhoeas and fever, represent nature's effort to remove from the system some morbid matter, some virus or poison which is dangerous to health or life."

Unity of Cure. The body's natural state is of perfect health. The current of life flows through every living thing--plants, animals and man. What this mysterious force of life is, nobody knows. But the principle of nature cure is that the life-force, or life-energy, in every living thing always strives for perfect health. The body possesses its own inherent self-curative forces and there are sufficient resources of vitality within every living body to overcome temporary disabilities. As soon as the dietary and other conditions necessary for its restoration to health are provided, the body immediately carries out its plan of regeneration, and good health follows.

By recognizing the unity of disease and the unity of cure, the nature cure system of therapeutics is based on the firm foundation of "principle" instead of ever-changing doctrines like other forms of medicine.

Fundamental Principles of Nature Cure

There are three fundamental principles of nature cure:

1. All forms of disease are due to the same cause, i.e. the accumulation of waste materials and bodily refuse in the body. These are fully removed from healthy bodies through the organs of elimination. But when the rate of the accumulation of these waste products is in excess of the body's capacity to excrete them, they putrefy within and begin to poison the system. This condition, known as "toxaemia" in medical parlance, is the fundamental cause of ill-health.
2. All acute diseases are attempts by the body to flush out the accumulated toxic waste within. If these are continuously suppressed or treated symptomatically, chronic diseases develop.
3. The body contains the power to cure itself, provided proper methods are employed.

Naturopathic Teaching and Treatment

Naturopathic teaching seeks to make every person aware that it is possible to maintain and sustain good health by believing in the curative powers of the life force, by obeying the laws of nature, and by maintaining a constructive and healthy mental attitude.

Nature cure maintains that the fundamental biological requirements necessary to maintain life exist both in nature and within ourselves. Nature cure lays a good deal of emphasis on "preventive methods". At the time of treatment, the nature-cure physician first attempts to analyse the cause of the disease and then prescribes remedies that aid the restoration of health without producing any injurious reaction in the body.

Therefore, the approach to the problem of health and disease from the nature cure point of view is based on two fundamental principles.

1. "Vis Medicatrix Natura"--the healing power of nature.
2. "Non Nocere"--the measures employed to treat disease must do no harm.

Principles and Philosophy of Nature Cure

To summarize, the principles and philosophy of nature cure are:

(a) Healing is from within.

(b) Trace the cause or causes of disease instead of concentrating on its symptoms alone.

(c) Treat the body as a whole, and treat both the body and the mind.

(d) Auto-intoxication or toxaemia is one of the principal causes of disease.

(e) Without cleansing, there can be no cure.

(f) The treatment should not be worse than the disease.

(g) Return, not back to Nature, but back to the fundamentals of nature cure.

(h) Prevention is better than cure.

(i) Know thyself. If you know the truth, it shall free you.

(j) Heal thyself. Your personal health is your personal responsibility.

Naturopathy and Human Potential

Naturopathy teaches that man is a microcosm, a universe within himself. He is a child of the cosmic forces of the external environment, the macrocosm. His individual existence is indivisible from the total cosmic manifestation. Naturopathy views health and "disease" in holistic terms, taking into account the inherent relationship between the individual and the cosmic spirit, the individual and cosmic consciousness, energy and matter.

According to the teachings of Naturopathy, every person has four biological and spiritual instincts: religious, financial, procreative and the instinct toward freedom. Balanced good health is the foundation for their fulfilment. By the proper balance of bodily energies, the processes of physical deterioration and disease can be impressively reduced. A person's capability for self-healing is the basic principle of naturopathy. Naturopathy helps the healthy person to maintain health, and the diseased person to regain it. It is a medical-metaphysical healing life science, the mother of all healing arts. The practice of Naturopathy is designed to promote happiness, health and creative growth. By studying the teachings of Naturopathy, anyone may acquire the practical knowledge of self-healing.

Naturopathy and the Western Mind

Western medicine and thinking tend to generalize and to categorize individuality. For instance, by the Western yardstick, what is common in a majority of people constitutes the norm. Naturopathy on the other hand holds that normality must be evaluated individually, because every human constitution manifests its own particular and spontaneous temperament and functioning. In the East, the key to understanding is acceptance, observation and experience; in the West, it is questioning, analysis and logical deduction. The Western mind generally trusts objectivity, while the Eastern gives more emphasis to subjectivity. Eastern science teaches one to beyond the division between subjectivity and objectivity. This difference in approach may explain why some Westerners experience difficulty in comprehending the methodology of Naturopathy.

Many statements made in this introductory text on Naturopathy may evince questions of "How" and "Why". Such questions, though inevitable, are not always answerable. Even in modern Western medicine, some concepts are proven to "work" without the reasons behind the phenomena being fully understood : e.g., though antibiotics are used to destroy the bacteria which form toxins in the body, no adequate explanation exists to explain how and why toxins are formed from bacteria. Furthermore, Naturopathy is truly a holistic science, one in which the sum of many elements comprises its Truth. To question details before a comprehensive overview of the whole science is acquired will prove unproductive and discordant. The reader is therefore respectfully advised provisionally to accept statements that may at first appear to lack adequate explanation, until he has begun to master the body of Naturopathic knowledge as a whole.

Naturopathy comprehensively illuminates the basic laws and principles governing life on earth. To understand Naturopathy is to understand the forces that engender our well-being as well as those that lie at the root of disease. This brief introduction has been an attempt to introduce the reader to this life science in a concise and informative way. The basic concepts of Naturopathy have been introduced here, yet the reader may still have unanswered questions about this science of life. In fact, this book may have raised more questions than it has answered. This may be unavoidable when one treats, in an introductory manner, an ancient system of wisdom that encompasses that vast horizon where human consciousness merges into Cosmic Consciousness.

CHAPTER II

Nature Cure Through The Ages

The origin of nature cure goes back to the arrival of Man on earth, when natural methods were the only methods for curing disease. Nature cure is essentially the accumulation of knowledge pertaining to the natural methods of living and healing that have been successfully practised through the centuries.

All living beings (including animals) practise nature cure by instinct. A sick dog will automatically fast. Cats and other felines know the importance of a sun bath. Aboriginal races have fewer diseases than civilized societies. This is because they live more naturally.

Since the beginning of history, evidence of the employment of sunshine, fresh air, heat, water, baths and fasting as agents of cure have been recorded. Early Egyptians used massage to cure certain ailments; the ancient Jews had strict rules of diet and hygiene which were given religious significance; the Greeks created a "physical" society in Sparta; and the Romans advocated the extensive use of baths of all kinds. In those ancient days, people realized the value of water, sunlight, fresh air and their effects on the health and well-being of mankind, and used packs and massages for curing diseases.

Long before Hippocrates, who lived in 450 B.C., there was a great advocate of methods of treatment in accordance with natural laws. He was called Ascutaptes, and was described by Homer as a "blameless physician".

Hippocrates' ideas on the use of water were taken up by Gallenus Paracelsus, another great healer, born in 1493 in Switzerland, who was renowned for his natural methods. He reinstated the old water cures with great success. Paracelsus said, "It was the book of nature which I studied and not those of scribblers, for each scribbler writes down all the rubbish that may be found in his head." Another prominent naturalist of the mid-fifteenth century wrote, "Nature's language is not learned in a stinking schöol atmosphere, nor at the corpses of the dissection rooms, nor by studying the tortured animals in the vivisection laboratories, but in nature herself."

Revival of Naturopathy

Over a century ago, like many other worldwide revolutions and reformations, nature cure resurfaced as a science in Germany, in Grafenburg, a small village in the Silesian mountains. Vincent Priessnitz, the father of the natural healing movement, decided that his pharmacopoeia would consist not of pills and potions, but of plenty of exercise, fresh mountain air and water treatment in the cool sparkling pools of rural Germany and simple wholesome country food.

Because of his success with water cure, the idea of drugless healing began to spread throughout Germany and later all over the civilized world. Priessnitz gathered a vast following of students from several countries. Medical practitioners from America and other nations crossed the ocean to become his students. Each of these doctors later enlarged and enriched different branches of natural healing. Some researched and propagated water cure and natural dietetics, while others delved deep into various systems of manipulative treatment, etc.

Louis Kuhne cured cases by sunshine, steam and sitz baths. His slogan was, "Only cleansing can heal." For his diagnosis, he depended almost entirely upon observing facial expressions. Kuhne's doctrine of the Unity of Disease is the bedrock of modern nature cure. Father Kneipp, another follower of Priessnitz, was a great advocate and practitioner of water treatment and the use of medicinal herbs and plants.

Dr. Henry Lindlahr, a student of Prissnitz, was the most successful exponent of the nature cure movement in the United States. He propounded the fundamental doctrine of nature cure which every naturopath now subscribes to–"Every acute disease is a healing effort of nature." He was the first nature cure physician to coordinate the different forms of natural treatment into one exact and complete science.

Additions to the methods of natural healing were thereafter made very rapidly. Dr. Stall made a valuable addition to natural methods of treatment by the invention of osteopathy, a system of scientific manipulation of the body structure, muscles, nerves and nerve centres. The work of Dr. Tilden on the subject that wrong feeding is one of the main causes of disease, is highly commendable. Dr. Palmer introduced chiropractic, a system of spinal manipulation to relax contracted tissues, reduce dislocated bones, liberate and stimulate the flow of the blood and nerve impulses, thereby removing the mechanical causes of disease. Dr. Kellogg, a physician of high repute, introduced hydrotherapy on a rational and scientific basis.

The eighteenth- and nineteenth-century pioneers of nature cure thus inaugurated a worldwide movement to propagate and practise more simple and rational ways of living and treating ailments. From limited beginnings, today the school of nature cure covers not only the original basic practice of nature cure, but also includes all that has been found to be beneficial in modern drugless and bloodless therapy.

Nature Cure in India

Naturopathy is one of the gifts of the ancient Indian civilization to the world. Centuries before Plato, Aristotle and Hippocrates, Indian yogis and sages had discovered the benefits of nature cure. It was mainly practised by philosophers, holy men and their disciples on themselves for the purification of the body, mind and soul and to help them in their long hours of meditation. This in turn called for great will power and self-control. Fasting, dieting, hydrotherapy, massage, etc., were all means to that end. When they experienced how significant the benefits of these practices were, they wished to place them within the reach of the humblest of men. The most effective means of doing so was to give them the sanctity of religion which they did. And it worked. Even today, Hindus fast, bathe and diet with reverential zeal.

Among the great naturopaths of India was no less a person than the Father of the Nation, Mahatma Gandhi. After his various long fasts, which he undertook for political or other reasons, he discovered that his intellect became sharper and his stamina improved. This set him thinking about how to bring these benefits within the reach of the poorest villagers, as he was greatly concerned by the high cost of modern medical treatment. To accomplish this, he opened a naturo cure centre in a moderately sized village, about 240 km from his ashram at Sabarmati, where the villagers were treated free of cost.

There are currently two schools of nature cure. The first takes into account only the five elements of nature: sunlight, air, fire (heat), water and earth (food). Their whole science is based on this doctrine, and this is how it was practised by the pioneers. This basic group considers that any aid taken beyond this is not proper nature cure. The other group, which might be called the eclectic group, includes the practices of electrotherapy, osteopathy, chiropractic, and other modern treatments, which also conform in every respect to the philosophy of nature cure. This group considers that methods which are constructive, not repressive, and which have no harmful after-effects, rightly come within the sphere of naturopathy.

Today, naturopathy is regarded as being primarily and fundamentally drugless and bloodless, yet in its broader aspects it does admit of the use of both natural medicines and surgery when there is no alternative to their use for saving lives.

The advanced naturopathic system has been broadly classified into threefold aspects. These are: (a) psychological--man's emotional, mental and psychic nature; (b) physiological--the body, its anatomy and functions; and (c) chemical--the chemical substances which compose the body cells and tissues, etc. The means employed for healing in these three fields are :

(a) *Psychotherapeutic*--Constructive suggestions to correct wrong habits and psychosomatic treatment for guiding the reciprocal influences of mind and body.

(b) *Physiotherapeutic*--Spinal and muscular manipulations, massages and vibrations, exercises, orthopaedic gymnastics, hydrotherapy, neurotherapy, zone-therapy, sunlight, air, water, earth, heat and cold therapy, light and colour ray therapy, electrotherapy, etc.

(c) *Chemical and Material*--Nutritional control, dietetics, external applications, minerals, cell-salts, vitamins and herbs.

The progressive system of natural therapeutics combines the best features of such methods as fasting, the proper combination of natural foods, curative diets and other dietetic measures, massage, curative gymnastics, physical exercises, osteopathy, chiropractic, spondylo-therapy, baths, scientific relaxation, mental and magnetic therapeutics and so forth. Modern naturopathy therefore, consists of a combination and selection from everything that is good, practical and efficient, all that conforms to the fundamental laws of cure and has no harmful or destructive after-effects.

As no single remedial adjunct of naturopathy or its forms of treatment is broad enough in its scope to be efficacious as a cure for every disease and condition that is met with in practice, the progressive naturopathic physician selects from his large therapeutic store-house, the particular form of treatment best suited to the needs of the case in hand. Naturopathy has consequently kept pace with the progress made in other fields of science, so that some of its methods today differ materially from those of the great pioneers. The individual modalities and techniques employed vary with the degree of intelligence, training and clinical experience of a practitioner. The ultimate objective, however, remains the same--to eliminate the disease from the body. This unchanging fundamental truth will always remain the bedrock of naturopathic practice.

Has Naturopathy Scope for Further Development?

The scope of the science of naturopathy is vast. It includes three classes of people: (1) those who are well; (2) those who think they are well; and (3) those who are ill.

Those who are well. Few individuals enjoy perfect health. However strong their constitution or however perfectly well they may be, even they cannot expect to remain healthy for long, if their habits of living are not in consonance with the laws of health and if they abuse their system.

Those who think they are well. Many boast of their good health. But on questioning, they admit to being afflicted with headaches, problems in digestion, pains and aches in the body, constipation and other chronic ailments. When asked whether they call these disorders concomitants of perfect health, they answer in surprise, "Why, everybody suffers from such things. Surely they are not diseases?" The fact is that "disease" has become so nearly a universal phenomenon among people of so-called civilized countries that they have come to think that they are enjoying perfect health, as long as they are not sick in bed.

Those who are ill. As a rule, people do not take to nature cure when they fall ill until their acute and sub-acute ailments have drifted into so-called incurable or chronic conditions. All diseases can be treated independently by nature cure except where surgical intervention becomes necessary or the case is beyond repair. It is generally found, however, that only medical rejects or "last resort" patients try naturopathy and expect miracles.

The various therapies known up to now, based upon the laws of science, have limited applications. It is possible that further research on the subject and standardization of conditions, will widen the scope of nature cure. Naturopathy has a great but relatively unexplored medical potential. The world cannot stand still and neither can the healing art. Nature cannot be improved upon, but all of us can improve our methods of utilizing the healing forces of nature. Funds are needed for research centres, study aids and proper training in teaching institutions and public hospitals where qualified naturopathic physicians can have a free hand to administer the many successful methods of nature cure treatment. For all this, government cooperation is essential.

Is Nature Cure Scientific?

The dictionary meaning of the word scientific is "investigations according to rules laid down in science for testing the soundness of conclusions that appear." In common parlance, science means "knowledge" but the modern usage of the term covers only certain kinds of knowledge. The scope of each of these is now so vast that no one can have a grasp of more than a minute fraction of any of them. Even the kinds of knowledge regarded as scientific are so diverse that it creates much misunderstanding about the term "scientific". The acceptance of our usage of the term "scientific" follows closely the growing prestige of research and investigation, as today, science has become completely equated with research. The fundamentals of modern naturopathy should not be branded as unscientific merely because they do not have an impressive array of modern research to prop them up.

Nature cure has a scientific background. Several methods of treatment in modern medicine are mostly old, well-accepted truths that were labelled in the past unscientific, but when adapted by other cults with a change of name and verification by modern medical research, and put before the world with a somewhat mysterious cause over them, began to be considered as scientific and hailed as new discoveries. Science is today finding in its research, confirmation of truths that were discovered by nature cure many decades ago. For example, the use of vitamins and the value of organic salts were mentioned by early naturopathic physicians like Otto Carque, Dr. Henry Lindlahr and others. Osteopathy and chiropractic adjustments, manipulative techniques (now known as manipulative surgery), massage, corrective exercises, heliotherapy and electrotherapy or heat treatment in some form or other, now known as physiotherapy or physical medicine, were always incorporated in the practice of naturopathy by nature cure pioneers. Nature cure is nothing new. It merely carries out the dictum of Hippocrates, the Father of Medicine, who declared, "Nature cures, not the physician".

The scientific chapters in the history of modern nature cure were written by several eminent allopaths. In America Dr. Kellogg, MD, FRCS, Dr. Henry Lindlahr, MD, Dr. Benedict Lust, MD, and others, systematized the science of nature cure. Dr. Kellogg, a physician of high repute, introduced hydrotherapy on a rational and scientific basis. Dr. Lindlahr, a stalwart of the nature cure movement, was the first naturopathic physician to combine the various drugless methods in a systematic and scientific way. Dr. Lust gave up his practice in medicine and took to nature cure. He became an internationally renowned nature cure physician.

In Germany, medical doctors were told by the government that they should join the nature science practice and a joint Congress of Naturopathic Physicians and Practitioners of regular medicine was convened by the government for documenting the various healing therapies of nature cure. It was financed by the government in the interests of public health and for the improvement of the country's economic and social conditions. Germany now recognizes natural methods as being extremely vital for the prevention and cure of disease. The country which gave the world a scientist like Einstein, a philosopher like Kant, a poet like Goethe, the originator of homeopathy in Hahnemann, the inventor of the biochemic system of medicine in Schussler, could not have made a statement wanting medical practitioners to join hands with nature cure if it was an unscientific discipline.

Nature Cure and Other Systems of Healing

Naturopathy teaches man to think in terms of health rather than disease. Naturopaths are trained to see the body as a self-sustaining entity that has the power to manufacture within its own marvellous laboratories all the necessary forces, ferments, secretions and chemicals in the proper proportions to maintain health and life, as long as there is correct coordination within it.

Allopathy, homeopathy, ayurveda and nature cure are the four main systems of medicine practised in India. Naturopathic physicians do not need to feel antagonistic toward the other schools of healing as all of them coexist harmoniously.

Allopathy regards each disease as a separate entity requiring specific drugs for its cure. Allopathic medicine has gone to great lengths to establish a name and a specific cause for almost every disease or condition that affects the body, in the belief that only by an exhaustive study of this nature can a knowledge of healing be gained. The parts affected by each ailment are minutely studied. Allopathy has produced a vast amount of knowledge of disease-based therapy, but gives little knowledge of health. Under allopathic treatment, certain drugs are given for certain symptoms, i.e. only the symptoms of the disease are treated, and not the body as a whole.

Homeopathy works with the laws of cure, not against them. "Similia similibus curantur"--"Like cures like"-- is the guiding principle of homeopathy. In practice, this means that a drug which is capable of producing a certain set of disease symptoms in a healthy body when taken in large, physiological doses, will relieve or 'cure' a similar set of symptoms in the diseased organism when it is given in small, homeopathic doses. True homeopathic medicines in high potency doses are so highly refined that they cannot possibly produce harmful results or suppress nature's cleansing and healing efforts. On the contrary, if they are prescribed according to the laws of homeopathy they assist in producing acute reactions of 'healing crises', thus aiding Nature in the work of purification. "Similia similibus curantur" is only another way of stating the fundamental law of nature--every acute disease is the result of a cleansing and healing effort of Nature. If a certain set of disease symptoms is the result of a healing effort of Nature and if a remedy which produces the same or similar symptoms in the system is given, it is aiding Nature in her attempts to overcome the abnormal conditions. In such cases, the indicated homeopathic remedy will not suppress the acute reaction, but will help it along, thus accelerating and hastening the curative process. If the remedy is well chosen, the very first homeopathic aggravation will be followed by speedy readjustment.

There are two fundamental doctrines of homeopathic medicine--the first is that the body contains repairing processes within itself, the second is that the physician treats the patient as a whole, taking all signs and symptoms into consideration. These doctrines more or less conform with those of nature cure. Homeopathy is therefore often recommended as a complement to nature cure.

If sugar or milk pellets are recommended by homeopaths why do they not prescribe allopathic drugs as well? The main difference between the same remedy prescribed in homeopathic doses and in allopathic drugs is that the latter suppresses acute bodily reactions, thus interrupting Nature's efforts to cleanse, heal and cure. Nature's healing processes are interrupted and suppressed by allopathic medicines, changing acute inflammatory healing efforts into chronic destructive disease, whereas homeopathy assists Nature in removing all the encumbrances from the cells. Disease resides in the body cells. The well-being of the organism as a whole is dependent upon the health of the individual cells of which it is composed. To restore the cells to health, we must free them of all their encumbrances. Elimination of toxins must begin in the cells themselves, and not in the organs of deputation. The organs of elimination do not make waste products--these are generated by the body tissues. Stimulating the activity of the kidneys or the skin with drugs does not neutralize and oxidize the morbid materials in the rest of the cells and tissues.

Dr. William Schussler, a homeopathic physician of long experience, conducted research and experiments on biological healing principles and succeeded in formulating a new and simpler method of healing known as *Biochemistry*. Biochemistry is a system of scientific treatment which restores impaired health by supplying to the body the cell-salts that it is deficient in. Cell-salts are the inorganic constituents of our tissues. They are supplied by nature in a pure and atomized form in certain proportions in all the tissues of our bodies, in all plants and in all our food, and they are abundantly available in their crude and impure state on the earth.

The invisible natural forces within us are the most effective guardians of our health. But even these great natural forces are unable to keep the complicated human structure in good working order if the blood does not contain the materials required for the building of new, healthy cells. This fact, together with other important discoveries made by renowned scientists relating to cellular pathology, regarding the constitution and functions of that wonderful fluid organ, the blood, furnished Dr. Schussler with the inspiration for his new, practical system of medicine. One of its striking features is that it requires only twelve remedies, the composition of which corresponds with the principal inorganic elements found in the body. These twelve biochemical remedies (often called mineral salts or tissue-salts) are absolutely harmless. They are not drugs in any sense of the word. They simply provide the system with its deficient inorganic elements, prepared homeopathically, in an extremely finely subdivided form which ensures their ready assimilation and a speedy restoration of that balance and harmony in the system which spells health and happiness. There is nothing miraculous in the action of these remedies. Their virtues are derived from the application of principles based upon the laws of nature. They are to the ailing what food is to the starving.

Ayurveda is as old as the world for it was bestowed by the Creator (Brahma) on the immortals, by the immortals on the sages, and by the sages on us. Life or *ayur* is the combination of the physical body, the senses of knowledge and action, the mind and the soul. Ayurveda therefore is a science which is prescribed for the betterment of life. As the body and the mind are the abode of diseases, they acquire certain indices of health at birth along with other instincts, faculties and characteristic properties. These are found both in the mind and in the body and are called sattva (purity), rajas (energy) and tamas (inertia). The equilibrium of these three states results in a sound mind and body, and their unbalanced condition, due to either the subnormal or abnormal state of any one of them, results in disease. According to Ayurveda there are just three indicators of health called vayu, pitta and kapha, also known as tridoshas or the three humours. The aim of Ayurveda is to keep the three humours in equilibrium for only then can perfect health be attained and maintained. Imbalance of the tridoshas leads not only to impaired health, but also to an impaired mental condition, because the mind's health is dependent on the body's health.

Nature Cure Approach for Eradicating Epidemics

Nature cure does not disregard modern scientific knowledge; neither does it deny the existence of 'disease germs'. But nature cure teaches that germs multiply only in bodies which are heavily encumbered with and weakened by wrong food, drink and drug poisons, and from morbid artificially developed disease products such as sera, antitoxins, calcine, etc. No disease is 'caught' unless there is already a breeding ground in the body in which its germs can flourish.

The only rational way to eradicate diseases and epidemics is to secure hygienic and sanitary conditions--both personal and general, with emphasis on preventive measures like educating people to become more health conscious. The people should be taught how to take personal care of the body and how to pay special attention to food, cleanliness, clothing, work, rest, morals, self-control and so on. Besides, the government should give priority to matters of sanitation, such as the management of sewers, the safeguarding of milk, water and food supply, etc., and various other schemes and activities that maintain and improve public health. Cleanliness goes hand in hand with the purification of the internal organs to ensure 'natural immunity'. More time and money should be spent on improving and checking conditions that will prevent the outbreak of epidemics rather than on methods of combating the disease germs with the administration of countless vaccines and drugs, which are at times not only unnecessary but definitely injurious.

Every person has the inalienable right to decide for himself whether or not to be vaccinated. He may be a conscientious objector, provided, of course, that he himself leads a hygienic and healthy life and rightly follows the mandate of nature cure's philosophy and principles.

If the vaccine is efficacious, then non-vaccinated people cannot be a source of injury to their neighbors who have been vaccinated. When people who have been vaccinated get smallpox, they are told that their vaccination could not have been properly done or that the lymph glands were not active or that the marks were too faint or that the vaccination was too old or too new. It is a case of "Heads I win, tails you lose."

Good medicine needs no policeman. Why have a police force, or something similar, to compel healthy people to be vaccinated? Changes in ideas can come not from the ignorant masses but from the government and the authorities who enforce this compulsion on so-called scientific and medical grounds, without actually investigating such matters very deeply. The conscientious objectors to vaccination should be respected, but the public health officials are unable to do so because they have been brainwashed about the necessity of vaccination. Even smallpox vaccinations are still required by governments even though this disease has been virtually eradicated. These vaccinations cause several side-effects that can lead to illness and even death, ranging from brain damage, post-vaccinal encephalitis, foetal infections, skin rashes and blood diseases. Some naturopaths even suggest that vaccine and sera are responsible for causing dangerous diseases like cancer and heart ailments.

Man's real freedom comes from being allowed to pursue his own good in his own way, so long as he does not attempt to deprive others of theirs, or impede their efforts to obtain it. Each individual is the proper guardian of his own health--whether bodily or mental and spiritual.

Whenever vaccination has been enforced, many naturopaths have come out with an anti-vaccination campaign. This also is wrong when the masses are deprived of proper hygienic and sanitary conditions, both externally and internally. Therefore, the question of vaccination will still remain a question mark for both the country and the masses in emergency situations. From an orthodox viewpoint, however, no sound case can be made out for mass immunization, and early childhood vaccination cannot be justified. Also, if adult vaccination programmes are kept to an absolute minimum, there will be no risk of spread of death.

The unorthodox view is that hygiene, cleanliness and the isolation of cases have brought about a reduction in the incidence of the diseases that we are vaccinated against. This is also felt to be the case with diseases such as diphtheria, scarlet fever, whooping cough and the complications caused by these illnesses. The need, above all, is therefore, for a programme of medical tests for diagnosing natural immunity against these illnesses. For instance, children may be tested for tuberculosis in general and when they show failure of immunity they should be closely watched, tested and perhaps X-rayed at intervals instead of introducing the BCG vaccine (anti-tuberculosis) as a routine and then discovering a high susceptibility to the vaccine which has been known to cause severe tubercular encephalitis and a great many resultant complications.

Changes in attitude about the routine need for vaccination under the guidance of the World Health Organization are under way and it is now not compulsory to be vaccinated except in cases where one is travelling to an endemic area. Some of the vaccinations and immunizations which travellers undergo before visiting countries are legally compulsory while others are not compulsory but are considered advisable. Hence, the question of vaccination and immunization is a difficult one. One has to weigh all the pros and cons before undergoing them, for there is much evidence that they are harmful to the system and the only way to clean their harmful effects from the system afterwards is by natural methods.

We gather from the report of the Official Blue Book of Sanitary Measures in India that the last two ten-year series of statistics afford no evidence that vaccination affects the usual epidemic courses of the disease, and hence this fact, in the face of extensive vaccination work during the present and past years, appears to lead to the conclusion that in its epidemic form, smallpox can be countered by improving the people's sanitary conditions. We conclude, therefore, that the only common factor in any country where smallpox is virulent, is the poverty of a great mass of the people, and the filthy conditions in which a considerable section of them are forced to live.

Medical opinion is strongly in favour of vaccination because a doctor's training begins in his youth and the doctrines of the older professionals are firmly implanted in the students even before they start their formal study of medicine. Anti-vaccination books are always excluded from orthodox medical college libraries and curricula. Actually, opinion in the medical profession itself is divided on the issue. Most of those who are anti-vaccination were once in favour of it and turned against it after tragic experiences in their practice led them to study both sides of the question. Others find their professional status bound up with the belief in vaccination. They cannot break away from it without jeopardizing their career. The favourite argument of believers in vaccination is that the sweeping smallpox epidemics which used to wipe out thousands have virtually vanished since the advent of vaccination against it. In reply, we may mention that even today, the only countries which still have smallpox epidemics are those which have compulsory vaccination against it like Italy, Egypt, Mexico and India, whereas smallpox has declined rapidly in the countries where vaccination has been abandoned and conditions of sanitation, hygiene and nutrition were improved.

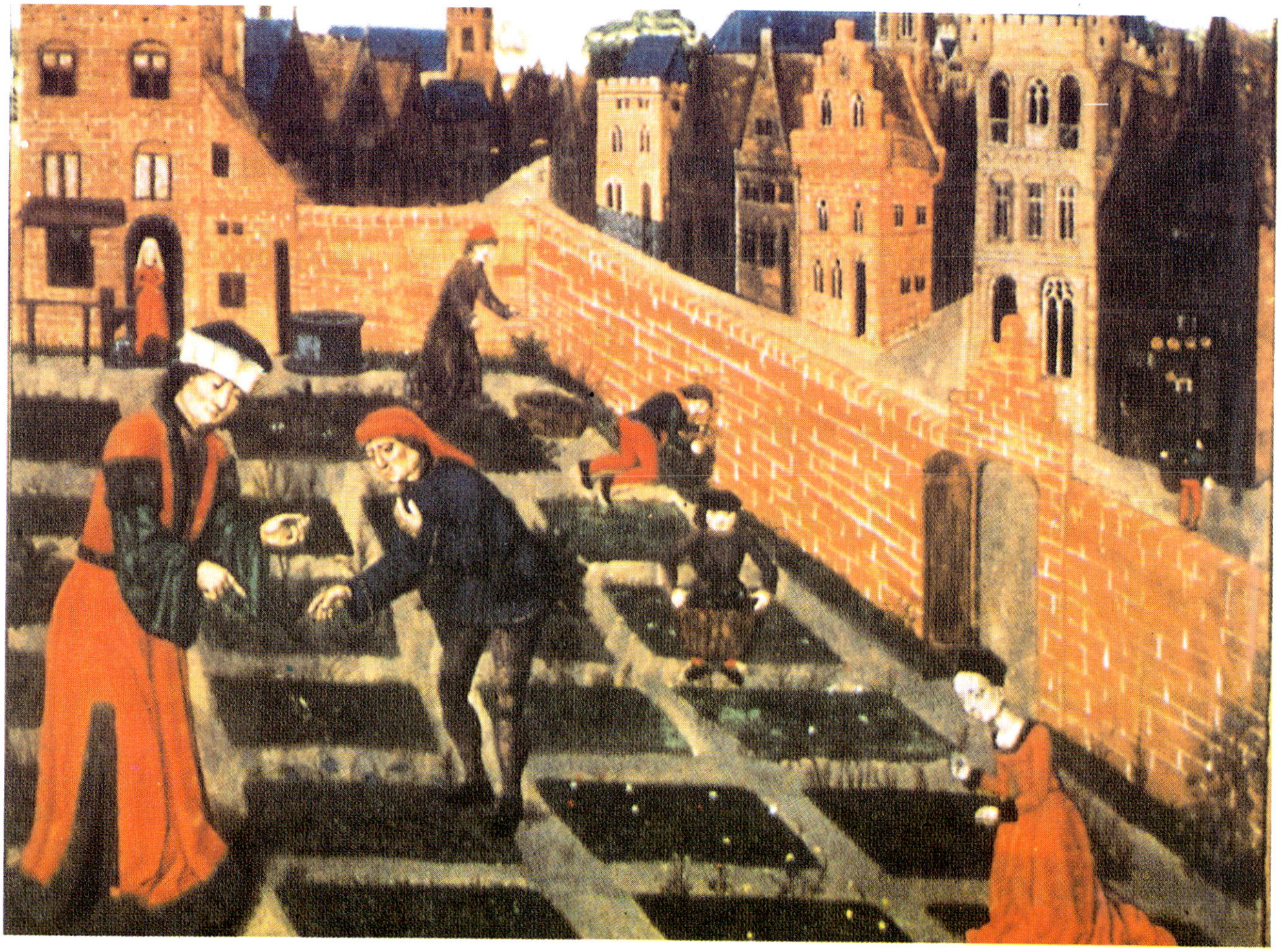

A PAINTING of a 14th Century herb Garden, Showing the formality of the geometric design Papular in Medieval time.

CHAPTER III

Fundamentals Of The Indian Philosophy Of Naturopathy

The Five Elements and Man

Naturopathy evolved in the meditative minds of the seers of truth, the rishis. Originating in cosmic consciousness, this wisdom was intuitively received in the hearts of the Rishis. For thousands of years their teachings were transmitted orally from teacher to disciple, and later they were set down in melodious Sanskrit poetry. Though many of these texts have been lost over time, an abundant body of naturopathic knowledge still survives.

The Rishis perceived that consciousness was energy manifested into the five basic principles or elements-- ether (space), air, fire, water and earth. This concept of the five elements lies at the heart of the science of naturopathy. The rishis perceived that in the beginning the world existed in an unmanifested form. In that state of unified consciousness, the subtle vibrations of the cosmic soundless "aum" were manifested. And from these vibrations, there first appeared the element of ether. This ethereal element then began to move and its subtle movements created the air, which is ether in action. The movement of ether produced friction, and through that friction heat was generated. Particles of heat-energy combined with each other which created intense light and from this light the fire element manifested itself. Thus, ether manifested into air, and it was the same ether that further manifested into fire. Through the heat of the fire, certain ethereal elements dissolved and liquified, manifesting the water element, and then solidified to form the molecules of earth. In this way, these manifested into the four elements of air, fire, water and earth. From earth, all organic living bodies, including those in the vegetable kingdom such as herbs and grains, and those in the animal kingdom, including man, are created. Earth also contains the inorganic substances that comprise the mineral kingdom. Thus, out of the womb of the five elements all matter was born.

Five Elements the Organs of the Sences and their actions

Element	Senses	Sense Organ	Action	Organs of Action
Ether	Hearing	Ear	Speech	Organs of Speech
Air	Touch	Skin	Holding	Hand
Fire	Seeing	Eyes	Walking	Feet
Water	Taste	Tongue	Procreation	Genitals
Earth	Smell	Nose	Excretion	Anus
Fire	–	Eyes		
Earth	–	Nose		
Water	–	Tongue		
Air	–	Skin		
Ether	–	Ear		

These five basic elements exist in all states of matter. Water provides the classic example. The solid state of water, ice, is a manifestation of the earth principle. Latent heat (fire) in the ice liquefies it, manifesting the water principle; and then eventually it turns into steam, expressing the air principle. The steam disappears into ether, or space. Thus the five basic elements, ether, air, water and earth, are present in one substance. All five originated in the energy issuing from cosmic consciousness; all five are present in all matter in the universe. Thus, energy and matter are one.

Man as a Microcosm

Man is a microcosm of nature and so the five basic elements present in all matter also exist within each person. In the body, there are many spaces which are manifestations of the ether element, such as the spaces in the mouth, nose, gastro-intestinal tract, respiratory tract, abdomen, thorax, capillaries, lymphatic system, tissues and cells.

practices of Yoga and Tantra is liberation, although only certain disciplined individuals are able to achieve this ultimate goal through these practices. Naturopathy can, however, be practised successfully by anyone for the achievement of good health and longevity.

In the spiritual evolution of a man, Naturopathy is the foundation, Yoga is the body and Tantra is the head. It is necessary first to understand Naturopathy in order to experience the practices of Yoga and Tantra. Thus, Naturopathy, Yoga and Tantra form an interdependent Trinity of life. None of these practices stands alone. The health of the body, mind and consciousness depends on the knowledge and practice of these three in daily life.

The Indian System of Naturopathy

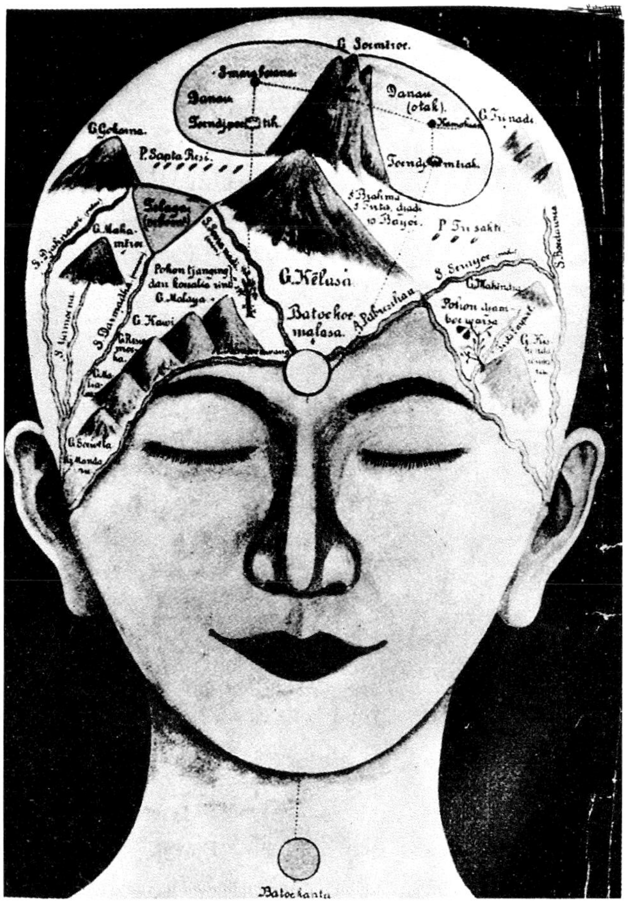

According to Indian naturopaths, there is a triplicate life system working in the body, which consists of--(a) the nervous system or vata; (b) the digestive system or pitta; and (c) the lymphatic system or kapha. These three elements regulate the entire human system and are considered to be its sole supporters. They are also called the three humours. Vata, the nervous system, governs all the functions related to the limbs, and because of it, we experience the sense of feeling. Pitta supplies warmth which governs the function of digestion. It provides body heat, lustre, intelligence, etc. Kapha keeps the joints in place and thus performs the cohesive, nutritive, development and stabilizing functions of the body. As long as these three elements retain their balance, the body keeps fit. But when their balance is lost in the event of internal or external disorders the body becomes diseased.

In addition, the body consists of the following major functional aspects--

(a) Five main elements--Earth, Water, Fire, Wind, Sky.

(b) Seven physical elements--Plasma, Blood, Flesh, Fat, Bones, Marrow, Semen.

(c) Five physical activities--Hands, Legs, Mouth, Penis (uterus), Anus.

(d) Five senses of perception--Eyes, Ears, Nose, Tongue, Skin.

(e) Four Other Subtler Senses--Mind, Intellect, Supreme Mental Power, Merciful Sense of the Heart.

(f) Three Excrements--Excrement, Urine, Perspiration.

It is necessary to understand the interelationship among these six elements and how the power of digestion maintains a delicate balance between them. The digestive power is almost a synonym of life. Its prime manifestation is in the digestive fire of the stomach. It acts in five ways; viz. digestion, pleasure, amusement, vision-promotion and elimination. It transforms the energy of food that we eat into the cells required by the body. When the digestive power in the stomach degenerates and becomes unbalanced, a process of deterioration begins and a series of diseases arise. Subsequently, if this process continues unchecked, the three humours get spoiled and they in turn spoil the six elements. Therefore, the cause of all diseases lies in an imbalance of the above elements, and when this imbalance continues over a prolonged period of time, the diseases are said to become chronic. Naturopathic treatment re-creates a balance between these elements and restores them to their natural and proportionate forms through Panchkarma, that is, the Fivefold Method of Diagnostic Treatment. Panchkarma usually results in an extraordinary success in the treatment of chronic diseases in a short span of time--something that other system of medicine are generally unable to achieve.

Kinds of Disease

According to modern science, there are 231 diseases in the head and the upper part of the body and 789 diseases in the rest of the body. Of these, 57 diseases come under the category of cancer--32 of them occur in the mouth and 19 of them are incurable.

Naturopathy, however, recognizes only five main categories of diseases--

(1) Diseases due to variation in the proportions of wind, bile and phlegm, i.e. the three humours in the body.

(2) Diseases arising out of natural causes.

(3) Diseases arising as a punishment for actions done in past (i.e. karma).

(4) Fleeting diseases that result from accidents.

(5) Diseases created by the strong chemicals and toxins of allopathic medicines.

These diseases can have physical and/or mental manifestations and can be treated by regulating the quality and quantity of natural foods consumed. No medicines are given in naturopathy.

Fever is the king of diseases. There are thirty kinds of fever. All fevers except those which are stress-induced, can be cured by fasting. Fasting is prohibited in fevers due to stress and anxiety. Allopathic treatment brings down fevers very quickly. Naturopaths believe this is detrimental to the body as it causes a tremendous strain on the physical system and leads to weakness. Naturopathic methods bring fevers down slowly but surely, and in the process also remove their causes.

Typhoid is considered to be the most severe fever by naturopaths because it lasts twenty-one days. Any fever that lasts longer is called a "worsened fever", visham fever or jirna-jwara. Tuberculosis and cancer are forms of jirna-jwara.

All fevers can be cured by panchkarma (five modes of treatment) without resorting to surgery. This has been borne out by scientific experiments. Panchkarma is also the only remedy in the world for curing cancer.

The main operating tenet of naturopathy is the following: "A disease can be expelled only by a suitable diet, which is prescribed in accordance with the principles of naturopathy. It cannot be fully removed even by consuming hundreds of medicines, in the absence of a wholesome natural diet."

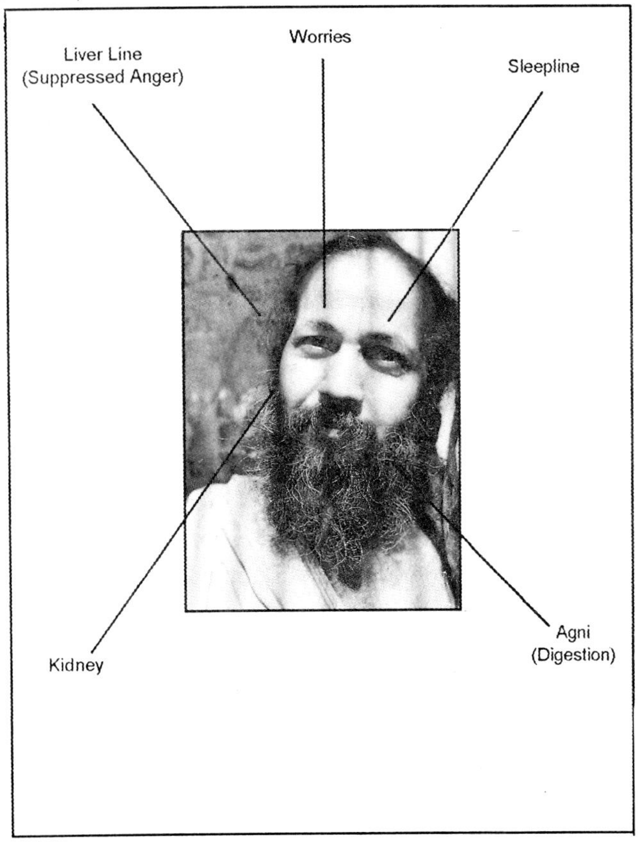

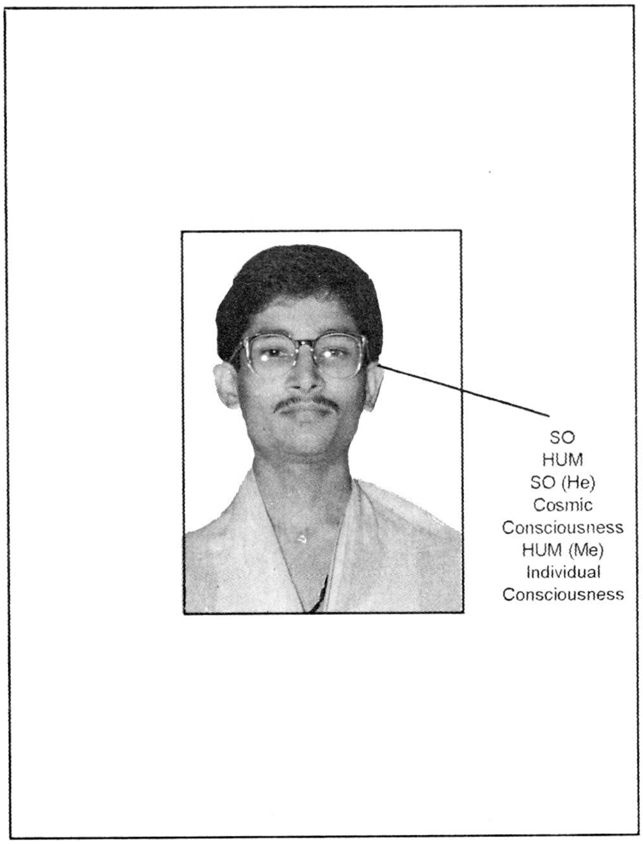

Chapter IV

Health And Disease

Prerequisites for Natural Health

In spite of the advance of science and knowledge, disease and sickness are on the increase. Could it be because there is something radically wrong with the conventional methods of living and treating ailments? The truth is that our civilization is encouraging life-styles contrary to the principles of healthy living. Custom and fashion are at war with Nature. The principles enjoined by modern living and the indulgence that they foster are steadily lessening our physical and mental strength, thereby increasingly burdening the very process of our survival.

Natural or positive health is the only true prophylactic, or means of immunity against disease. It is the duty and privilege of every intelligent person to acquire sufficient knowledge of the principles of healthy living in order to lead a happy, healthy and successful life. How strange it is that we know much less about things near at hand than about things at a distance. Nothing is more intimately part of us than our body, but there is perhaps nothing else of which our ignorance is so profound and our indifference so complete.

Health is a normal and harmonious vibration of the elements and forces comprising the human entity on the physical, mental, moral and spiritual planes of being, in conformity with the constructive principles of Nature applied to individual life. Health is the result of living in accordance with the natural laws that operate in the mind, emotions and body. To build and maintain the optimum level of health, every habit must be correct and every law of life observed, to the extent possible. The basic principles of healthy living are:

- fresh air and sunshine;
- deep breathing;
- regular exercise;
- correct posture;
- rest, relaxation, recreation and sleep;
- proper food and regulated diet;
- external and internal cleanliness and proper elimination;
- right mental attitude.

Fresh Air and Sunshine

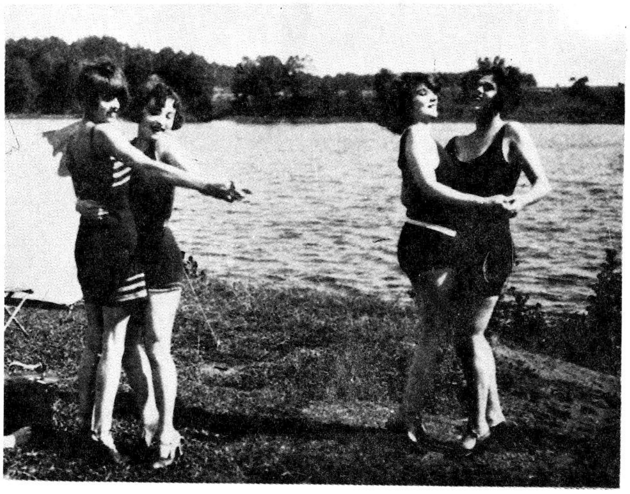

Fresh air and sunshine are as necessary for good health as food, water and breathing. Oxygen, received into the body from the air, is necessary for every bodily function. One of its most important yet least recognized functions is its role in burning up the body's waste materials. It is impossible to have good blood, active nerves and a high level of metabolism if fresh air is denied, so avail yourself of all you can get. Live, work, play and sleep in the open as much as possible and secure an ample amount of fresh air when indoors.

While taking an air bath, we expose the entire body to the air, bathing it in the air, so to speak. An sir bath gives the skin a chance to breathe if its pores are not clogged with debris. It keeps the pores active and promote the elimination of waste. But more than this, it has a most soothing and invigorating effect upon the nervous system, particularly when the air is cool or cold. At the time of an air bath, it is essential that the body is comfortably warm.

The sun, the great sterilizer and life giver, has to be given its proper place for aiding health. The sun is a great nutritional agent and sunlight is an essential factor for maintaining health. Sunlight has tremendous curative and health-giving properties. Injurious bacilli on the skin are rendered innocuous by sunlight. It also induces the production of vitamins D and E, both essential for healthy living. Although sunlight cannot manufacture vitamin A by its action on the skin, it induces changes by which the least amount of this vitamin will serve to maintain growth and health.

The regenerative action of the sun on the skin is due to its light rays and not its heat rays. Therefore, the cold rays of the sun should be availed of as far as possible since unaccustomed over-exposure to the heat of the sun may be injurious. The best times, therefore, for having a sunbath early morning and late evening when the rays of the sun are diffused. Small doses of sunlight do not injure the skin or create any other adverse effects.

Deep Breathing

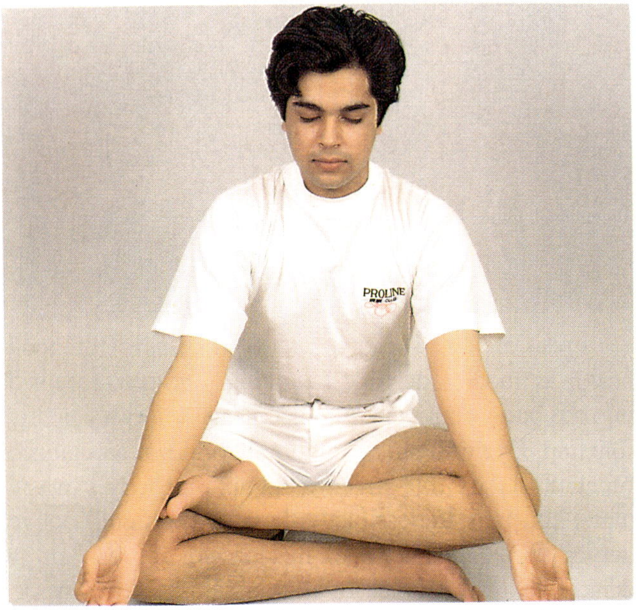

We can go without food for many weeks and without water for several days, but without air we cannot live for even a few minutes. Breath is life. Taking a deep breath is like blowing at a smouldering fire, because it brightens the vital flame of life. By taking a full breath, we inhale a large quantity of oxygen and by retaining it a while, we stir and purify the air which always remains in the lungs. On exhaling, we expel carbon dioxide and other poisonous gases.

Not only does physical health improve with correct breathing, but mental power, happiness, self-control, clear-sightedness, moral and even spiritual growth can be increased by proper breathing or Pranayama. Deep breathing is an effective method by which the respiratory organs can be developed. It has the additional advantage of putting extra oxygen into the blood and, therefore, of securing a richer tone for the blood, which in turn, means an offer of richer material to the system for its consumption. Proper breathing also helps to wake one up. It is a good preparation for the morning exercises or bath, and energizes all the bodily functions for their routine of daily duties. Remember never to neglect your systematic breathing while walking, exercising, sitting or resting.

Nature has made oxygen the primary element for the survival of all living beings. In natural and outdoor surroundings one can freely breathe in an abundance of this oxygen. We also get oxygen from water and food, but the life-sustaining source of oxygen is the air.

Man, in his natural state, has no need of instruction in breathing and like animals and children he breathes naturally and properly just as Nature intends him to do. But civilization has taken him away from the natural states of existence and has changed not only his breathing, but also the other aspects of his physiology. He has adopted improper methods and postures of walking, standing and sitting, all of which have robbed him or his birthright of natural and correct breathing. The habitat of modern-day man, which consists of temperature-controlled rooms, forces him to breathe stale air with a low oxygen content. Also, the tensions of work and anxieties of living produce an apathy of the nerves and muscles that control breathing and hence there is an insufficient supply of health-giving oxygen in most of them. Man has paid a high price for civilization.

Breath should be inhaled from only the nostrils, because among the organs of respiration, only the nostrils have a protective filter apparatus or dust catcher, i.e. their numerous tiny hairs. Also the long, narrow, winding passage of the nostrils is filled with warm mucous membranes which warm the inhaled air so that it can cause no damage to the delicate organs of the throat and the lungs. Inhaling through the mouth deprives us of this protection. People who breathe through their mouth in sleep awaken with a parched feeling in the mouth and a dryness in the throat.

The best time to do breathing exercises is in the morning, just before or after rising, and in the evening, but not just before or after retiring. In the morning, the stomach is empty and there is plenty of room for full expansion of the lungs.

Exercise

Exercise is essential to life and health. The body can be efficient only as long as its muscular system is in shape. The muscle tone depends upon the elasticity and compactness of individual muscles, and also upon their ability to expand and contract. Normal muscles alternately contract and relax. Contraction forces blood out of the muscles and relaxation forces more blood to come to them. The return flow of venous blood depends on the intermittent pressure of this action and reaction.

Exercise tones up muscles. Active, vigorous exercise requires the complete coordination of the nervous, cardiovascular and respiratory systems. The muscles derive their energy from oxygen in the blood, and to a lesser extent, from the fats, carbohydrates and proteins in the body. They transform potential energy into kinetic energy. Vigorous active exercise may require as much as five to ten times the amount of oxygen consumed during rest. To ensure that the respiratory system supplies this an increased amount of blood is pumped into the heart, which then contracts more vigorously and quickly. The blood pressure also rises correspondingly and there is also a marked increase in the activity of the central nervous system. The more the oxygen consumed, the greater the increase in the hydrogenation concentration in the blood passing through the respiratory centres, and the greater is the increase of nervous impulses. This accelerates the activity of the lungs. The heart and diaphragm share in this process and there is a consequent increase in energy due to a greater coordination of the nerves, the muscles and the circulatory and respiratory systems.

Violent or unaccustomed exercise should never be indulged in by sedentary persons or those suffering from any ailment or infection as it can result in severe injury or even death. It is essential that the body is completely healthy before any exercise is prescribed.

Exercise may be for physical training or for therapeutic purpose. Exercise undertaken for physical training or education is further subdivided into athletic sports and ordinary gymnastics. Therapeutic exercise--also known as medical gymnastics--is prescribed for correcting various deformities, diseases or injuries.

"Walk more, ride less". Walking is the greatest of all exercises. It is an exercise that can be taken by everybody--strong as well as weak. No matter what form of muscular activity you may be using, walking should be included. For walking to be beneficial, it must be graceful. If one walks in a slow, slovenly manner the improvement will be much less than if one moves briskly with an elastic step.

Correct Posture

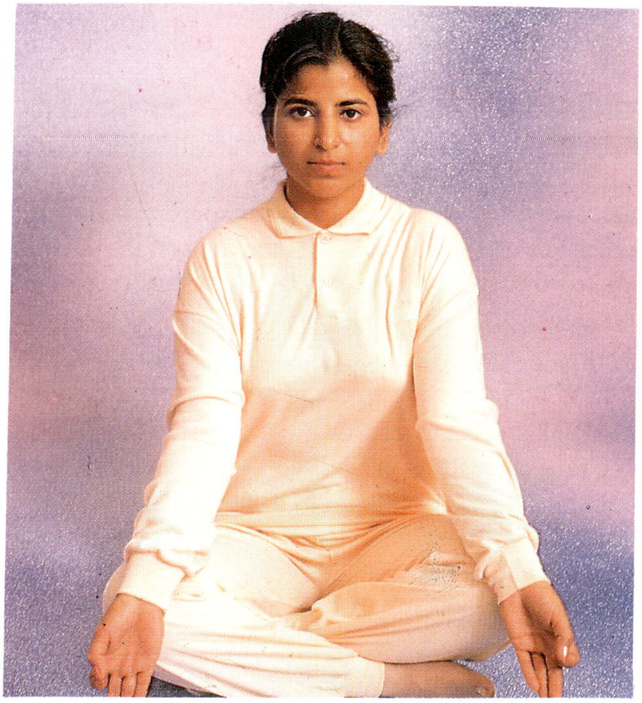

Man is the only animal that walks erect and the only animal whose spine bends forward in old age.

Hold the chest up when sitting, standing and walking and, as far as possible, at work. Maintaining an erect spine is physiologically important. The mechanical arrangement of the spine is such that if it is held erect, the important nerves that emanate from this central 'bureau' to all parts are able to function perfectly. When there is pressure on these nerves, their functioning is bound to be impaired, affecting the organs concerned. An erect carriage also maintains the proper position of the vital organs. When the body is held erect, the chest is full, round and somewhat expanded, leaving plenty of room for the heart and lungs. The stomach, liver and intestines all tend to sag when the body bends forward and their functioning then becomes impaired, just as a machine malfunctions when its parts are distorted.

From the cradle to the grave, gravity affects man's posture. He has to resist this force while awake and even when resting. He must also improve his working habits so that he can assume a normal posture at every opportunity. Mother nature has generously endowed man with the chemical and material factors of life and the mental ability with which to obtain them. But when the body structure is mis-aligned, the full ability to use these factors is lost.

Abnormal posture affects the spine, producing rotations, curvatures, hyphosis (humps) and lordosis (abnormal sways). These spinal distortions interfere with the normal motion and produce pressure on the nerves which emanate from between the vertebrae and lead to various parts of the body. When the spinal muscles are weakened the individual vertebrae become distorted easily and abruptly, thereby producing serious nerve pressure, pains, disease and malfunctions in the body. Many of these spinal distortions, especially curvature related, cause mechanical pressure effects and twists upon the internal organs, thus interfering with their drainage and other functions.

Among the bad habits that produce a distorted posture is the habit of putting more weight on one foot than the other. This practice causes the longitudinal-transverse arch to become lower or more collapsed in one foot than in the other. This leads to the sacrum, the big bone at the base of the spine, tilting to that side. The resulting spinal rotations and curvatures may balance themselves abruptly enough at certain points of the column to produce serious nerve pressures.

Rest, Relaxation, Recreation and Sleep

Exercise is necessary for health, but relaxation is equally necessary. One cannot be constantly active. It is important to take proper rest by a change of stressful activities and recreation and to endeavour to sleep well by going to bed early and getting up early.

Rest means an absence of effort; it is counterbalancing of work. *Recreation* is a physiological term which denotes a change of effort. Recreation balances the output of energy by exercising physical and mental energies which have not been at work. In other words, recreation is an activity which calls into action parts of the body and brain not ordinarily used, or which uses parts that were previously active in a different manner. Recreation thus refreshes the body by a change of activity. *Relaxation* denotes muscular limpness. It is important to learn to relax both mentally and physically, because only if there is complete relaxation can the muscles work more efficiently. Relaxation completely relieves fatigue in a very short time as it promotes venous blood circulation throughout the body.

The best method of relaxation is to practise the "dead-man's pose", the *shavasana*. When we lie down to rest in a waking condition our muscles remain slightly contracted. Even this slight contraction is overcome in Shavasana.

Sleep provides conditional or partial rest to the human machine. Nature has provided sleep as a means of alternating activity and rest and thereby securing health. One cannot really rest unless the demand for rest has first been created by activity. The natural process of body and tissue repair takes place during rest and relaxation. Muscles are not built during exercise; it is only when they are at rest or during muscular relaxation that the building process takes place.

The purpose of sleep is to repair the losses and damage which are caused by work. Every nerve centre, every cell in fact, is a storage battery. Work discharges this battery while sleep recharges it. Sleep must be sound, deep, regular, timely and refreshing. For sleep to be good and refreshing, it must be sound; for sleep to be sound it must be regular, i.e. it should occur at pretty much the same time every day. Alternate sleeping and waking, during the same hours on successive days, can render sleep difficult, uneasy and insecure.

A state of unconsciousness, or simulated sleep produced by drugs is a dangerous counterfeit, as it induces a state of abnormal muscular lethargy and weakness which are as debilitating as fatigue. The activation of the subconscious while we are asleep is essential for a sound and refreshing sleep.

Regulated Diet

This deserves a chapter by itself and is treated in Chapter VIII.

Internal and External Hygiene

One's well-being is the sum total of the care of all the different and vital organs of one's body, both individually and collectively, plus the necessary precautions and observances of general hygiene. The term "hygiene" denotes individual cleanliness. Sanitation generally refers to municipal cleanliness, the main items of which are water supply, drainage, etc. Both hygiene and sanitation are important for health.

Personal hygiene does not apply to merely washing

the outside skin or wearing clean clothes but also to the cleaning of the teeth, the hair, the nose, the eyes, etc. Filth breeds disease. Cleanliness is a strong defence against disease--whether contagious or self-generated. Cleanliness involves everything with which we come in contact. It should be observed not only at home, but must involve all our surroundings and environment. The condition of the internal organs depends, to a great extent, upon the cleanliness of the body.

The body has an ever-flowing stream of healthy blood. Any impurities or abnormalities in the blood because of toxic conditions in the body lead to discomfort and disease. Self-poisoning, also known as auto-intoxication, is poisoning from within. The worst is intestinal auto-intoxication because it affects every organ and tissue of the body.

The colon serves as a waste receptacle or sewer and, like every other sewer, means must be provided for its flushing. The first important step in keeping the colon clean and healthy is to eat a diet consisting of wholesome and natural foods, instead of merely eating to please the palate or the stomach and then depending upon purgatives to clear away the garbage. The colon's normal mode of functioning, its natural rhythm or periodicity must be considered and given its rightful place in the day's programme. The functions of the colon cannot be neglected or postponed with impunity.

Many think themselves to be in good health because their bowels move once a day. But their bowels may be incompletely evacuated, and consequently they may suffer from a foul breath and coated tongue and other indications of auto-intoxication. Constipation is called the "mother of all diseases". It should be avoided, not by strong purgatives and pills but by regulating the diet, by exercise and in short, by observing the laws of health.

Right Mental Attitude

Just as gymnastic exercises, faithfully practised, develop bodily health and strength, mental training is indispensable to increase the health and efficiency of the mind. Both the body and the mind need to have routines for their activities and rest if they are to function properly.

Thinking is not merely confined to the brain. The whole body participates in this thought process. We feel and think with our bodies, and sensations arising in the body in turn express themselves through what we call thoughts or feelings. In turn, the mind, and especially the emotions, are among the most powerful influences which affect the body. Joy, sorrow, anger, fear and other emotional states may exalt or depress bodily functions as quickly and as powerfully as the most potent of drugs or the most active of physical agents. Certain emotions poison the body. Hate, envy, scorn, jealousy and fear actually create poisons, not merely psychological poisons, but also powerful toxic chemicals which poison the life force and the blood. Under their influence, the body weakens and all the bodily processes get disturbed. It is therefore important to be calm and content, and avoid worrying and depressing or exhausting emotions.

Since mind and body are inextricably linked, if either of them get out of order the whole system suffers. It is an illusion to believe that the mind can be cultivated at the expense of the body. The two are so closely interwoven and interdependent, that any effort to develop one at the expense of the other will defeat itself. A highly developed mind is an outgrowth of and not a substitute for a well-developed bodily life.

The growth of man and civilization should be parallel. Reason, intelligence and mind must rule all civilized men. Yet this is not so because all the so-called civilized men of today do not agree that both brain and brawn should be developed side by side.

The belief that the new mechanical sources of power and energy render the physical development of man unnecessary and that man's contribution to the mechanism of civilization is wholly mental is a serious error. For man's mental dynamo is charged from his physical health. When the wheels of his physical being slow down, the electrical energy of his mind will correspondingly weaken and decay. Physical weaklings are incapable of directing the machinery of civilization.

Success in life largely depends upon mental health, which in turn cannot be maintained without a good foundation of physical development. The well-being of the body must be first developed to pave the way for the well-being of the mind. This is the natural order of development. Neglect your body, and your whole life will become a failure. Without a sound knowledge of the principles of health, therefore, no one can be prepared for life's responsibilities. Rightly the ancients said, "*Mens sana in corpore sano*"--A healthy mind in a healthy body.

A healthy mind is the result of eliminating fear, conquering worry, avoiding anger, omitting depression, shunning hate, studying cheerfulness, cultivating hope, developing courage, exhibiting confidence, assuring success, living simply, maintaining buoyancy, controlling one's self, and thinking of health as one's due. When tranquillity is undisturbed by keeping serene, one's mental powers are at their best.

Longevity

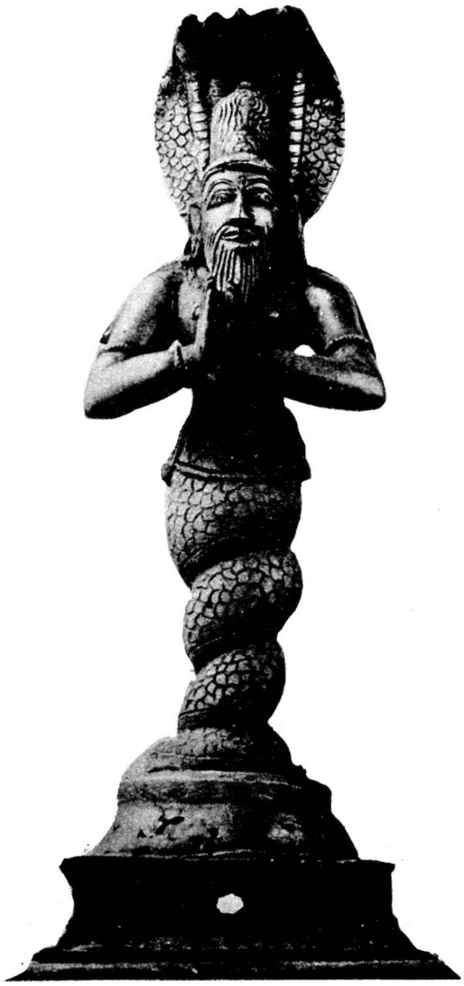

The body is engaged in a continuous struggle against the ageing process. Because continuous breakdown of the bodily tissues and organs at the cellular level causes deterioration and degeneration, it is at the cellular level that rejuvenation must take place.

The tridosha of vata, pitta and kapha are of prime importance in the maintenance of cellular health and longevity. Kapha maintains longevity at the cellular level. Pitta governs digestion and nutrition. Vata, which is closely related to pranic life energy, governs all life functions.

At a deeper level, to combat ageing it is necessary to balance the three subtle essences (dhatu) within the body--prana, ojas and tejas. Their functioning corresponds, at a subtler level of creation, to the functioning of vata, kapha and pitta, respectively. Proper diet, exercise and life-style can create a balance among these three subtle essences, ensuring long life.

Prana is the life energy that performs respiration, oxygenation and circulation. It also governs all the motor and sensory functions. The vital pranic force enkindles the central bodily fire (agni). The body's natural intelligence is expressed spontaneously through prana. For example, if a child has a deficiency of iron or calcium, the body's natural intelligence, governed by prana, will lead the child to eat mud which is a source of these minerals. The head is the seat of prana, which governs all higher cerebral activities such as memory, thought and emotions. The functioning of the heart also is governed by prana; from the heart prana enters the blood and thus controls oxygenation in all the dhatus and vital organs.

Prana governs the biological functions of the two other subtle essences, ojas and tejas. A disorder of prana may create an imbalance of ojas and tejas and vice versa. In the foetus, prana enters mainly through the umbilical cord.

Ojas is the vital energy that controls the life functions with the help of prana. It is the essence of the seven dhatus or bodily tissues and is the vital energy that governs the hormonal balance. Ojas contains all the vital substances of the bodily tissues and is responsible for the auto-immune system and for mental intelligence. The superfine element of shukralartav, which is the essence of all dhatus, is located in the heart.

Ojas being related to kapha, aggravation of kapha displaces ojas and vice versa. Displaced ojas creates the kapha-related disorders of diabetes, looseness of the bones and joints and numbness of the limbs. Decreased ojas will create vata-related reactions such as fear, general weakness, reduced sense perception, loss of consciousness and death. Balanced ojas is necessary for biological strength and immunity.

Ghee helps to enhance ojas. In infants, mother's milk promotes it. Ojas travels into the fetus from the body of the mother during the eighth month of pregnancy. This is why premature birth may endanger an infant's life. This shows the importance of ojas in the maintenance of life functions and for longevity.

At the psychological level, ojas accounts for compassion, love, peace and creativity. Through pranayama, spiritual discipline and tantric techniques, one can transform ojas into spiritual strength. This powerful spiritual energy creates a halo around the crown chakra. A person with strong ojas is attractive, with lustrous eyes and a spontaneous and calming smile. He is full of spiritual energy and power. Spiritual practices and celibacy enhance ojas. Those who over-indulge in sex and masturbation dissipate ojas at the moment of orgasm. The resulting weakness of ojas directly affects the immune system, rendering the individual susceptible to psychosomatic ailments. Tejas is the essence of a subtle fire that governs metabolism through the enzyme system. Agni, the central fire in the body, promotes digestion, absorption and assimilation of food. The further transformation of nutritive elements into subtle tissues is governed by a subtle level of energy of agni, which is tejas. Tejas is necessary for the nourishing and transformation of each dhatu. Every dhatu has its own tejas, or dhatu-agni. This essence is responsible for the physiological functioning of the subtle tissues.

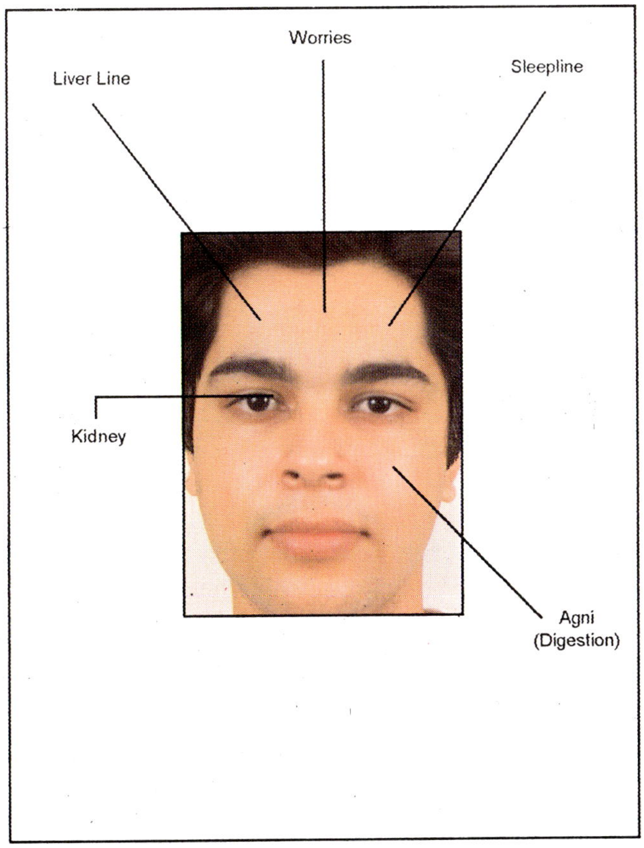

Tejas, if aggravated, burns away ojas reducing immunity and over-stimulating pranic activity. Aggravated prana produces degenerative disorders in the dhatus. Deficiency in tejas results in tumorous tissue and obstruction of the flow of pranic energy.

Just as it is essential for health to ensure balance among the three humours (vata, pitta and kapha), the dhatus (prana, ojas and tejas) and the three bodily wastes (malas--excrement, urine and perspiration), it is also important for longevity that prana, ojas and tejas remain in balance. Improper diet, bad living habits and overuse of drugs cause an imbalance in tejas. Hot, sharp and penetrating substances directly enhance tejas, creating an imbalance.

Rejuvenation must take place on the physical, mental and spiritual levels. Before starting the physical rejuvenation programme, the body must be cleansed. A dirty cloth will not take the right colour when dyed; so also the body will not profit from rejuvenation unless it has first been cleaned from inside. A rejuvenating herb, taken orally, passes through the stomach, small intestine and large intestine before entering the bloodstream. All these physiological pathways must be purified for the herb to reach the deeper bodily tissues where the rejuvenation process begins.

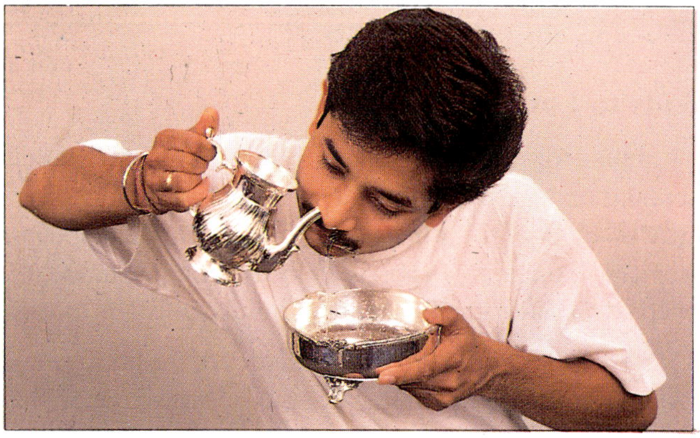

Bodily cleansing is accomplished through Panchkarma (five actions or processes): vomiting, purgatives, medicated enemas, nasal administration of herbs and purification of the blood. Vomiting cleanses the stomach which is the seat of kapha; purgation purifies the small intestine, the seat of pitta; medicated enemas cleanse the large intestine, the seat of vata; and nasal administration of herbs clarifies the mind and consciousness. To purify the blood, blood-letting is necessary; this treatment cleanses the blood so that the blood plasma may carry the rejuvenating nutrients of the herbs to the deep tissues.

Mental rejuvenation involves calming of the mind. A quiet, meditative mind also helps longevity. To this end, one must learn to witness all mental activities, thoughts and emotions, remaining detached from the experience.

To promote mental peace, one naturopathic recommendation is isolation and avoidance of worldly affairs and society. Since this approach is not practical for most people, naturopathy recommends a second method, in which one learns to be in the world but not of the world. With this approach, he observes his attachments to determine which of them creates stress. A life without attachment and stress is the happiest, healthiest and most peaceful, enhancing longevity. Celibacy and spiritual discipline are useful for rejuvenation as are yogic practices. These disciplines lead to spiritual understanding and a rejuvenating way of living.

Modern medicine has developed the technology to sustain bodily life even after the body's communication with the emotions and the spirit has ceased. Although naturopathy supports the extension of life, it also teaches that there may be karmic limitations to life. Naturopathy respects both life and death and their intimate bond; the science of life, it also suggests ways in which one can meet death peacefully. According to naturopathy, death is a friend of man. The body dies but not the individual consciousness (soul): it is eternal.

Aids to Longevity

Freedom presupposes discipline. The naturopathic foundations of discipline are a careful diet and a balanced way of living. Discipline of the body, mind and spirit--and consequent freedom--is gained through pursuit of such traditional practices as yoga, pranayama and tantra.

Yoga. If naturopathy is the science of the body, yoga is a science of the spirit. They are sister sciences. According to naturopathy, the practice of yoga is an important, natural, preventive measure to ensure good health. In India, it is traditional to study naturopathy before taking up the practice of yoga, because only when the body has become fit through the study of naturopathy is the individual considered ready to study the spiritual science of yoga.

The father of yoga, Patanjali, described eight limbs of yoga and yogic practices as follows: the natural regulation of the nervous system; discipline; cleansing; postures; concentration; contemplation; the awakening of awareness; and the state of perfect equilibrium. Yogic exercises have both preventive and curative value. They bring man to the natural state of tranquillity, which is equilibrium. Yogic practices help to bring natural order and balance to the neuro-hormones and the metabolism and improve the endocrine metabolism and thus fortify one against stress. Yogic practices for the treatment of stress and stress-related disorders (such as hypertension, diabetes, asthma and obesity) are remarkably effective.

Yoga is the science of union with the Ultimate Being. Naturopathy is the science of living, of daily life. When yogis perform certain postures and follow certain disciplines, they open up and move energies that have accumulated and stagnated in the energy centres. When stagnant, these energies create various ailments. Yogis may temporarily suffer physical and psychological disorders because in the course of yogic cleansing of the mind, body and consciousness, disease-producing toxins are released. Employing naturopathic diagnosis and treatment, the yogis deal effectively with these disorders.

Naturopathy indicates which type of yoga is suitable for different constitutions. For example, a person of pitta constitution should not perform the headstand posture for more than one minute. If he does, mental disorientation may result. Similarly, a person of vata constitution should not perform the shoulder stand as it exerts too much weight on the seventh cervical vertebra. This vertebra is sensitive and the delicate bone structure of vata may cause a shift in the spinal column. Repressed anger will shift the cervical vertebra to the right side and repressed fear will shift it to the left. The person of kapha constitution should not perform the hidden lotus posture too long because this pose causes direct pressure on the adrenal glands.

Breathing (Pranayama). Breathing exercises, called pranayama, are a yogic healing technique that can bring about an extraordinary balance in consciousness. In practising pranayama one experiences pure Being and learns the true meaning of peace and love. Pranayama cleanses the lungs, heart and other organs and purifies the nadis which are pranic currents of energy in the body. Pranayama has many healing benefits and also affects creativity. It can bring joy and bliss into life.

Naturopathy indicates which pranayama exercises are suitable for different constitutional types. A person of pitta constitution should perform left nostril breathing--inhale through the left nostril and exhale through the right, using the thumb and middle finger to close and open alternate nostrils. This exercise cools the body by enhancing female energy. A person of kapha constitution should do right nostril breathing, inhaling through the right nostril and exhaling through the left. This exercise heats the body by stimulating male energy. A person of vata constitution should perform alternate nostril breathing. As vata is an active force, alternate nostril breathing brings balance.

An obese person should perform the yogic breathing exercise called the 'breath of fire'--sit in a comfortable position, take a deep breath and exhale quickly and forcefully through the nose. Inhalation will happen naturally after each exhalation. This exercise aids in metabolizing fat. It should be performed for one full minute followed by one minute of rest and then another minute of breathing exercise for a total of five minutes. This exercise is equivalent to running two miles. (An overweight person doing this breathing exercise will sweat and become thirsty. He should, however, avoid a chilled drink, because chilled drinks increase the build-up of body fat.

Pranayama, executed correctly, can cure disease; but will create disease if done improperly. The reader should not begin pranayama without the guidance of an individual who has experience in this system of healing.

Mantra. Mantram (singular of mantra) is a Sanskrit term denoting a word or group of words that carries certain phonetic vibrations and energy. Certain sacred Sanskrit words carry tremendous energy and chanting them in a prescribed manner releases this energy. A mantram should be chanted aloud first so that one can listen to the sound. The vibration of the mantram penetrates deeper and deeper into the heart and finally one may remain silent, working internally with the supersonic sounds. The energy of a mantram helps one to achieve balance in the body, mind and consciousness. Just as food for the body should be chosen according to the constitution, so also with mantram whose purpose and effective action is to nourish the individual soul.

Meditation. Meditation brings awareness, harmony and natural order to life. It awakens the intelligence to make life happy, peaceful and creative. The awakening of this creative intelligence is the benediction of meditation.

A single, simple method of meditation is to select free time, in the early morning if possible, and sit quietly. Allow your eyes to survey the surrounding environment, your ears to receive its sounds. Relax your muscles. After spending some time observing this external world, close your eyes and bring your awareness from the outside to the inside. Begin to notice the movements of your thoughts, desires and emotions. From the bank of consciousness observe the movements of the river of thoughts. Do not try to stop, change or place judgments on this experience. Through this internal observation, you are being cleansed of distractions; you are arriving at the beginning of a radical transformation. As unobstructed awareness increases, you will begin to enjoy increased relaxation and the store-house of energy will unlock within you: these are the benedictions of meditative practice.

Another form of meditation also brings great blessings. Sit quietly and observe your breathing. Breathing is the movement of prana. Prana is life-force and life-energy which has two polarities: inspiration and expiration. Inspiration is cold and expiration warm. Together they create a natural biorhythm. Through breathing, you will become aware of the vibration of cosmic sound. This cosmic sound, which is the soundless sound "aum", has a male manifestation and a female manifestation. The male manifestation is "hum" and the female energy is "so". During inhalation, you will feel the vibration of the cosmic sound "so" and during exhalation, the sound "hum".

In "so-hum" meditation, individual consciousness unites with Consciousness. Listen to the "so-hum", "hum-so" sound through the breath. These vibrations are sound-energy which is one with the life-energy of the breath. Your breathing will become quiet and spontaneous and you will go beyond thought, beyond time and space, beyond cause and effect. Limitations will vanish; your consciousness will empty itself, and in that emptying, consciousness will expand. This merging of individual consciousness into the Cosmic Consciousness brings samadhi, the state of highest equilibrium. In that state, peace and joy will descend as a benediction. Your life will change and daily living will become a new and fresh experience. Life will become meditation, for meditation is not separate from life but a part of life. Life is meditation and meditation is life. Creative intelligence will begin to operate in your body, mind and consciousness. All problems will dissolve in this new expanded awareness. Keep in mind, however, that all the beneficial results of meditation are the fruits only of committed and regular practice.

CHAPTER V

Diagnostic Methods

The progress of nature cure, despite its wonderful achievements, has been greatly retarded by the perpetuation of the old idea that diagnosis is not necessary. Many naturopaths still maintain that it is only necessary to intensify elimination and neutralize toxemia and then nature cure will take care of the rest. This is not always so, and the physician who has been practising for any length of time soon comes across cases that require specific diagnostic investigations. The fact that naturopaths treat their patients symptomatically does not render diagnosis superfluous. Adopting diagnostic means does not necessarily mean imitating allopaths. It means progress, or being true to our patients, and it also means an end to being the laughing-stock of other practitioners. Only by being or attempting to be scrupulously correct in all these clinical activities will naturopaths win the esteem of medical practitioners and patients alike.

Proper examination and diagnosis gives the physician a much better understanding of the abnormal conditions with which he must contend, and thereby greatly facilitates efficient treatment. Moreover, the patient is entitled to a correct diagnosis of his case and to a rational and reliable prognosis. It is only with correct diagnosis and specific treatment that the risk of malpractice can be avoided.

In a disease, many conditions are hidden deep down in the body's recesses which laboratory and other fine tests are often unable to reveal. The diagnosis of a disease is important but what is more important is a diagnosis of the condition of whole body--physical, mental, emotional and spiritual. Only when nature cure physicians, scientists and astrologers will have reached a friendly understanding, will health be universally enjoyed, for mankind will be taught how to live properly and thus avoid suffering and sickness. Then the doctors will be just as anxious to keep people well as they now are to help them to recover from disease.

In the West, the term diagnosis generally refers to identification of the disease after it has manifested. In naturopathy, however, the concept of diagnosis implies a moment-to-moment monitoring of the interactions between order (health) and disorder (disease) in the body. The disease process is a reaction between the bodily humours (tridosha) and the tissues. The symptoms of disease are always related to derangement of the balance of the tridosha. Once we understand the nature of the imbalance, balance may be reestablished through treatment.

Naturopathy teaches precise methods for understanding the disease process before any overt signs of the disease have manifested. By detecting early symptoms of imbalance and disease reaction in the body, one can determine the nature of future bodily reactions. Day-to-day observation of the pulse, tongue, face, eyes, nails and lips provide subtle indicators. Through these, the student of naturopathy can learn what pathological processes are occurring in the body, which organs are impaired and where dosha and toxins have accumulated. Thus, by checking the body's indicators regularly, pathological symptoms can be detected early and preventive measures taken. Naturopathy teaches that the patient is a living book, and, for understanding and physical well-being, he or she must be read daily.

The methods used for examination and diagnosis, from the nature cure view point, are a combination of all those that have been proved to be true and efficient in all systems from the oldest to the most advanced, whether orthodox or unorthodox, provided they conform to the fundamental laws of cure. This is what makes nature cure philosophy and practice a true eclectic system of treating ailments.

The progressive naturopathic physician employs some of the means generally adopted in medical practice for making his diagnosis, and in addition, osteopathic and spinal diagnosis. This practice often reveals causes of functional derangement which are not normally discoverable by other methods of examination.

According to naturopathy, the following five steps should be adopted while diagnosing any ailment--

1. *Case history*, i.e. the full medical history of the patient.
2. *Pre-condition*, i.e. details of all the symptoms prior to the onset of present disease.
3. *Present form*, i.e. complete details of the symptoms of the current ailment.
4. *Allayment*, i.e. the meals, medicines & situations in and by which the patient gets relief from the symptoms of his present ailment.
5. *Total change*, i.e. how has the disease affected his body as a whole.

Experienced naturopathic physicians can diagnose any of the 1020 diseases of the body very quickly by following this diagnostic procedure. The key bodily indicators which naturopaths examine before arriving at a diagnosis are given below.

Examination of the Radial Pulse

The radial pulse is felt with the index, middle and ring fingers. The doctor faces the patient and takes the pulse of each wrist. The indicators of the pulse vary between the two sides of the body, so it is best to check the pulse on both sides. The pulse should not be taken after exertion, massage, eating, bathing or sex. The pulse will also be affected by sitting near heat or by taking strenuous exercise. The pulse may be taken at other points on the body as well.

To check your own pulse, keep your arm and wrist slightly flexed. Place your three fingers lightly on the wrist just below the radial bone (wrist bone) and feel the throbbing of the pulse. Then decrease the pressure of the fingers slightly to sense varying movements of the pulse.

The position of the index finger denotes vata dosha. When vata is predominant in the constitution, the index finger will feel the pulse strongly. It will be irregular and thin, moving in waves like the motion of a serpent. This type of pulse, called the "snake" pulse, indicates aggravated vata in the body. The resting place of the middle finger denotes pitta. When pitta is predominant in the constitution, the pulse will be stronger under the middle finger. It will feel active and excited and will hop like a frog. Called the "frog" pulse, it denotes aggravated pitta. When kapha is predominant, the pulse under the ring finger throbs strongly. Its movement resembles the floating of a swan. It is therefore called the "swan" pulse.

Not only the constitution, but the status of the organs also can be determined by examination of the superficial and deep pulsations. The beats of the pulse not only correspond to the heartbeat, they also reveal something about the important meridians that are connecting pranic currents of energy in the body. These currents circulate through the blood, passing through the vital organs such as the liver, kidney, heart and brain By feeling the superficial and deep pulsations, a sensitive examiner can detect the conditions of these various organs. Each finger rests on a meridian of the element associated with the dosha of that place. For example, the index finger which rests on the vata dosha detects bodily air; the middle finger which touches on pitta detects fire; and the ring finger which feel the kapha pulse, water.

The index finger rests on the patient's right wrist at the site for feeling the activity of the large intestine with a superficial touch; when deeper, firmer pressure is applied, the activity of the lungs may be sensed. If very prominent throbbing is felt when the index finger on the right side is applied superficially, then vata is aggravated in the large intestine; if the deep pulse is strong and throbbing, there is congestion in the lungs. The middle finger resting on the right wrist can detect the status of the gall bladder with superficial touch and the liver with deeper pressure. The ring finger senses the pericardium (outer covering of the heart) when applied superficially; and, with a deep touch, the harmonious relationship of vata-pitta-kapha is detected.

The index finger resting superficially on the patient's left wrist monitors the activity of the small intestine, while the heart is monitored by deep pressure. With superficial pressure of the middle finger, the activity of the stomach is observed; and deep pressure reveals the status of the spleen. The ring finger applied superficially reveals the condition of the bladder while deep pressure checks the functioning of the kidneys. To learn this technique of examination of the pulse requires attention and day-to-day practice.

You can feel the variations in your pulse at different times of the day. You can also note changes in the pulse after urination, when you are hungry or when you feel anger. Observing such changes, you will begin to learn how to read the pulse

Facial Diagnosis

The face is the mirror of the mind. The lines and wrinkles in your face are revealing. If disorder and disease are present, they will be indicated on the face. Observe the different parts of your face carefully in the mirror. Horizontal wrinkling on the forehead indicates you have deep-seated worries and anxieties. A vertical line between the eyebrows on the right side indicates your emotions are repressed in the liver. A vertical line between the eyebrows on the left side indicates your spleen is holding in emotions.

When the lower eyelids are full and puffy, it indicates that the kidneys are impaired. A butterfly-like discoloration on the nose or on the cheeks just below the cheek bones means the body is not absorbing iron or folic acid and the digestive metabolism is malfunctioning because of low agni.

Generally, a person of vata constitution cannot gain weight. Therefore, his cheeks become flat and sunken. A person of slow metabolism (kapha constitution) will retain water, fat and the cheeks will be plump.

The shape of the nose can indicate the constitution. A sharp nose may denote pitta; a blunt nose, kapha; and a crooked nose, vata.

Iridology

Naturopaths frequently use "iridiagnosis", which is a method of diagnosing bodily conditions by an examination of the iris. In the normally functioning body, there are no discolorations or marks in the iris. The average individual's iris presents almost every conceivable colour, although there are two fundamental colours--blue and brown. Bodily conditions, racial characteristics and climatic conditions have mixed many other shades of brown, greyish blue, inky blue and hybrid shades. One iris may be brown and the other blue or one iris may have one part brown and the other the other part blue, etc. The iris contains many minutely pigmented cells, muscular fibres, vessels and filaments or nerves, which through the optic nerves, optic thalami, the sympathetic nervous system, and the spinal system, connect the iris with every body part. This enables it to receive impressions from every part, and because of its delicate structure, it produces pigments and lesions that reflect the changes that have taken place in the organs. These changes can be recognized by the various colours deposited in the layers of fibres of the iris. Sluggishness and atrophy of nerves and other bodily structures can be recognized in their respective stages--such as acute, chronic and destructive by examining the iris. The more degenerative the condition, the deeper is its impression in the layers of the iris.

Nature proves to us through the eyes that all substances which cannot be assimilated or be absorbed in any form and remain in the body become toxic. It is often noticed that the diagnosis obtained from the iris of the eye independently describes the same lesions in the eyes which the spinal therapist discovers in the spine and nerve centres, and which the physician finds through his physical examination and which is confirmed by laboratory and radiology findings as well. When the purification of the whole system takes place as a result of the elimination of body contaminations and toxins, the result is immediately reflected in the eyes. The diagnosis from the iris is of great interest and importance, not only because it gives accurate information about diseases which cannot be diagnosed in any other way, but also because these wonderful records confirm the fundamental principles of the philosophy and practice of nature cure.

Other Diagnostic Methods

Nadi Vidya (the science of the pulse) is the system of diagnosis by feeling the pulse. It is practised by the old school of Ayurvedic physicians and should be included in the practice of nature cure.

Those interested in rational methods of treatment, whether conservative or progressive, feel that ***astro-medical analysis*** if judiciously employed, can and should play a role in the understanding of diseases and the scientific cultivation of health. Astro-diagnosis is the science and art of obtaining scientific knowledge regarding diseases and their causes and the means of overcoming them by studying planetary configurations and movements. Latent ailments can always be foreseen astrologically.

The zodiac is the broad belt of space in which the sun and planets seem to travel around the earth. It is divided into twelve segments, each being related with some body part. Thus the first segment, Aries, is related to the head; the second, Taurus, to the neck and so on. These divisions follow in regular order down to the twelfth and last, Pisces, which corresponds to and sympathizes with the feet. Any one or more of the planets can occupy various portions in the zodiac, depending upon where their orbital revolutions take them at any given moment, and their position *vis-a-vis* the earth as it rotates on its axis, and according to the manner in which each planet thus located combines its rays favourably or adversely with the other planets. Thus, the influences of the zodiac, either for good or for evil, are manifested in the body parts that correspond to each of its signs. In astro-pathology, special importance is attached to malefic planetary influence. Thus, the fiery Mars can cause fevers and acute diseases, while the chronic Saturn can cause obstructions, Uranus can cause spasms, etc.

To be accurate, all these details have to be computed from data collected by the astronomical observatories, and then interpreted in accordance with the accepted rules of astrology. By determining the date, place and time of a person's birth, we can get a map or picture of the position of the stars that influence him and the fundamental asteroidal forces at work in his system. Such a map is likely to indicate any weak parts or organs. Constitutional tendencies are thus discoverable, and can then be suitably dealt with. By more detailed and complicated analysis, we can also estimate the astral influences that operate for any given year. Thus astrology makes it possible to diagnose a patient's symptoms which can otherwise only be discovered by the usual methods of physical examination.

The twelve zodiac signs govern different body parts and are related to its cell-salts. Their position in a person's birth chart plays an important role in predisposing his body to certain types of ailment. The parts that the twelve zodiac signs influence are as follows:

Aries, the ram, rules the head. Its chief constituent is kali phos (potassium phosphate).

Taurus, the bull, rules the neck, throat and cerebellum. Its chief cell-salt is natrum sulph (sodium sulphate).

Gemini, the pair of celestial twins, rules the lymphatic and respiratory systems. Its cell-salt is kali muriaticum (potassium chloride).

Cancer, the crab, rules the solar plexus and the chest. Its cell-salt is calcaria fluor (calcium fluoride).

Leo, the lion, rules the heart and motor nerves. Its cell-salt is magnesia phos (magnesium phosphate).

Virgo, the virgin, rules the abdominal region. Its cell-salt is kali sulph (potassium sulphate).

Scorpio, the scorpion, rules the hips. Its cell-salt is calcaria sulph (calcium sulphate).

Libra, the scales of justice, rules the urinary and sexual organs. Its cell-salt is natrum phos (sodium phosphate).

Sagittarius, the archer, rules the thighs. Its cell-salt is silica (silica oxide).

Capricorn, the goat, rules the bones and legs up to the knees. Its cell-salt is calcaria phos (calcium phosphate).

Aquarius, the water bearer, rules the calves up to the ankles. Its cell-salt is natrum mur (sodium chloride or common salt).

Pisces, the fish, rules the feet and blood (chiefly the red blood corpuscles). Its cell-salt is ferrum phos (phosphate or iron.)

Each of these twelve cell-salts is a natural product of the earth. Their production is increased in the whole organic kingdom when the sun enters each sign of the zodiac, i.e., when the earth comes between the sun and each sign of zodiac.

Astrology not only helps in diagnosing the physical characteristics of an ailment but also the character and disposition of the patient, whether he is weak, whether he is negative or emotional, etc.

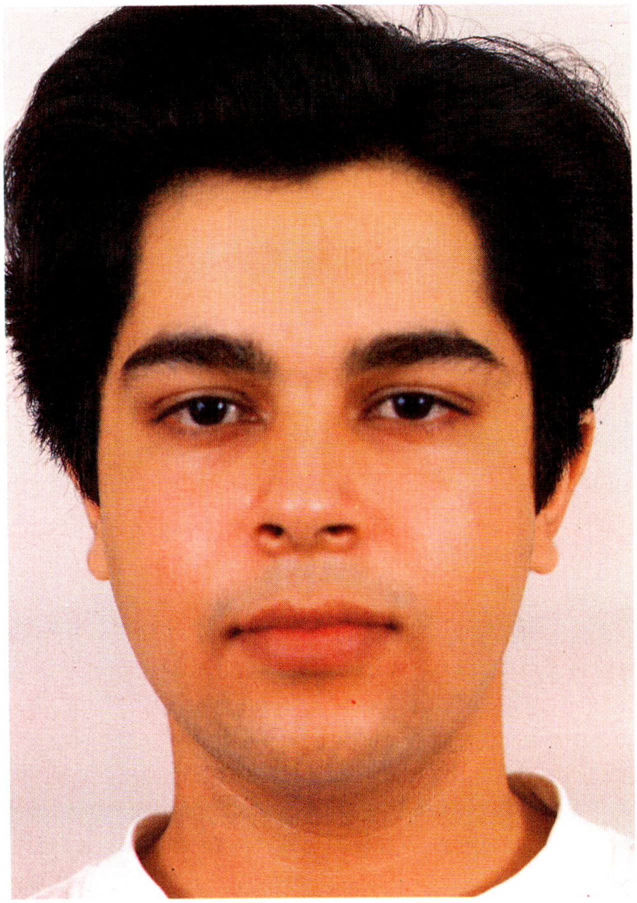

CHAPTER VI

Treatment

All naturopathic treatment attempts to establish a balance between the bodily humours--vata, pitta and kapha. Disease results when these three are out of balance on account of the accumulation of toxins in the body. The initiation of any form of treatment (whether medication, acupuncture, chiropractic, massage, allopathy or any other) without first eliminating the toxins will only push these poisons deeper into the tissues. Superficial treatment may result in symptomatic relief of the disease process, but the fundamental cause of the illness will not be affected and the problem will therefore manifest again in the same or another form.

There are two types of naturopathic treatment, i.e. (a) elimination of toxins and (b) neutralization of toxins. These treatments may be applied on both the physical and emotional levels.

Emotional Release

Anger, fear, anxiety, nervousness, jealousy, possessiveness and greed are common emotions. Yet most people learn not to express these negative emotions in childhood. As a result, one begins at an early age to repress the natural expression of these feelings. The science of naturopathy teaches that one must release these emotions because, if they remain repressed, they will cause humour imbalances resulting in the creation of disease-causing toxins.

The naturopathic technique for dealing with negativity is observation and release. For example, when anger appears, one should be completely aware of it; watch this feeling as it unfolds from beginning to end. From this observation, one can learn about the nature of the anger and then let the anger go, release it. All negative emotions may be dealt with in this way. Naturopathy teaches that through awareness all negative emotions can be released.

Fear is associated with vata; anger with pitta; and greed, envy and possessiveness with kapha. If one represses fear, the kidneys will be disturbed; anger, the liver; greed and possessiveness, the heart and spleen.

Physical Treatment--Panchkarma

Panchkarma ("five actions" or "five processes") is very useful in eradicating toxic matter from all parts of the body. It is naturopathy's efficacious treatment for numerous ailments such as excess mucus in the chest, bile in the intestines, kapha in the stomach or gas accumulation in the large intestine. The processes of Panchkarma cleanse the body, mind and emotions. The five basic processes of Panchkarma are--vamana (vomiting); virechana (purgatives or laxatives); basti (medicated enema); nyasa (nasal administration of medication); and rakta-moksha (purification of the blood).

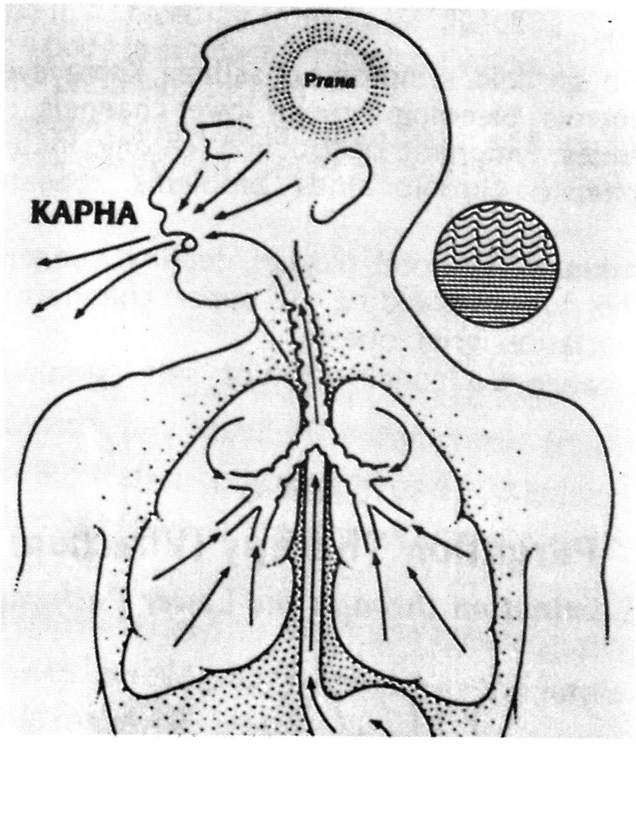

Vamana (therapeutic vomiting). When there is congestion in the lungs causing repeated attacks of bronchitis, cough, cold or asthma, the naturopathic treatment is therapeutic vomiting (vamana), to eliminate the mucus-causing excess kapha. One method of accomplishing this is to administer three or four glasses of licorice or calamus root tea and then stimulate vomiting by rubbing the tongue. Alternatively, before brushing one's teeth in the morning, one may take two glasses of salt water, which will aggravate kapha and then rub the tongue to induce vomiting. Once the mucus is released, the patient will feel instantly relieved. Congestion, wheezing and breathlessness will disappear and the sinuses will become clear. Therapeutic vomiting is also indicated for skin diseases, chronic asthma, diabetes, chronic cold, lymphatic obstruction, chronic indigestion, edema (swelling), epilepsy (between attacks), chronic sinus problems and repeated attacks of tonsillitis.

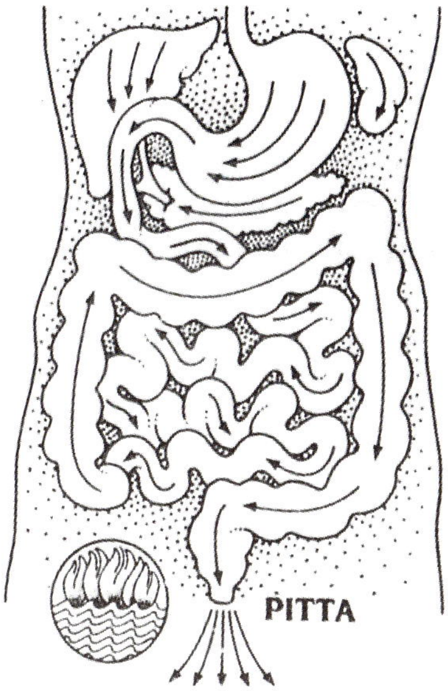

Virechana (purgatives). When excessive bile is secreted and accumulated in the gall bladder, liver or intestines, an allergic rash or skin inflammation such as acne or dermatitis, as well as chronic fever, ascites, biliary vomiting or jaundice may result. The naturopathic treatment for this condition is administration of purgatives or laxatives. A number of fine herbs can be used for this treatment. For example, senna leaf tea is a mild laxative. In people of vata constitution, however, this tea might create griping pain, since its action aggravates the peristaltic movement in the large intestine.

An effective laxative for persons of vata or pitta constitutions is a glass of hot milk to which two teaspoons of ghee have been added. This laxative, taken at bed time, will help to relieve the excess-pitta-induced bile disturbance in the body. Such purgatives can, in fact, completely cure the problem of excessive pitta. Purgatives should not, however, be given to persons with low agni, acute fever, diarrhoea, severe constipation, anal bleeding or lung cavities. Nor should they be administered when a foreign body is present in the stomach, after enema, or in cases of emaciation, weakness or prolapsed rectum.

When purgatives are used, it is important to check the diet. The patient should not eat foods that will aggravate the predominant humour or cause the three humors to become unbalanced.

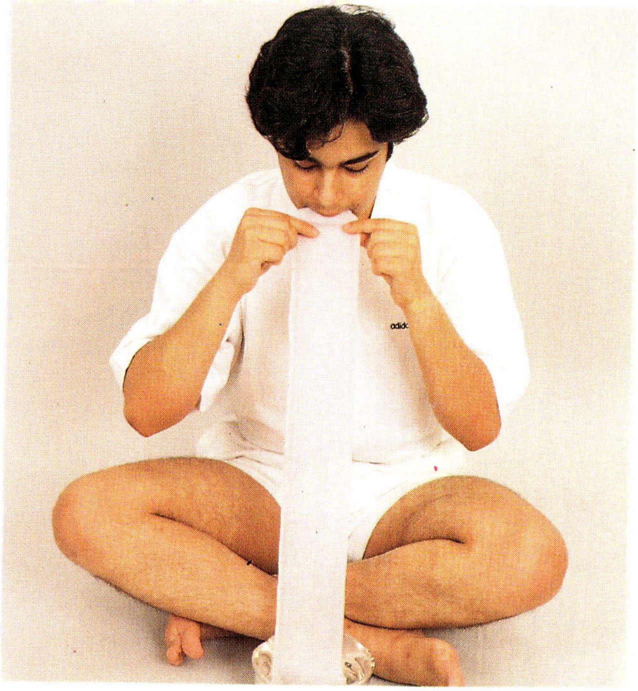

Basti (enema). Naturopathic enema treatment involves the introduction of medicines such as sesame oil, calamus oil or herbal decoctions in a liquid medium into the rectum. Medicated enemas are regarded as being the complete treatment for all vata disorders. Vata is a very active principle in pathogenesis, and there are at least eighty different vata-related disorders. Basti is a complete treatment for eighty per cent of these diseases. It alleviates constipation, distension, chronic fever, common cold, sexual disorders, kidney stones, heart pain, vomiting, backache, neck pain and hyper acidity. Many vata disorders such as sciatica, arthritis, rheumatism and gout can also be treated with enemas.

Medicated enemas should not be given if the patient is suffering from diarrhoea or anal bleeding. An oil enema should not be given to persons with chronic indigestion, cough, breathlessness, diabetes or severe anaemia; nor to the aged or children below seven years of age. Decoction enemas (herbs boiled in water) should not be given for acute fever, diarrhoea, cold, paralysis, heart pain, severe pain in the abdomen or emaciation. Oil or decoction enemas should be retained for a minimum of thirty minutes, and longer if possible.

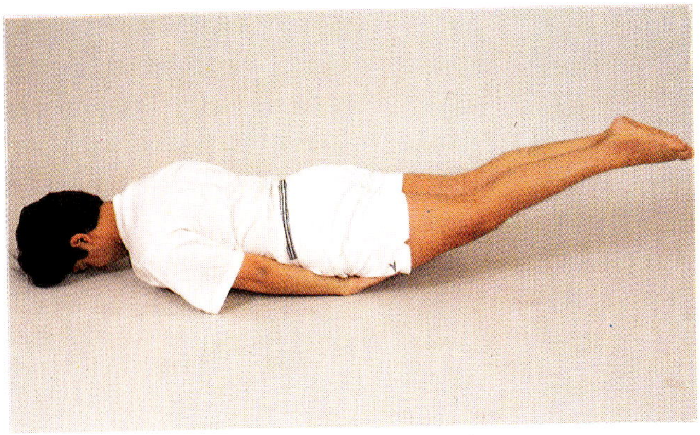

Nasya (nasal administration). The nasal administration of medication is called nasya. An excess of bodily humours accumulated in the throat, nose, sinus or head is eliminated by means of the nearest possible opening. The nose is the door to the brain and to consciousness. Prana or life energy enters the body through the breath inhaled through the nose. Prana maintains the sensory and motor functions. Nasal administration of medication helps to correct the disorders of prana which affect the higher cerebral, sensory and motor functions.

Nasal administration is indicated for dryness of the nose, sinus congestion, hoarseness, migraine headache, convulsions and certain eye and ear problems. In general, nasal medication should not be administered after a bath, food, sex or drinking alcohol, nor should it be applied during pregnancy or menstruation.

Breathing also can be improved through nasal massage. For this treatment, the little finger is dipped in ghee and inserted into the nose. The inner walls of the nose are slowly massaged, going as deeply as possible. This treatment will help to open the emotions. (Nose tissue is tender and for this application the fingernail must be kept short to avoid injuring the delicate mucous membranes). Since a lot of people have a deviated nasal septum, one side of the nose will be easier to penetrate and massage than the other. The finger should not be inserted forcibly. The massage should proceed by slow penetration, the finger moving first in a clockwise, then in a

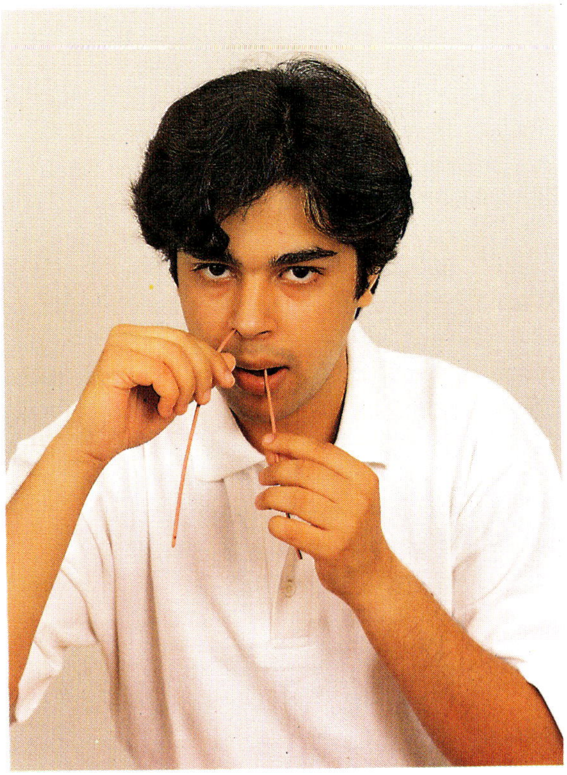

counterclockwise direction. By this means, the emotions that are blocked in the respiratory tract will be released. One may administer this treatment every morning and evening. In this way, breathing patterns will change as the emotions are released and the eyesight also will improve.

Rakta Moksha (blood-letting). Toxins absorbed into the bloodstream through the gastro-intestinal tract circulate throughout the body. They may manifest under the skin or in the joint-spaces, creating disease. In such cases, elimination of toxins and purification of the blood is necessary.

For repeated attacks of skin disorders such as urticaria, rash, eczema, acne, scabies, leucoderma, chronic itching and hives, blood-letting (rakta moksha) is indicated. It also is effective in cases of enlarged liver and spleen, and for gout.

Pitta is manifested in the waste products of the blood, so in many pitta disorders, such as rash and acne, toxins are circulated in the blood system. Thus, for many pitta ailments, extracting a small amount of blood from the vein relieves the tension created by the toxins in the blood. (This procedure should be administered only by a physician.)

Blood-letting also stimulates the production of antitoxin substances in the blood, which in turn help to develop the immune mechanism of the blood system. Thus, the toxins are neutralized enabling radical cures of many blood and bone disorders.

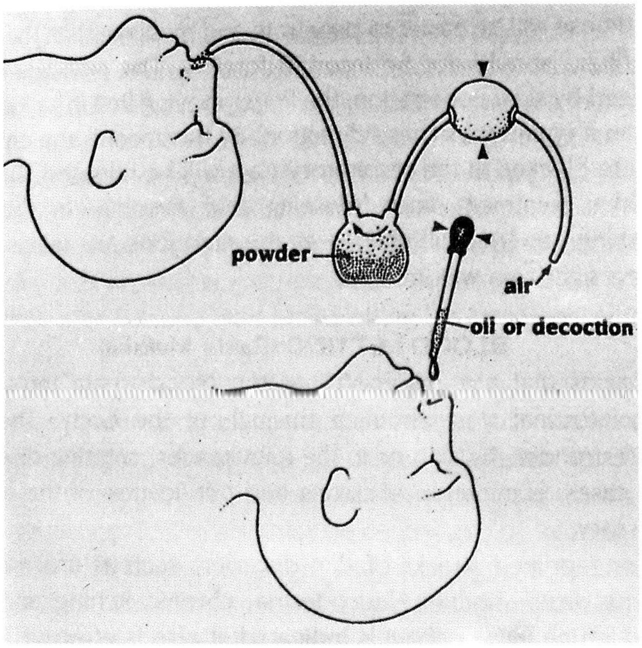

Blood-letting is contra-indicated in cases of anaemia, edema and weakness. This treatment is not recommended for young children or the aged.

Some substances such as excess sugar, salt, yogurt and sour tasting foods are toxic to the blood. In certain blood disorders, to keep the blood pure, these substances should be avoided.

Burdock root tea is the best blood-purifier. For blood-carried disorders such as allergy, rash or acne, the patient should take a milk laxative and the next evening begin burdock root tea therapy. The tea is made from one teaspoon of powder in one cup of hot water. If taken every night, the action of the herbs will begin to purify the blood. Other blood-purifying herbs are saffron, sandalwood powder, turmeric and calamus root powder. Pomegranate juice, orange juice and asparagus root are also beneficial for blood ailments. These may be used after blood-letting has been performed.

Palliation

Following Panchkarma treatment to eliminate the more serious toxins, the process of palliation (shaman) is employed. Palliation involves neutralizing the toxins by enkindling aging and stimulating the digestion through fasting. Toxins also may be neutralized by internal use of hot, pungent herbs such as ginger and black pepper. Sustained hunger and thirst, exercise, sunbathing and sitting in the fresh air are other means of neutralizing toxins.

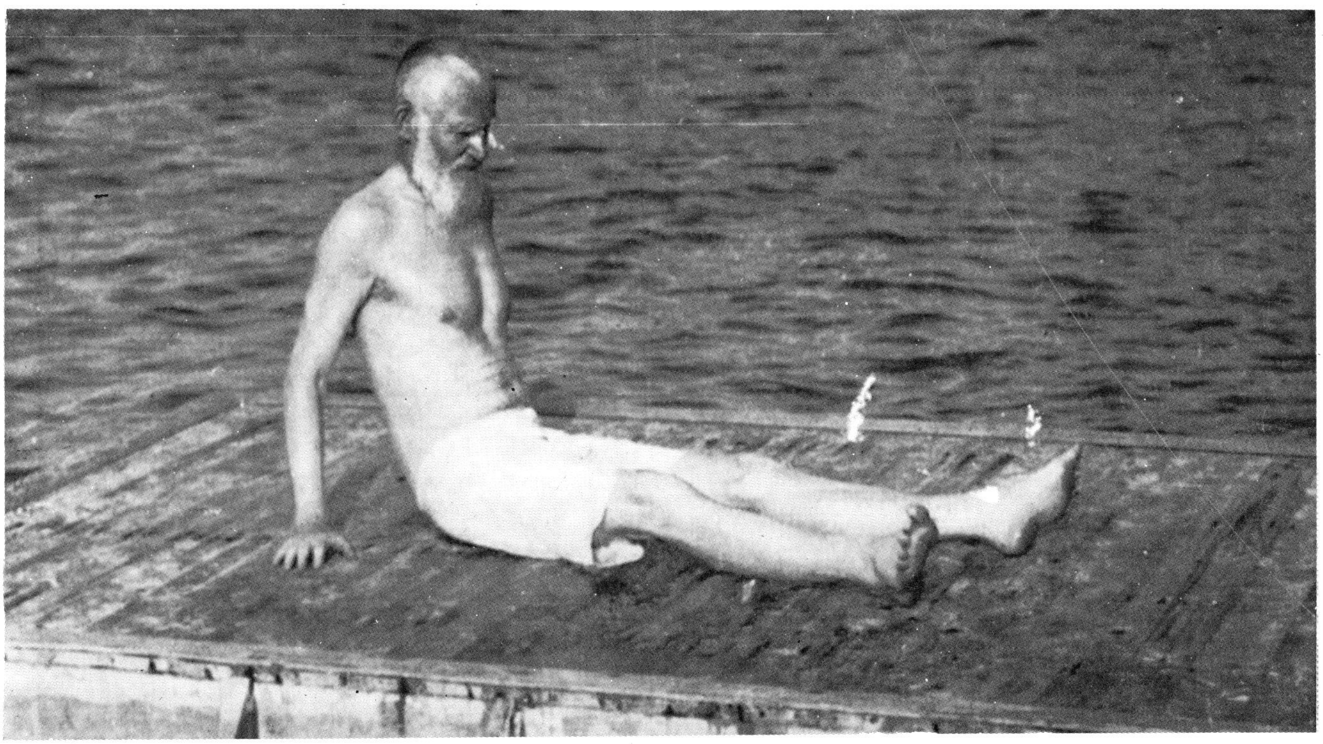

Mr. Bernard Shaw is an enthusiastic sun-bather.

CHAPTER VII

Drugless Therapy

Naturopathy combines the various systems of drugless therapeutics into a correlated system of general practice that brings man into harmony with nature. The various systems of drugless healing used by naturopaths are: hydrotherapy, electrotherapy, ultra-sound, heliotherapy, chromotherapy, chiropractic, osteopathy, vibro-therapy, orificial therapy, spondylo-therapy, zone-therapy, exercise, massage, traction and psychotherapy. These are described in the following paragraphs.

Hydrotherapy

Hydrotherapy or water treatment includes the use of water in every possible form and method--internally as a beverage, externally as a bath, through breathing as vapours or steam, as a cleansing agent in douches and enemas, as hot and cold water baths, as an ingredient in mud baths and clay packs, and as a therapeutic exercise medium in swimming pools--to treat ailments. Water is the oldest of all remedial agents. The earliest medical literature refers to it. The habits and customs of ancient civilizations, which have been brought to light in recent years by the study of the old Assyrian and Egyptian records, also disclose this fact. The ancient Egyptians, Hebrews, Greeks, Persians and Indians all employed water in the treatment of disease, as do their descendants even today.

The popularity of hydrotherapy has waxed and waned during the centuries, but its use has continued. The modern popularity of water as a remedy is largely owing to the enterprise and ingenuity of Vincent Priessnitz, who has been called the Father of Water Cure. In the United States too, hydrotherapy attained great popularity towards the end of the last century through the efforts of Dr. Simon Baruch. Dr. John H. Kellogg, of Battle Creek, Michigan later set up a large nature-cure sanatorium, which specialized in hydrotherapy. He pioneered the development and systematic application of various forms of water treatment with great success and presented his results before the medical profession.

Water possesses four remarkable properties, all of which render it very valuable for healing purposes:

1. Great power in absorbing and communicating or giving up heat.
2. Great solvent properties--water is the one universal solvent.
3. Availability in three forms--liquid, solid and gaseous (Steam).
4. Great flexibility in method of storage--it takes the shape of any container it is stored in.

No other therapeutic agent possesses so many admirable qualities as water. It is the most flexible medium for producing any thermic and mechanical effect desired, and can be applied both to a limited area and to the whole surface of the body. No other substance is capable of absorbing so much heat as water does. It also gives up this heat readily. It can therefore be used for either abstracting heat from the body or for use in the form of an enema or colonic irrigation. Water is of great use in the elimination of urea and uric acid, harmful body salts, excessive sugars and many other blood and food chemicals that are waste products. Apart from the thermal effects, the mechanical effect of water (pressure) also enhances the therapeutic effect of water application.

Several vital reactions and organic changes can be brought about by the periodic application of hydrotherapy. The nerve centres, the heart and blood vessels, the voluntary and involuntary muscles, the digestive system, and in fact, every organ, every tissue, every cell and every function, is effected by the proper application of water.

While water is usually applied to the body, in both health and disease, in its liquid form, there are conditions in which the application of vapour form (i.e. steam) has superior advantages. There are still other conditions in which its solid form (i.e. ice) is extremely convenient and more serviceable.

Cold water increases muscular tension and therapy improves the tone of the muscles and blood vessels. Warm water causes relaxation, brings on muscular dilation and a consequent reduction of muscular tone. Water is therefore a natural tonic.

Cold Water. Cold applications have several beneficial effects on the body. A localized cold application contracts the capillaries in that area and produces pallor and coldness. But as soon as the application is over, blood rushes to the area, and the area is suffused red. Hence, if the patient's vitality is high, the secondary effect of a cold application is increased vigour, because of the force with which blood rushes to the cooled parts. But if one's vitality is low, even short cold applications may cause fairly prolonged depression as the parts to which the applications were made soon return to their previous state of subnormal activity. In such cases, cold applications will not have any beneficial effect. To conclude, cold water application on the body results in the apparent paradox of deriving a stimulating or tonic effect from an action which primarily depresses the activity of the skin and its surrounding tissues. This clearly shows that it is not the effect of the cold that one seeks to produce in most cases, but the after-effects induced by cold sensations.

Hot Water. One of the chief values of the application of hot water on the skin is that it prepares the body for the application of cold water. The reactive power of cold water is greatly increased if a certain degree of preliminary heating has taken place. In cases of fatigue, rheumatism, anaemia or enfeeblement, such a preliminary heating of the body is of considerable importance.

Hot baths have, in many respects, just the opposite influence of cold baths. Hot baths relax the tissues while cold baths energizes them. Hot water is soothing and is invariably effective in relieving pain.

Hot water can also be used to excite or depress the nervous system. High temperature baths should not last very long or they will over-excite the nervous system and produce nervousness, headaches, dizziness, nausea, etc. Water-induced heat, if continued unduly long, may also produce exhaustion and fatigue.

On the other hand, a prolonged neutral bath (that is, with water slightly below the body's temperature), if continued for half to one-and-a-half hours, produces a complete insulation of the nerve centres and acts as a delightful sedative.

Alternative Hot and Cold Application. One of the most stimulating of water applications is the alternate hot and cold bath. This is a most efficient means of stimulating nutrition and of overcoming local congestions and anaemias, without causing any disturbance in the body's heat balance.

The Body's Capacity to Tolerate Heat. The body's internal mucous membranes can tolerate water ten to fifteen degrees hotter that can the external skin temperature. This is why we drink liquids comfortably which are hot enough to scald the skin. The hot water of an enema or rectal irrigation may be comfortably borne in the rectum while its contact with the skin passage would be painful. In steam or vapour baths, a temperature up to 120 F is generally employed for most patients, but for some who can remain in hotter baths a temperature of 145 F is given for a short time. In Turkish or hot air baths the usual temperature is much higher and ranges from 140 F to 180 F. In special cases, it can even be raised to 220 F to 250 F without injury.

A sweat box, which includes steam baths, radiant heat or hot air and sauna baths, is a most convenient means of inducing perspiration. The chief therapeutic value of these baths is elimination. They are generally employed for treating rheumatism, gout, urticaria, toxaemia, diabetes and obesity.

Several newer applications, uses and procedures of hydrotherapy are being discovered every year across the world. Two of the most recent advances have been the development of whirlpool baths and underwater exercises. They are extensively employed today, especially in the treatment of poliomyelitis. It has been shown that partially paralysed patients can move with very little effort in water because of its buoyancy which increases the possibility of movement in all planes.

Whirlpool baths were first employed during World War II in the treatment of painful stumps after amputation. Such baths have also been found to be of value in the management of other conditions such as sprains, dislocations, peripheral vascular diseases, arthritis, and infected wounds of the extremities. These baths are extremely useful in treating fractures of the extremities, especially at the time of the removal of a limb from a cast or a splint. They are almost ideal in all such cases for improving circulation, relieving pain and stiffness and for preparing the limb for subsequent massages and exercises.

It is fortunate that this great healing agent has been systematized and made into a science, for its improper applications may prove more detrimental. Water is a double-edged sword. While it is a most simple and natural remedy, it is also a most powerful destructive agent.

Electrotherapy

There are a multitude of indications for the use of electricity in therapeutics. Electricity produces mechanical, chemical, thermic, actinic and psychic effects on the body. The application of different electrical currents and modalities causes powerful muscular contractions of both the voluntary and involuntary muscular fibres, stimulates damaged nerves and restores them to normality, produces profound sensory effects, relieves pain or over-irritation and inflammatory conditions, dilates or constricts cutaneous blood vessels without producing heart depression, corrects faulty metabolism, hastens the elimination of waste products such as urea, uric acid, carbon dioxide, solidified lime deposits, etc., hardens or liquefies the body tissues; and produces anaesthesia and artificial respiration, introduces various remedies through the unbroken skin directly to the seat of pain.

Also, employing electrotherapy in diagnosis enables us to differentiate between the different forms of paralysis by ascertaining whether it is due to a brain lesion or a lesion in the spinal cord, to test muscular degeneration, locate foreign bodies, identify structural dislocations and malpositions within the body and so on.

The use of electricity enables the nature cure physician to obtain quick results. Some of its applications are in the form of currents like galvanic, faradic, sinusoidal, high frequency currents, diathermy of the long and short wave varieties, radiant heat baths, etc. Electricity does a function that water cannot in heat treatment. Heat induced by methods like hot water, hot air, steam bath, hot compresses, hot air douches, etc. produces only surface heating. Electricity is the only technique of heating the innermost tissues and organs. By means of electric diathermy, heat can be produced at any desired depth and place inside the body.

Ultra-Sound

A recent introduction in electric heat application is the ultra-sonic or ultra-sound process. Just as ultra-violet light cannot be seen by the human eye, ultra-sound is inaudible to the human ear. Sound vibrations can pass deep into tissues through the skin, muscles and bones and bring about strong movements in the tissue particles. Such movements are accompanied by friction, and friction produces heat. In fact, warmth is instantly felt in the tissues through which the ultrasound waves pass. Some diseases which are treated by diathermy over a long period without result can be cured quickly and effectively by using ultra-sound. It has a lasting effect especially in nervous diseases like neuritis, neuralgia, sciatica and other similar illnesses.

Until a few years ago, all kinds of diseases were sounded somewhat desultorily, resulting in reactions that were not always welcome. Systematic research and application has made it possible to control the results more satisfactorily.

Electrotherapy is not a cure-all, and is not a substitute for other methods. But it is a single broad spectrum remedial agent and there is scarcely a condition or disease for which it cannot be used in some form, either as an adjunct or as a remedy.

Heliotherapy

Sunlight is a fundamental biological need, and in importance ranks alongside oxygen, water and food. Natural sunshine and artificial sunshine are both of extreme value in therapeutic work as auxiliary healing agents. Used in conjunction with other measures like fasting, dieting and exercises, they form a very useful and successful means of healing.

In India, with its abundance of sunshine, heliotherapy can go a long way in providing medical relief to the teeming masses. An Institute of Ray Therapy (Solarium) has been established in Jamnagar in Gujarat, where systematic research on heliotherapy is done. Large number of cases are being treated there, especially those of rheumatism, surgical tuberculosis and skin sensitivity.

A therapeutic sun bath utilizes a wide range of wave energies. Of all these, the short ultra-violet waves are the most therapeutic. The other longer heat waves are also beneficial, but it is the shorter waves that stimulate various life processes and destroy bacteria.

Radiation is a broad term which includes X-ray, radium emanation, ultra-violet, visible rays and infra-red rays. Strictly speaking, only that portion of the spectrum which we see, i.e. the visible region, is light. Though heliotherapy is commonly known as light therapy, it is more correct to refer to heliotherapy as ultra-violet and infra-red radiation rather than of ultra-violet and infra-red light.

The benefits of sunlight are intimately related to climate and altitude. The most beneficial results are attained on a seashore. The least beneficial location is flat, low altitude countryside because the dust, smoke, gases and water vapour in low lying inland regions obstruct the passage of sunlight.

Ultra-Violet Radiation. Ultra-violet rays have a low penetrating power. They draw blood outwards, towards the surface of the skin. The skin also undergoes a series of changes in response to exposure to potent ultra-violet radiation. In uncontrolled exposure, after a latent period of one to six hours, the well-known phenomenon of sunburn (erythema) appears, its severity varying with the length of exposure, the intensity of the radiation and the sensitivity of the individual. Sunburn is followed by pigmentation or tanning.

Ultra-violet rays are of considerable value in treating rickets, a disease in which there is a softening of the skeleton and a posture deformity as a result of the deficiency of vitamin D. This vitamin facilitates the absorption and depositions of calcium and phosphorus in the bones. Ultra-violet rays are the most effective anti-rickets rays. They are of great benefit in treating anaemic patients. Their radiation imparts an increased appetite, better sleep, an increased sense of well-being and also has a bactericidal action.

Infra-Red Radiation. The local effects of infra-red radiation are much the same as those of other types of heat. Infra-red rays are absorbed in the most superficial layers of the skin, dilating the smaller vessels in it and increases the rate of blood flow, capillary pressure and lymph drainage. These result in increased blood pressure and carbon dioxide tension because of increased tissue metabolism, and local leucocytic migration. Phagocytes and immunity are thus greatly increased. In addition to these local effects, if small applications of infra-red radiation are regularly given for some time, there is a sustained general peripheral vaso-dilatation of reflex origin.

It is apparently due to the action of the body's heat regulating mechanism, that the heat absorbed in one area is not transferred elsewhere, so that the overall body temperature does not increase. Therefore, if radiation is applied to a specific reflex area, only the vessels of the related organ will be dilated and its musculature will get relaxed through the connecting muscular reflexes.

Chromotherapy

Chromotherapy is a method of treating diseases by means of sunlight and colours. In it the chemical rays of the sun are applied through coloured glass, to preserve health and increase energy, and to cure diseases in accordance with nature's laws of healing. In obstinate cases, the patients are placed in a room where everything is coloured according to need and the coloured rays of sunlight can be directed towards the patient's body by fixing coloured glass pieces in the windows through which the sun's rays can radiate into the room.

Even pure water, if kept in coloured bottles and subjected to the rays of the sun for three or four hours, will acquire healing properties and can be used medicinally. Food or drink can also be charged with ultra-violet rays to fortify it with vitamins and minerals that help to cure diseases.

Chiropractic

Chiropractic is the study of the spine. Chiropractors work with the spinal column exclusively.

The spine is formed of thirty-three vertebrae--seven in the cervical (neck) region, twelve in the dorsal region (from the lower neck to where the small of the back begins), five in the lumbar region (the small of the back), five in the sacral region (the flat bone near the end of the spine), and the last four in the coccygeal region, and together form the coccyx. The last nine vertebrae in the spinal column unite in the adult and form two bones. The coccyx occupies the very end of the spine and has no definite nerve centres as the spinal cord does not extend below the second lumbar vertebrae. However, we also treat the area above the lower lumbar region and the sacrum as the spine, because the tail of the spinal cord is located there.

The different parts of the body and their functioning are controlled by different spinal centres. Thus, the dorsal section of the upper body--i.e., the stomach, kidneys, intestines, liver, bowels, pancreas and spleen, all have their control centres in the dorsal spine. The lower body, i.e., the legs, bladder, rectum, ovaries, and uterus, are controlled by nerves in the lumbar spine.

For years, it used to be believed even by medical experts, that displacement of the vertebrae, in the absence of fractures was practically impossible. This theory has been proved incorrect by research during the last fifty years.

Chiropractic concerns itself with abnormalities in the spinal tissues and the correction of these abnormalities and spinal lesions called sublimations. Chiropractic is founded on the theory that any vertebra can become subluxated, that is to say, a slight displacement of its opposing articular surfaces may occur at any time. As a consequence of this subluxation, an impingement is produced on the nerves which pass through the intervertebral formation corresponding to the vertebra involved in the displacement. The pressure upon the nerves blocks the production of impulses at this point, and the organs that it controls do not receive their full quota of ? intervation. Since the functional activity and organic integrity of all body parts depends upon their levels of nervous ?intervation, any withdrawal of this ?intervation constitutes a predisposing cause of diseases.

Subluxation or slipped disc means a slight shifting in the position of one of the surface areas of two adjacent vertebrae as opposed to dislocation, which means the complete dis-alignment of one or more vertebra. Chiropractic deals with subluxation. Subluxations can also easily be palpated by those who have been trained for this work. Chiropractors can easily demonstrate that, following adjustments of a subluxated vertebra, all abnormal conditions in the organs and tissues controlled by its nerves disappear.

Osteopathy

The basic premise of osteopathy is that the body is a vital mechanism subject to derangements, structural alterations and functional changes as a result of violence or injury on the physical plane, as well as disturbances on the psychic and biochemical planes. Hence osteopathy is inclusive of psychological and physiological preventive, palliative and curative measures. Osteopathy is the collective term that means all rational methods or systems of healing.

Osteopaths believe that disease is caused by abnormal changes in the tissues of the ligaments, muscles and organs as well as in the position and mobility of the bones. Osteopathy teaches that the structural integrity of the body mechanism is the most important factor in restarting and maintaining the well-being of the living organism. Its chief therapeutic measure is the adjustment of the body tissues and body structures. It also embraces all the biological, chemical and surgical measures which have been proven to be of restorative value.

Health is regulated through nerves. The nerves control the body's actions. Through the nerves, nature gives each of these parts the ability to keep itself strong and healthy. Through the blood, every bodily part receives new material for building and repairing itself as well as oxygen for its vital chemical processes. Through the lymphatic system, the nerves direct the elimination of impurities and keep the body free from their harmful effects.

When nerve reactions are impaired, the body is prevented from curing itself. Osteopathy seeks to find these interferences and remove them. Nature is thus empowered to begin her own effective campaigns against the body's ailments.

Difference Between Chiropractic and Osteopathy

The main differences between these two systems of healing are the manipulative techniques they use and the methods of their application. The chiropractor makes the spine the focus of treatment for all common and uncommon ailments. The chiropractic philosophy is defined as an adjustment of luxated or subluxated vertebrae, which cause all the physical ills known to mankind. Thus, the prime objective of all chiropractors is to restore these vertebrae to their normal state. As soon as their normal state is re-established, health is restored. Chiropractors claim that the entire body is supplied with energy emanating from the spine, that the spinal nerves control every tissue and function of the body, and that when these spinal nerves are free from pressure or interference, the body is in a normal or healthy condition.

Diagnosis of all conditions in chiropractic are made by what is commonly understood as 'palpation' or the location of deviations in the spinal cord by physically feeling it with the fingers. When all its vertebrae and nerves are in 'line', the patient is in a state of health but if even a slight deviation exists, a person is regarded as being diseased. The only treatment of diseases in chiropractic consists of the physical manipulation of the vertebrae of the spinal cord. The methods that chiropractors use for adjusting the spine differ from those used by osteopaths. Chiropractors use quick and sudden methods or means of manipulating the spine, because they believe that sudden movements, if done at the exact point where the adjustment is required, lead to instantaneous results. Osteopaths on the other hand, manipulate the spine slowly and gently. Osteopaths require from fifteen minutes to an hour to treat a patient, while the chiropractor requires from one to five minutes to both palpate and adjust the spine. The science of osteopathy and its philosophy consists of the physical manipulation of all parts of the patient to remove blockages in the circulation of blood and other body fluids. Osteopaths adjust bones and remove dislocations in any body part and also relax its muscular system and the limbs, whenever these are necessary for treating an ailment. Thus, osteopathy does not confine itself to any single part of the body and uses techniques such as the massage of a muscle, the treatment of the spine, the articulation of a joint, the flexing of a limb, the stretching of a muscle or bone formation, or a general going over of the entire body. The manipulation of muscles by pulling, stretching and pummelling them frees the system from everything that is supposed to cause disease.

Whether osteopathy is superior to chiropractic is an open question. The fact that they both serve very useful ends in the field of drugless therapy cannot be denied. Some practitioners prefer osteopathic movements to chiropractic ones because they are comparatively more gentle (as far as the spine is concerned) and the patient naturally feels better about this, as he is not in fear of pain or injury. On the other hand, perhaps the results from osteopathy are not as quickly discernible as those from chiropractic treatment.

Osteopathy is an older science than chiropractic and when the later came into vogue, it probably was merely an improved and extended study of Swedish movements and massage. It later embraced the treatment of the vertebrae by adjustments which are peculiarly osteopathic in nature. All said, the two sciences can be blended and used to advantage in many cases. Therefore naturopaths have a good deal to gain by being familiar with both of them as this will ultimately benefit their patients. Spinal manipulation, both osteopathic and chiropractic, is very frequently used in nature cure. Nevertheless as the sciences of osteopathy and chiropractic are also practised independently of nature cure science, a naturopathic physician who wishes to practise osteopathy and chiropractic as adjuncts to other nature cure methods, should get himself qualified for this purpose. When both osteopathy and chiropractic are combined with other forms of natural treatment, they are very efficacious indeed in bringing about quick and long lasting results.

Before the functions of the intra-vertebral disc were discovered by modern medical science, doctors treated slipped disc cases in same manner as lumbago, sciatica, and backache. They treated their patients with anti-rheumatic pills and pain-killers, which was unnecessary medication. Now that they are aware of what a slipped disc is they send their patients to appropriate specialists like neuro-surgeons, orthopaedic surgeons, osteopaths or chiropractors. Osteopaths, chiropractors and bone-setters have been practising manipulations and mechanical adjustments of the spine for many generations to treat cases of 'out of alignment' or a 'misplaced vertebra' and were far more successful than medical practitioners.

In India, bone-setters have been treating strains, sprains, fractures, dislocations and subluxations of the spine since time immemorial. These bone-setters usually belonged to a set of practitioners who learned this art from their fathers and forefathers. Their families have transmitted this art from father to son for many generations.

Spondylo-therapy

Spondylo-therapy is a system for the removal of impingements on the special nerves. It consists of stimulating one or more of the spinal nerve centres by means of concussion (light hammering), deep pressure or electricity, thereby creating an effect upon its peripheral organs and tissues. Thus every organ can be either contracted or dilated by spondylo-therapy. Spondylo-therapy seeks to stimulate spinal reflexes. A spinal reflex is a change in the tone, size or functional activity of an organ or blood vessel that follows the stimulation of the spinal tissues to which it is connected. Any stimulation of a spinal tissue or a body part which is supplied by the sensory nerves that are intertwined with the spinal cord produces a movement (i.e. a motor impulse). Spondylo-therapy, therefore, consists of the practice of manipulating segments of the spinal cord. This produces changes in the organs or body parts which are directly connected with the nerves that emanate from that particular segment of spinal vertebrae. Spondylo-therapy does not believe in subluxations. Hence it should not be considered as a part of chiropractic, but as an adjunct to it.

The methods used in spondylo-therapy are pressure, concussion and electricity. *Pressure* is applied on both sides of the spine by the tips of the thumbs or a blunt instrument. The fingers are generally placed behind the vertebrae, or just below the transverse sections of the vertebra. Their pressure should be heavy enough to produce a feeling of pain and tenderness and should not be continued more than thirsty seconds at any single treatment. When pressure is used only for the relief of spinal or visceral pain or tenderness, less force in used and the treatment is continued from three to five minutes. *Concussion* can be administered by the hand or with a wooden mallet. The blows should be on the tips of the vertebrae given with the mallet or clenched fists. When concussion is administered with the hands, the second finger of the left hand should be placed on the other hand. When a mallet is used, a small block of soft rubber should be kept on the vertebrae to protect their tissues from injury. It is of course important that the vertebra to be treated should first be properly located.

Vibro-therapy

Vibration has been mainly used to treat chronic osteopathic conditions. However, it is also useful in treating many other acute diseases, where it is employed with caution by trained vibro-therapists. Vibration is a valuable adjunct to various other forms of naturopathic treatment. It aids most of the physiological restorative processes in a perfectly natural way and this expedites the alleviation of disturbed functions. Whether it is applied to nerve centres, lymphatics or to their peripheries, it always produces blood and energy circulation changes. Vibro-therapy either stimulates or inhibits the circulation system depending upon the type of vibrator used, the time factor and the manner in which the operator adapts the technique to the personal requirements of different patients.

Orificial Therapy

Orificial therapy is a system of treatment that emphasizes that the bodily orifices undergo various pathological alterations in a diseased body. It seeks to normalize all ailments through digital, mechanical and electrical treatment of the orifices.

Every tube or passage in the body is controlled by the nervous system. Ailments create imbalances in the flow of energy in the voluntary and involuntary passages of the nervous system. The orifices have terminals of both the voluntary and involuntary nervous system, and are therefore the first centres of the body to change pathologically in illness of any kind. A lesion at the orifice of any tube exerts an influence of considerable magnitude in preventing the normal functioning of the body parts near the orifices, or by reflex action, the functioning of other parts. Orificial therapy, therefore, is a method based on the theory that many morbid or abnormal conditions are due to reflexes originating at the external orifices, such as the mouth, nostrils, ears and eyes in the upper part of the body, and lower orifices such as the anus or rectum, vagina, urethra and uterus (cervix). It seeks to normalize the energy supply to these through digital, mechanical and electrical measures.

Orificial therapy thus aims at relieving impingements on all the nerve terminals at the bodily orifices. As a result, the blood supply to the orifices is improved, and its capillaries are flushed. The entire body is benefited in its turn. Orificial therapy thus favourably affects every organ and every function of the body.

Zone-therapy

Zone therapy is effective in curing or greatly relieving several cases of chronic disorders that have resisted most known forms of treatment. It involves providing relief from pain and curing various disorders by applying pressure directly below the seat of the trouble or at some point on a finger, toe, knee, elbow or ear which is remote from the seat of trouble, but in the same zone. The zone-therapy theory divides the body arbitrarily into ten longitudinal zones, running from the tips of the toes to the tips of the corresponding fingers, and even to the corresponding zones of the head for this purpose. The duration of pressure in therapy ranges from half-a-minute to anywhere up to ten minutes or even more, depending upon the patient's tolerance level. Pressure is usually applied with a sharp-pointed instrument, the thumb and finger-nails or a metal comb, or with elastic bands or even with ordinary spring clothes-pins.

Zone-therapy is mostly a means of relieving pain caused by a 'nerve block', i.e. a condition in which the nerves affected become less capable of forwarding the impulse of pain to the headquarters of sensation. This sometimes allows the patient to relax sufficiently to get the necessary physical recuperation which then enables his own internal organic forces to overcome local difficulties themselves.

Exercise

The first law of life is activity: Use or lose. Any bodily part that is not exercised will gradually atrophy. This applies to the brain and muscles, and to the voluntary and involuntary parts alike.

Early man had to exercise to survive. He had to be able to run from an enemy, hunt for his food, climb trees and mountains and cross rivers. Every moment of life was filled with physical effort. In short, the physical struggle to stay alive was exercise enough. In the modern day and age, apart from dietetics, exercise, both active or passive, is the most valuable therapeutic agent. All exercise must have a definite purpose apart from productive labour and recreational play.

Exercise may be classified into two main groups, i.e., exercise for eliminating disease and regaining health and exercise for development.

Exercise for eliminating disease. When the body is clogged with waste material as a result of over-eating and under-activity, a feeling of sluggishness and fatigue results, which cannot be overcome by rest and sleep. Exercise in this case must be for one purpose only: to increase individual vitality--to promote blood circulation so that more heat will be generated and more air will be taken into the system, thereby oxygenating the blood stream. The eliminating organs then become more active, and metabolism will increase. Such exercise should be done with little expenditure of nerve energy. Simple mechanical movements or walking are enough.

Exercise for development. The cells in a sick body have no energy to carry out the normal bodily processes of development and growth, so its whole force is used for eliminating its toxic, morbid elements. When this has been accomplished, we may begin to exercise for development. Muscular exercise has a remarkably stimulating and rejuvenating influence on the system. Health and strength are by no means synonyms. If an individual is healthy, his body will assume the proportions best fitted for his special occupation.

Exercise is one of the most powerful preventive techniques of staving off the disabilities of middle and old age, and is also an important therapeutic tool in repairing the ravages of disease. Not only is it necessary for maintaining health and for building up a shapely and capable body, but it also has, in many instances, a specific curative value. There are a number of deformities, which are acquired through faulty postures, and the aftermath of disease, for which exercise, in conjunction with curative measures, has to be specially prescribed.

Massage

Massage signifies a group of systematic and scientific manipulations of bodily tissues which are best performed with the hands, to improve the nervous and muscular systems and general blood circulation. Scientific massage ranks among the most valuable therapeutic resources with a practically unlimited scope of action.

Massage is used as one of the means to treat numerous abnormal conditions and is often combined with electrical or light therapy. A passive form of exercise, it is a useful adjunct to the more important treatment by exercise. Massage relaxes hardened and congested body tissues, and forces out the stagnant and impure blood collected in them, thereby stimulating the inflow of new arterial blood laden with oxygen and food materials, thus ensuring rapid combustion and perfect elimination.

Massage is an art. Rightly used, it can be a pre-eminent therapeutic method. But wrongly used, it may produce harm, even to the extent of preventing recovery. The touch of massage is not simply an ordinary contact of the hand with the body, but is a skilled or professional touch. It is a touch which is applied with intelligence and control.

Massage brings about movement of energy into the body. For maintaining health and to create balance among the three humours--vata, pitta and kapha--naturopathy recommends massage with various oils. The massage process and type of oil depend upon individual constitution. For an aggravated vata constitution, naturopathy suggests massage with sesame oil to calm and balance the body. Vata people have dry skin and closed follicles. Stroking against the grain of body hairs facilitates penetration of the oil into the hair follicles. Massage for pitta constitution should be with sunflower or sandalwood oil, which have cooling properties. For kapha constitution, corn or calamus root oil is recommended, or massage without oil.

Certain techniques apply to specific disorders. For example, for stagnation of blood and poor circulation, massage toward the heart. For muscle spasms, tightness and soreness, massage in the direction of muscle fibers. Massage should be done in the morning for kapha disorders, in the evening for vata disorders and in the afternoon for pitta disorders. For kapha people, deep massage is beneficial. A gentle massage is good for vata and pitta individuals.

Traction

The spinal column is more than merely the vertical axis of the body that supports its skeletal framework. The systems of spinal manipulation have popularized knowledge about the spinal column, and most people are aware that the nerves which emanate from the spinal cord connect all the organs that lie below the skull.

The spinal cord has twenty-three intervertebral discs, each between every two movable vertebrae. These discs are composed of fibre-cartilage, with more or less gelatinous centres. They are malleable like rubber, and serve as shock-absorbers, minimizing the effects of jolts, jars and concussions upon the spinal cord and the brain. Were it not for these discs, our motions would be slow, clumsy, very limited, and no doubt, rather painful. Apart from separating the vertebrae these pads also maintain suitable spaces for the spinal nerves and blood vessels to weave around them.

Through many years of improper posture, or on account of weakness, strains, jolts, jars and numerous other conditions occurring in everyday life, the connective tissues of the spinal cord which are composed of cartilages and ligaments become more or less damaged. This is particularly noticed in the intervertebral discs. Normally the spinal 'windows' or openings are so large that even accidents or shrinkage due to old age or other conditions, rarely permit direct pressure of the bones to fall upon the spinal nerves and vessels. But these conditions have such detrimental effect upon the structures, that these windows contract and squeeze the connective tissue fibres that pass through them. These in turn, apply pressure on to the sheaths covering the nerves and vessels that emanate from the spine.

As age advances, blood circulation diminishes, less heat is produced, the walls of the blood vessels contract, the glands secrete less, and all nutritional functions become weakened; elimination becomes sluggish; the joints and articulations lose their suppleness becoming stiff, which makes twists and sudden jerks and movements irritable or painful; the lubricating cells and tissues dry up; muscular and other tissues harden and contract, losing their tone and becoming otherwise impaired; organs shrivel up, and function barely enough to maintain life. In short, the body machinery gradually wears out and life becomes an increasing burden. Many of these changes may reasonably be considered to be the result of the shrinking of the spinal fibrous cushions and ligaments, inhibiting nerve impulses from the spinal cord to the vital organs and tissues.

Spinal traction opens up the spaces between the vertebrae and permits the discs to receive more nutrition. Because the discs are closely attached to the vertebrae immediately above and below them, traction pulls upon the fibres of these discs and directly stretches them, tending to restore them to their normal thickness.

Traction opens up spinal circulation channels, permitting a better flow of nourishing blood to the spinal cord, thus causing it to generate and transmit better and stronger nerve impulses. Traction helps to restore the normal forward-backward curves in the spine which are so necessary to prevent irritating jars to the spinal cord and brain; it helps also to restore normal posture and to elevate the ribs and make them more flexible--a condition necessary for full vigour. It stretches the muscles of the entire trunk, and the blood vessels in these muscles, thus serving as a valuable exercise and as a means of securing better nutrition throughout the body.

Psychotherapy

Psychotherapy also forms an essential feature of nature cure, as both the mind and body are inextricably linked. Any imbalance in one causes disturbance in the other. In nature cure, psychology is generally employed more as an integrating factor than as an analytical factor. Most psychological disorders can be traced to a person's failure to experience the joy of living--a common failing--and endless time is spent, both by practitioners and patients, to combat its results. As naturopathy attempts to deal with the causes rather than with symptoms in the physical structure, it also approaches the mental and emotional side of life through psychotherapy.

There is no single method for the treatment of ills. All or some of the various forms of drugless treatment should be combined and used as and when required.

Does nature cure condemn drugs?

Nature cure is not inclined to use drugs as they are generally poisonous and destructive and because they suppress nature's natural cleansing and healing efforts. But in so far as a 'drug' has been defined to mean any substance used medicinally or as a chemical ingredient for curing an ailment, the use of a 'drug' as such is not objectionable.

The objection to drugs by a naturopath is not based on prejudice. He realizes that many medicines have a proper place in the doctors art and knows that a certain percentage of diseases is strictly a medical problem and can be cured by administering the proper medicine. At the same time, a naturopath has to make sure that, except in extreme emergencies, a drug should not be used if its intrinsic danger outweighs the symptoms.

Nature cure also has a great respect for the art of surgery when it is practised in a constructive manner. He realizes that when conditions and circumstances demand surgical intervention and assistance, there is no substitute. At the same time, a naturopath should warn his patients against promiscuous and uncalled-for surgical interference. After the removal of the inflamed part of an organ, which is usually but a symptom of a disease, one should examine its cause or causes and give naturopathic treatment accordingly to avoid further recurrence and complications.

CHAPTER VIII

Dieto-Therapy

Food is given top priority in naturopathy. Food is naturopathy's greatest medicine. We cannot think about naturopathy without food induced body purification. Naturopathy purifies and heals the body as well its structure through a planned diet of natural foods and regulated fasting.

Life begins with feeding, continues with feeding and ceases when food stops. Food functions like petrol and oil in an automobile. The food burns in the body, giving it heat, building its tissues, and furnishing lubrication.

Diet is the key to health. Most of our health problems can be traced back to diet. It is being recognized as the most important single factor in promoting either health or disease. Wrong eating and drinking are the most prolific causes of disease and therefore regulation of the diet in harmony with nature's laws and principles is of prime importance in the treatment of acute and chronic diseases. Nearly all chronic disorders are associated in one way or another with wrong eating, and one cannot expect a permanent cure until one is educated along scientific dietetic lines. A balanced diet is the strongest defence against degenerative diseases. Not only must the person suffering from diseases have a proper diet, but healthy persons should also consume proper foods in the correct proportions if they wish to remain healthy. Naturopathy gives diet a prominent place in its therapy.

Dietology is perhaps the most difficult of all therapies, as well as the least investigated in relation to its potential. It should have the constant attention of every advanced practitioner. Dieto-therapy is both an art and a science. To obtain the desired results intelligently, extensive knowledge extending into many branches of science as well as into the practice of healing and the propagation of foods is required. Not only must the practitioner have a knowledge of foodstuffs and their break-up into various chemical components, but he must also have a complete knowledge of the physiology and pathology of the body. Most of us are totally ignorant about our foods and their effect on our bodies. Modern cooking places a greater emphasis on taste rather than health, and is therefore, in the long run, detrimental to our bodies.

The body is a chemical composition of sixteen primary elements. Four of these are gases: oxygen, carbon dioxide, hydrogen and nitrogen. The rest are minerals which are furnished by the earth. These are: calcium, phosphorus, sulphur, potassium, magnesium, chlorine, sodium, iron, iodine, fluorine, silicon and manganese. Each of these elements has a particular place in the body and plays a definite part in its construction and maintenance, similar to the way in which various elements and materials are used in building a machine or a house. When we fall ill on account of the deficiency of these natural elements in our body, doctors give us pills and injections of these elements.

Our bones and teeth are chiefly made of calcium and our blood contains a good deal of magnesium, phosphorus and iron. Calcium energizes our sense organs, our heart and veins and prevents the levels of the other alkalis in our body from dropping below normal. Calcium carries out these functions with the help of vitamin D. Sodium and potassium are present in the inner and outer fluid of the body cells. Sodium chloride, potassium carbonate and bicarbonate balance the water and the acid--alkali levels in the body. We normally excrete 20--30 grams of alkalis a day which consist chiefly of chloride, phosphates of sodium, potassium, magnesium and calcium. To facilitate the process of balancing the alkalis in the body, it is necessary that our everyday meals contain all these saline elements. Growing children, lactating mothers and pregnant women should take extra quantities of these elements to avoid symptoms of their deficiency.

Food Guidelines for Basic Constitutional Types

Note : Guidelines provided in this table are general specific, adjustments for individual requirements may need to be made, e.g. food allergies, strength of agni, season of the ear, and degree of dosha predominance or aggravation.

⇧ Aggravates Dosha	Vata		Pitta		Kapha	
⇩ Balance Dosha	No ⇧	Yes ⇩	No ⇧	Yes ⇩	No ⇧	Yes ⇩
FRUITS	Dried Fruits	Sweet Fruits	Sour Fruits	Swee Fruits	Sweet & Sour	Apples
	Apples	Apricots	Apricots	Apples	Fruits	Apricots
	Camberries	Avocado	Berries	Avocado	Avocado	Berries
	Pears	Bananas	bananas	Coconut	Banans	Cherries
	Persimmon	Berries	Cherries	Figs	Coconut	Cranberries
	Pomergranate	Cherries	Cranberries	Grapes (Dark)	Figs (fresh)	Figs (dry)
	Watermelon	Coconut	Grapefruit	mango	grapefruit	Mango
		Figs (Fresh)	Grapes (green)	Melons	Crapes	Peaches
		Grapefruit	Lemons	Organes (sweet)	lemons	Pears
		Lemons	Papaya	Pineapples (sweet)	Organes	Persimmon
		Mango	Peaches	Plums (sweet)	Papaya	Prunes
		Melons (sweet)	Pineapples (sour)	Pomegranate	Pineapples	Raisins
		Organes	Persimmon	Prunes	Plums	
		Papaya	Plums (sour)	Raisins		
		Peaches				
		Pineapples				
		Plums				
VEGETABLES	Raw Vegetables	Cooked	Pungent	Sweet & Bitter	Sweet & Juicy	Pungent & Bitter
	Broccoli	Vegetables	Vegetables	Vegetables	Vegetables	Vegetables
	Brussels Sprouts	Asparagus	Beets	Asparagus	Cucumber	Asparagus
	Cabbage	Beets	Carrots	Broccoli	Potatoes (sweet)	Beets
	Cauliflower	Carrots	Eggplant	Brussels Sprouts	Tomatoes	Broccoli
	Celery	Cucumber	Garlic	Cabbage	Zucchini	Brussels Sprouts
	Eggplant	Garlic	Onions	Cucumber		Cabbage
	Leafy Greens*	Green Beans	Peppers (hot)	Cauliflower		Carrots
	Lettuce*	Okra (cooked)	radishes	Celery		Cauliflower
	Mushrooms	Onion (sweet)	Spinach	Green Beans		Celery
	Onions (raw)	Potato (sweet)	Tomatoes	Leafy Greens		Eggplant
	Parsley*	Radishes		Lettuce		Garlic
	Peas	Zucchini		Mushrooms		Leafy Greens
	Peppers			Okra		Lettuce
	Potatoes (white)			Peas		Mushrooms
	Spinach*			Parsley		Okra
	Sprouts*			Peppers (green)		Onions
	Tomatoes			Potatoes		Parsley
				Sprouts		Peas
				Zucchini		Peppers
						Potatoes (white)
						Radishes
						Spinach
						Sprouts
GRAINS	Barley	Oats (cooked)	Buckwheat	Barley	Oats (cooked)	Barley
	Buckwheat	Rice	Corn	Oats (cooked)	Rice (brown)	Corn
	Corn	Wheat	Millet	Rice (basmati)	Rice white)	Millet
	Millet		Oats (dry)	Rice (white)	Wheat	Oats (dry)
	Oats (dry)		Rice (brown)	Wheat		rice (basmati, small amount)
	Rye		Rye			Rye

**These Vegetables are OK in moderation, with oil dressing.*

⇧ Aggravates Dosha ⇩ Balance Dosha	Vata No ⇧	 Yes ⇩	Pitta No ⇧	 Yes ⇩	Kapha No ⇧	 Yes ⇩
ANIMAL FOODS	Lamb Pork Rabbit Venison	Beef Chicken or Turkey (white meat) Eggs (fried or Scrambled) Seafood (small amount) Vension	Beef Eggs (yolk) lamb pork Seafood	Chicken or Turkey (white meat) Eggs (white) Rabbit Shrimp Vension	Beef Lamb Pork Seafood	Chicken or Turkey (dark meat) Eggs (Not fried Scambled) Rabbit Shrimp
LEGUMES	No Legumes except Mung Beans,		All Legumes OK excepts Lentils Tofu, Black & Red Lentils		All Legumes are good except Kidney Beans, Soy Beans, Black Lentils & Mung Beams	
NUTS	All Nuts are OK in Small Quantities		No Nuts excepts Coconut		No Nuts at All	
SEEDS	All Seeds are OK		No Seeds except Sunflower & Pumpkin (in moderation)		No Seeds except Funflower & Pumpkin	
SWEETENTERS	All Sweeteners are OK except White Sugar		All Sweeteners are OK except Molasses & Honey		No Sweetners except Raw Honey	
CONDIMENTS	Al Spices are Good		No Spices except Coriander, Cinnamon, Cardamom, Fennel, Turmeric & a Small Amount of Black Pepper.		All Spices are Good except Salt	
			No ⇧		Yes ⇩	
DAIRY	All Dairy Products are OK (in moderation)		Buttermilk Cheese Sour Cream Yogurt	Butter (unsalted) Cottage Cheese Ghee Milk	No Dairy except Ghee & Goatmilk	
OILS	All Oils are Good		Almond Corn Salflower Sesame	Coconut Olive Sunflower Soy	No Oils except Almond, corn or Sunflower in Small Amounts	

Certain foods contain adequate amounts of calcium but they also have a lot of oxylates. When these oxylates are mixed with calcium during the process of digestion, they are turned into insoluble calcium which is useless for the body. Sesame seeds, spinach and chowrai leaves are the chief sources of oxylates; there are also a lot of oxylates in tea and coffee.

In India, betel leaf or *paan* is generally eaten with lime (calcium hydroxide). *Paan*--eaters thus consume a lot of calcium hydroxide, which is useful for the body. Logically, therefore, lactating and pregnant women should eat *paan* to maintain an adequate level of calcium in their bodies.

Sometimes, an imbalance of the alkaline and saline elements in the body causes weakness and anaemia. These symptoms can also be caused by an iron deficiency. Anaemic patients cannot absorb iron if their bodies are deficient in copper, cobalt and vitamin B-12. Similarly, calcium and phosphorus are necessary for the absorption of each other in the body. Neither of them can be absorbed alone, and we should therefore eat natural saline and alkaline foods that contain them both in adequate quantities. Natural food items contain all the alkaline elements which make their simultaneous absorption possible. Fresh fruits and vegetables are abundant sources of natural salinity.

We should also return to Mother Nature all the elements that we take from her. Only then will the soil be able to give them back to us in the form of crops, fruits and vegetables. Just as various saline elements are useful in order to maintain the internal homeostasis of the body, rich soil, healthy plants, fruits and grains require these elements for their sustained nourishment as well. They are found in natural manure, dung manure etc., and should be regularly put into the soil in order to maintain its richness, productivity and freshness. If the soil lacks any of these elements it would be unable to supply them to the plants and fruits that grow in it, and would therefore, make them less nutritious.

Apart from these elements, the consumption of certain essential components of food like carbohydrates, fats, proteins, vitamins and cellulose are necessary for maintaining good health. *Carbohydrates* are the foods which provide the body with starch and sugar. They are composed largely of carbon, hydrogen and oxygen. The principal sugars which the body utilizes are cane sugar, malt sugar, milk sugar and dextrose. Starch is the principal component of carbohydrate-rich food. It is found in cereals, ripe bananas, certain nuts and in most vegetables. It mostly abounds in those vegetables which are roots and tubers like potatoes, beets, etc. Starch provides heat to the body and supplies it with the energy to work. Every movement in and out of the body, however slight or great involves the burning or destruction of carbohydrates. If an excessive amount of carbohydrates is consumed, it is necessary to utilize it immediately. Carbohydrates are usually stored in the body as fat or in the liver as sugars. This is a sort of residue which the body draws upon during starvation or in a fast. Reduction in weight is made possible by limiting the amount of carbohydrates consumed.

Proteins provide the body with nitrogen, sulphur and phosphorus which together with certain other substances, constitute body structure, the nerves, muscles, glands, etc. Examples of proteins in foods are the white of eggs, lean meat, curd and wheat gluten. Protein is essential in our diet, yet its excessive consumption is dangerous, as there is no provision for storing it in the body. A common result of consuming a high protein diet is that the excess proteins putrefy in the intestines, giving rise to gases, poisons and toxins.

We generally consume large quantities of proteins. All our meat, fish, eggs, cheese, pasteurized milk, various types of pulses and vegetables are protein-rich. In digestion, all the proteins are first turned into amino acids. After these have been digested, the remainder are turned into uric acid and excreted. Too many proteins in our food burden our intestines. The continuous intake of protein-rich food reduces the ability of our intestines to excrete them and the uric acid that should have been thrown out of our body gets absorbed into our blood-stream. Excessive uric acid in the blood, over a sustained length of time, causes rheumatism, heart disease and high blood pressure.

Fats are derived from animal and vegetable sources. Every animal produces a fat peculiar to itself. When a fat is consumed, it is deposited in the tissue in the same form as it was eaten. The fat into which excess of starch is converted differs from animal or vegetable fat. Man can live for months on a fatless diet, which shows that fat is not an essential element of food. Fat is, however, a desirable food element. In recent years, it has been ascertained that some vitamins, in fact all the growth-promoting ones, are associated with fats. They are found in abundance in butter and in many vegetable oils but not in lard. Fat produces a certain kind of satiety which is more than what any other kind of food generates. People who consume excess fats are susceptible to rapid weight gain and intestinal putrefaction. Such a diet may also give rise to acidosis.

Vitamins are invisible food elements whose existence has been definitely established scientifically, although their chemical composition is still unknown. Vitamins are necessary for growth and are an essential constituent of nerve tissue. If food does not contain enough vitamins, degeneration and paralysis sets in, because the vitamin constituent of the nerve tissues is lost. Vitamins abound in the bran of cereals, green and root vegetables and especially in citrus fruits. Virtually all green vegetables contain vitamins in a greater or lesser degree. Of course, one's diet should be varied in order to ensure adequate supply of each class of vitamins. Boiling, drying, sterilization and pasteurization destroy vitamins. Hence raw and uncooked vegetables and fruits should be included in the day's fare.

Cellulose is perfectly harmless food element and is also a laxative. Foods containing cellulose in considerable quantity are--whole wheat, cracked wheat, whole wheat bread, asparagus, beans, brussels sprouts, cabbage, raw carrots, steamed cauliflower, raw celery, raw cucumbers, knol-khol, lettuce, onions, parsnips, dried peas, baked potatoes, pumpkin, spinach, prunes, apples, plums, cherries, grapes, raspberries, blackberries, huckleberries, strawberries and cranberries.

The Basic Elements of Food

In the laboratory, hydrogen ion or pH norms are used to test acid and alkaline levels. The body's acidity (pH) levels range from 0.00 to 14.00. A pH level of 0.00 indicates absolute acidity, and a level of 14.00 indicates absolute alkalinity; a level of 7.00 indicates neutrality. Our body fluids and blood are somewhat alkaline in content as their normal pH levels range from 7.35 to 7.45.

To maintain the internal balance of acids and alkaline, our body has four "refuse dispersal systems" which are--

the organs of inhalation and exhalation, the perspiration system, the urinary system, and the excretory system. These systems regulate the body's acid-alkaline balance and thus continuously detoxify the body and the blood. This is why naturopathy endeavours to improve their functioning. Generally, body refuse in any of these forms is acidic in content. The other non-routine excretions from the body, such as tears and blood, are alkaline in content.

Once the body's blood and tissues have been cleaned through the process of purification its absorbing power begins to increase. This leads to a better assimilation of foods and thus results in better health. Purification and absorption are interdependent processes. At the outset, therefore, naturopathy prescribes foods with an alkaline content in order to reduce the levels of acidity in the body. Only after the level of acidity has decreased, can we concentrate on healing specific organs. All food can be divided into acid-based or alkaline-based. Foods which contain calcium, magnesium, sodium and potassium are considered to be alkaline, while those which contain sulphur, phosphorus and chlorine are considered to be acidic. The classification of foods as acidic or alkaline depends upon the predominance of either acids or alkalis in them. Most non-vegetarian foods like meat, fish, eggs, etc. have a high acid content, while foods like milk and milk products, vegetables and fruits have a high alkaline content.

Vegetarian Diet

Naturopaths prefer a vegetarian diet to a non-vegetarian one.

Vegetarianism means different things to different people. From the dietetic point of view, vegetarians in India are mostly lacto-vegetarians i.e. those who do not eat the flesh of animals but who consume a plentiful supply of milk and milk products, vegetables, fruits, nuts, pulses and cereals. Some include eggs in their diet. Others like Jains eat no food which grows underground like potatoes, carrots, turnips and the like.

Vegetarianism has become a mere habit among many in India--not as a result of understanding, but because considerable ignorance prevails amongst vegetarians about the kind of foods that they should eat. What is important is to encourage a balanced diet and the right quality of food rather than quantity. Cutting down on excess food intake should go a long way in helping to solve the problems of health and food scarcity. The vegetarian world has proved that life based on a vegetarian diet is not only possible but is also extremely healthy and can be maintained for generations.

Occidental prejudices against a vegetarian diet are born of preconceived notions which have no foundation. From the nature-cure point of view, it is considered that the underlying cause of most diseases is auto-intoxication, i.e. self-poisoning or poisoning from within. It has been scientifically proved that meat increases toxaemic conditions, while a balanced vegetarian diet leads to better health.

A well-balanced vegetarian diet, besides providing a balanced menu, is free from the adrenaline-rich matter that the flesh of animals abounds in because of their high levels of metabolism. It therefore obviates the extra burden which is thrown upon the excretory mechanism of the flesh-eater who is compelled to dispose of such noxious residues from his system. If these are retained in the body due to defective excretion, they result in various disorders and self-imposed suffering.

Flesh is often a carrier of disease germs. Diseases of many kinds are on the increase in the animal kingdom, making flesh foods more and more unsafe. The animal dragged to the slaughter-house is in the grip of intense fear, and its body secretes large quantities of hormones which remain in the carcass that is consumed by non-vegetarians. Non-vegetarians are therefore more prone to emotional outbursts than vegetarians.

Vegetarianism as a way of life thus has various aspects--aesthetic, ethical, moral, spiritual and humanitarian--apart from the dietetic and health view points. Much more, however, is needed than merely giving up meat. Unbalanced diet as well as conventional, unwholesome cooking are equally unhealthy.

The growing band of vegetarians all over the world have led to an upsurge in the demand for wholesome organic food, i.e. of fruits and vegetables grown by organic methods (composting) and not by using chemical fertilizers. Unprocessed foods are being increasingly preferred to those which are demineralized and devitalized by milling, refining, canning, preserving and colouring with chemicals.

McCarrison, a foremost authority on food, describes what he considers a perfect diet:

"A perfectly constituted diet is one in which the principal ingredients are milk, milk products, any whole cereal grain or mixture of cereal grains, green leafy vegetables and fruits. These are all protective foods. They make good the deficiencies of the other constituents in the diet, protect the body against infection and diseases of various kinds and their use in sufficient quantity ensures physical efficiency."

Leafy Greens

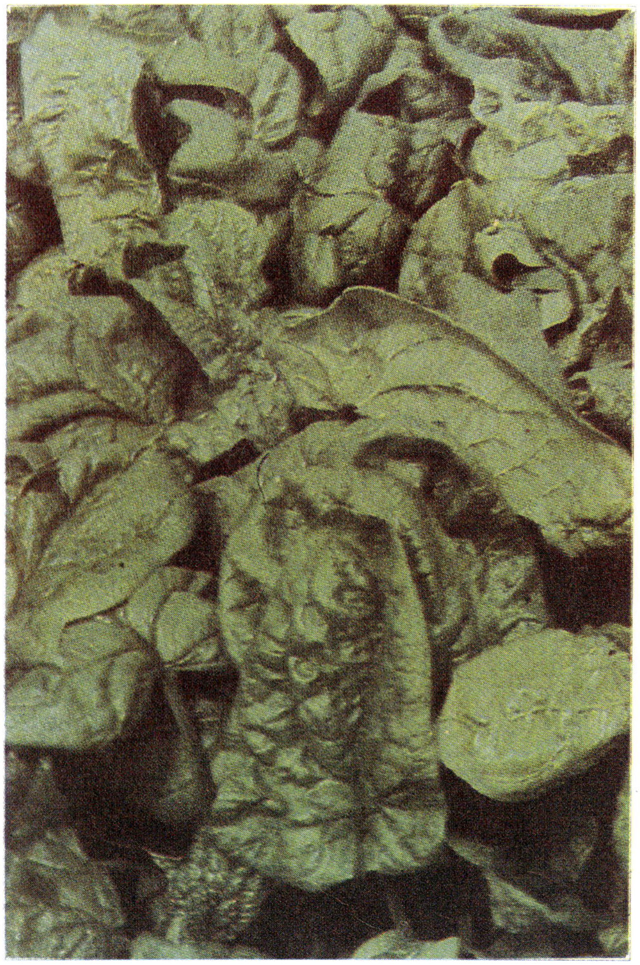

Leafy green vegetables like spinach, mint etc. are cheap and rich sources of alkalis. They are essential for the growth and protection of our health and are particularly important for pregnant women, breast-feeding mothers and children. Even if the intake of fruits is scanty, the body will not suffer if the intake of leafy green vegetables is sufficient.

The sun is the basis of creation and is the life source of everything in nature. The thin and soft leaves of vegetables absorb the sun's energy directly and store it in their branches, roots, fruits, and seeds. Men and animals are unable to absorb enough energy from the sun, therefore their intake of such vegetables is essential. Generally all types of vegetables are rich sources of alkalis. Vegetables also contain different quantities of minerals, as shown in the chart below.

Leafy Greens	Mgn.	Sodium	Potassium	Copper
Sulphur	Chlor.	Acid-base		
MI Acid	OIN Base			
Green leaves (Chulai)				
Kulfa-saag				
Green dhaniya				
Spinach				
Methi leaf				
Neem leaf (soft green)				
Ajwain leaf (fresh green)				
Lettuce				
Mint				

The Importance of Uncooked Food

As a naturopath with several years of experience, I have conclusively found that uncooked foods considerably decrease the length of time of treatment of chronic and "hard to cure" diseases like leprosy, asthma, paralysis, cancer etc. Just as a drowning man clutches at straws, all patients of such diseases crave for the symptoms of recovery, and as soon as they see even the slightest glimmer of a remission from their symptoms, their confidence in the doctor and their dedication to the treatment become stronger.

It is therefore necessary to first concentrate on making sure that patients can experience some alleviation of their symptoms as soon as possible. Very often, patients get fed up of hearing words like "improvement will take some time", and often stop the treatment in disgust if they do not see signs of recovery in the early stages of the treatment. Therefore, it is essential that naturopaths prescribe the proper kind of foods after studying the symptoms of their patients very carefully, to make sure that discernible signs of recovery present themselves as soon as possible.

In the ultimate analysis, the experienced dedication of a doctor alone is all that a patient requires. The prescription of raw and uncooked fruits and vegetables usually results in the rapid generation of symptoms of recovery, even in the most chronic diseases.

All the different elements of food are preserved in their balanced state only in uncooked foods. This balance is of the utmost importance in ensuring the proper digestion, absorption and excretion of food. Cooking destroys several of these elements and makes foods uneven, imperfect and difficult to digest. Our system does not have enough enzymes and gastric juices to digest excessive quantities of foods, therefore over-eating results in the clogging of our intestines with undigested foods which create toxins. This process acts as a catalyst of disease. Also, cooked foods have less natural minerals and elements and make us sluggish, while raw foods abound in them, and therefore make us feel more energetic and fresh.

From the standpoint of nature's laws, we commit a crime by murdering the living elements in food by cooking it in order to make it tasty. Also, since we tend to eat less when we consume raw foods, we act as preservers and conservers of the earth's flora when we eat such foods.

Germination makes raw grains far more nutritive. The consumption of germinated grains gives our bodies the greatest amounts of natural energy and increases its resistance and healing powers substantially.

When we mill gram or grain into flour, we destroy its germinating capacity and throw away its husk which has more food value and healing power than its kernel. The polishing of rice causes the same damage. When we make sugar, especially the white one, we throw out its salinity and molasses. The skins of carrots, potatoes, apples, and other fruits and vegetables which have the maximum amount of food value, are peeled and thrown away before we eat them. In this manner, we destroy the natural healing elements of our food every day in our kitchens.

Modern civilization stresses the gaining of an economic edge. The farmers, the food producers of the world, are also driven by the same motive: produce more to earn more. Since modern science suggests that artificial nature and pesticides enhance crop yields, farmers all over the world are using more and more of these, conveniently forgetting that the excessive use of artificial inputs--containing toxins like lead, arsenic, strychnine, nicotine, etc. and acids like benzoic, salicylic, nitric, boric and sulphuric--are absorbed by their crops. Also, these pesticides in the long run damage the soil. For most farmers, their short-term monetary gains outweigh the possible hazards that their practices may generate in the long term.

When we eat grains, fruits and vegetables grown in this manner, we consume the toxins they contain. The seeds of these foods are equally harmful because they contain the same toxins, and will therefore, grow into toxin--bearing plants and produce toxic grains, fruits and vegetables in the future. The only way to protect ourself from such toxic elements is to eat food grown without the use of chemical fertilizers and pesticides. Happily, the awareness of 'natural farming' (as this process of cultivation is called), is becoming more widespread. Natural farming will not only benefit us and our kith and kin, but will also protect the future generations from inheriting our toxic genes.

Preservatives used to keep foods fresh over long periods of time are also toxic. The ideal foods are those grown without pesticides and consumed immediately after they are plucked. Therefore fresh vegetables and fruits are always prescribed by naturopaths. Persons who consume such foods rarely fall sick. Pregnant women whose diet consists of large quantities of such foods deliver without much pain or trouble.

Fresh Foods and Smoking

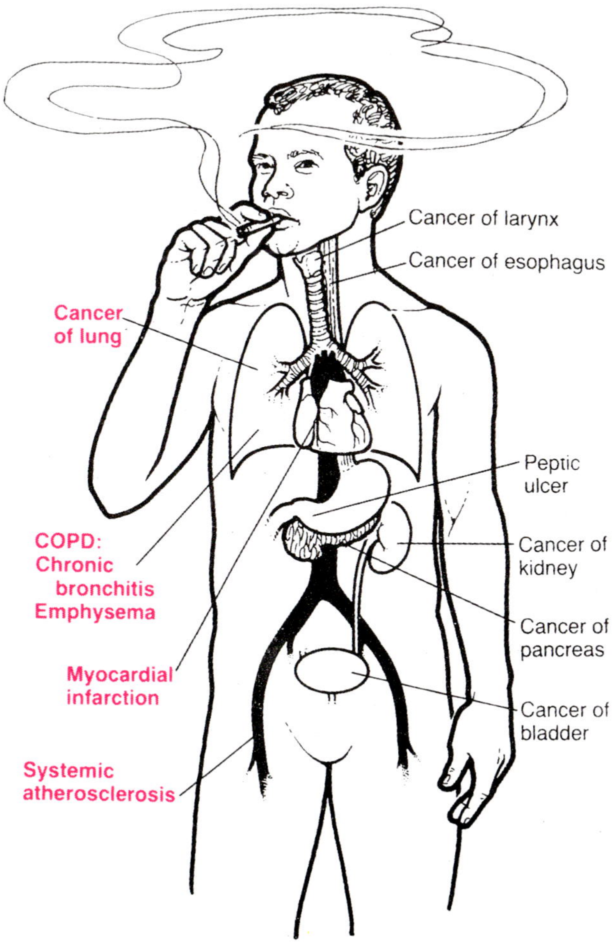

Tobacco, consumed in whatever form--smoking, chewing, or inhaling--contains a toxin called nicotine which irritates the heart, throat, tongue, lips, and cheeks. Over a period of time, this irritation can turn into cancer. It also causes various types of gastric troubles like intestinal inflammation, ulcers, etc. Heart diseases are also caused by the intake of tobacco. People who consume large quantities of fresh foods have a keen sense of smell, and generally cannot tolerate the smell of tobacco. The consumption of fresh foods is, therefore, the best method of getting rid of tobacco addiction.

Pre-Preparation for the Intake of Fresh Foods

Fresh fruits and vegetables should be consumed with care. People with healthy teeth can eat fresh vegetables and fruits by biting into them after washing them with clean water. People with poor teeth should eat them after cutting them up into small pieces or after grating them. It is most important that fresh food is thoroughly chewed. Also, its quantity should be restricted so that it does not create any digestive problems like diarrhoea, indigestion and the like. Soft foods like fruits and most vegetables do not generally result in such problems but hard, course grains can be problematic. Patients with gastritis, colitis or ulcers must consult a doctor before eating large quantities of fresh foods.

If fresh foods are grated or made into juices, they should be consumed immediately, because they oxidize as soon as they come into contact with the atmosphere. Oxidation destroys one-fourth of the vitamin content of food. Breakfast is the best time for consuming juicy fruits like lemons, pomegranates, grapes, etc. It is healthier to consume these fruits by sucking them rather than by squeezing their juice, so that our saliva can mix with their juice while it is fresh, and all its vitamins can thereby be absorbed into the body. Another benefit of sucking fruits is that we can consume them in small quantities, whereas if we drink their juice, we tend to consume a far greater quantity of them, which can create digestive problems. If juicy fruits are not available, we can take lemon water, honey or currants instead. Canned juices are not good for health because of the various preservatives they contain. These create toxins in the body and do more harm than good.

According to naturopathy, breakfast should always be a light meal. It is best to avoid it altogether and eat proper meals just twice a day. The midday lunch should ideally consist of germinated grains, uncooked vegetables, leaves and roots. Potatoes, if eaten, should be consumed with their skin as there is a lot of chlorine in their greenish part which lies just under their surface and it is good for preserving the enamel of teeth. People with poor teeth should eat germinated grains and dried nuts after grating them.

Dried nuts, almonds and green coconuts are more healthful than milk or milk-based products. These foods are of great value in curing colds, coughs and some hard-to-cure diseases like cancer. In any case, naturopathy prohibits milk for cancer patients. Milk is a mucous forming food and mucus stimulates the growth of cancer cells. Cancer patients can drink green coconut water and soybean milk instead of cow or buffalo milk. Eating 5 to 10 almonds a day mixed with honey, forms an integral part of the naturopathic treatment of cancer.

It is preferable that cancer patients avoid tea, coffee, cocoa, etc. as they produce uric acid in the body, which is well known to be a cancer--aggravating substance.

I lived with the renowned naturopath, Purushotamdas Tandon in my childhood. He had a recurring cough which he cured by discontinuing the consumption of milk, sugar and salt and instead drank a syrup of 5-7 almonds mixed with honey everyday. His cough was cured in just a few days with these.

Fruits

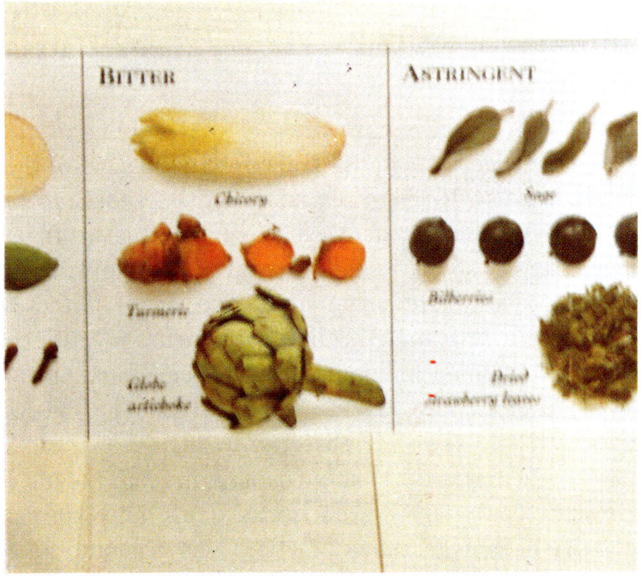

Dates, currants and other similar dried fruits should be eaten after they are washed and soaked in water for 8 to 10 hours, so that they swell up like fresh fruits. Small amounts of them should be eaten with the midday meal. Cancer patients should eat only fresh fruits and salads. Naturopathy recommends both a light dinner and a light breakfast for them. In case they feel hungry between meals, they can eat as many fresh fruits and salads as they like.

Cultivation of Vegetables

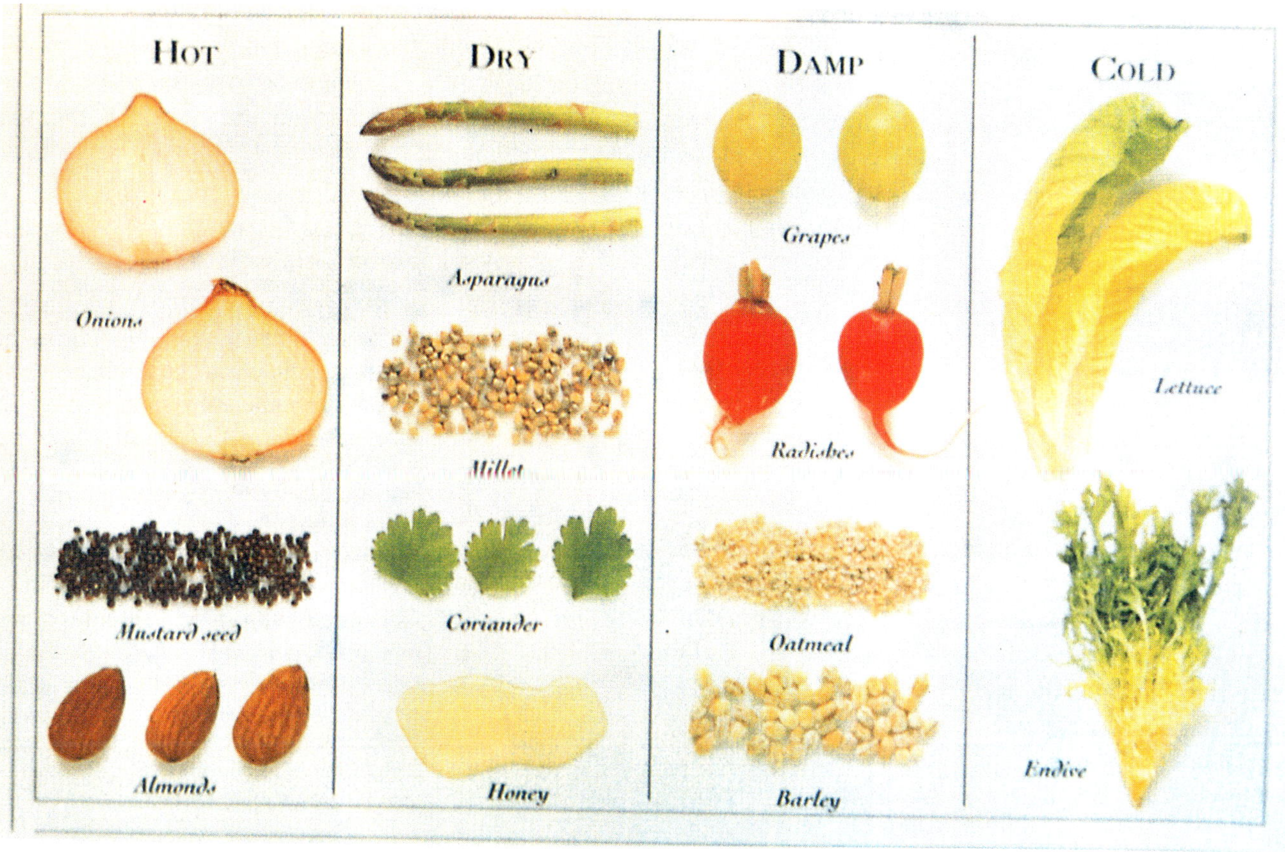

For those who have the space, the cultivation of a few vegetables in a small kitchen garden is extremely useful. This will enable them to come into contact with the sun and the soil and to also get fresh vegetables for their own consumption. This will also, in the ultimate analysis, benefit both their mind and their bodies. Also regular exercise in the kitchen garden would take their attention away from negative preoccupations and refresh their minds, in addition to ensuring a regular supply of fresh vegetables for their use. If their body can tolerate soft sunshine, they should wear scanty clothing while pottering around their kitchen gardens. This will enable them to have a sunbath and thus obtain the benefit of natural evaporation. Thereafter, they should have a cold water bath to refresh the muscles. A kitchen garden can thus become an excellent opportunity to remain in constant contact with mother nature and utilize all its life giving resources.

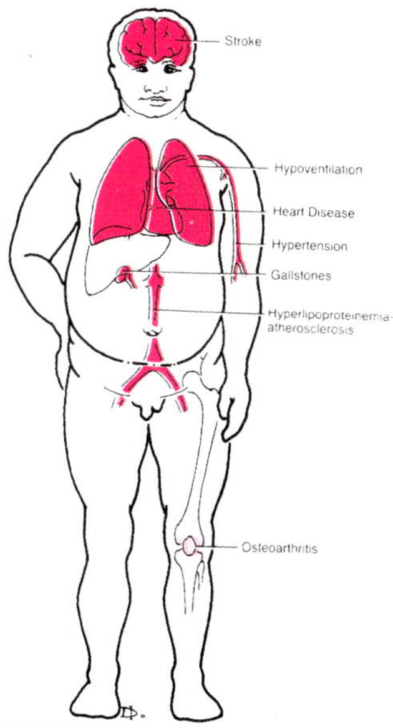

Fasting

Fasting is an overhauling process. It is a form of digestive or physiological rest during which the body can devote all its energies to eliminating the accumulation of poisonous wastes from the system. It is, of all methods of nature cure, the most natural and positive, and an effective short-cut to health--one that will completely restore the normal functioning of the various bodily organs. Fasting is constructive and health giving. In contrast, starvation is a destructive, fatal process, a slow suicide. We can starve on three meals a day if their contents lack the essential organic minerals and salts, and conversely we may fast our way back to health, for fasting is nature's own way of cleansing and regenerating the body and mind. Fasting, if properly conducted, is distinctly beneficial.

Fasting is as old as life and is instinctively resorted to by sick and wounded animals and man. Fasting can be undertaken for three reasons--for self-conquest, for spiritual reasons and for therapeutic reasons. The conquest fast is done to conquer oneself, to strengthen one's mind and will power and to perfect one's personality. It will be found that after fasting, clarity comes to the mind as never before, as not only one's conscious but also the unconscious self will undergo a complete rebirth and awakening. The spiritual fast is undertaken for religious reasons. Many great seers and saints have been devout apostles of fasting for illumination and spiritual revelation.

Fasting from the therapeutic point of view is done for the treatment of diseases or tendencies toward disease. There is hardly any diseased condition for which fasting cannot be used with benefit. Although we generally understand fasting to mean abstention from solid food, a strict fast means also going without liquids. In this way one obtains very quick results, for one lives entirely on one's own flesh, and all surplus of carbon, mucus, acids and the harmful elements of the system get burned up. In other words, one's body, if properly taken care of, will cleanse itself.

Many talk of fasting, but few seem to have the will power to go on a fast. This is because fasting requires an unusual measure of self-mastery, will power and personality.

Fasting is difficult only for the first three days. Thereafter the body adjusts itself to the changed conditions. The most effective method of fasting is not to gradually lessen the amount of food, but to stop eating altogether and to drink nothing but plain water. Drinking orange juice or pineapple juice makes a fast even more difficult to sustain, because the stomach nerves are continually being stimulated. In fact, consuming a diet of juices cannot even be called fasting.

The effects of fasting are enhanced by the cleansing of the bowels at an early stage of the fast. This is a regular feature of naturopathic practice and is usually carried out by enemas or colonic lavage (bowel wash).

Fasting is regarded as the only possible way of cleansing the body and its organs and tissues of accumulated toxins. This method is probably as near to nature as anything can be, as it overhauls the whole system and gives rest to its overworked vital organs. So necessary has this method of cleansing the system been to life and health and so reluctant have people been to practise it, that every religion on earth has incorporated its practice in its essential requirements. No theology has existed without it, and fasting has been practised for thousands of years.

Fasting should not be resorted to only when one is ill. A short fast for a day or two should be undertaken systematically for the prevention of disease. When fasting is continued beyond the stage of elimination of poisons, or when it ceases to be a cleanser, however, fasting begins to cause harm as it leads to starvation. Fasting is a double-edged sword. Long fasts should never be conducted without the supervision of an experienced nature-cure physician.

Over-eating or indiscriminate eating and drinking and lack of exercise is a universal vice. People keep their bodies constantly surfeited with food, forcing every organ to work overtime. Their nerves and glandular systems are overtaxed and their reserve forces are called upon to digest and assimilate this surplus food in order to eliminate the poisons that result from its decomposition in their intestines. A fast reverses all this. The surplus food is used up, the toxins are eliminated, the organs get a much needed rest and are able to repair themselves. There is no other means of obtaining total physiological rest. By abstaining from food, the stomach, bowels, kidneys, glands, heart, nerves and other tissues automatically rest and thus secure an opportunity to repair themselves. It is not merely the digestive organs which rest during a fast--its benefits extend to every part of the body. Hence the two chief purposes of a fast are to allow the body to catch up with its elimination process and to provide physiological rest.

Besides, the sick usually suffer from nervous fatigue (enervation) and are in need of rest and not stimulation. They suffer from redundancy of nutrition and require a fast rather than "plenty of good nourishing food to keep up their strength". Their organs get damaged from toxic irritation and overwork. Nothing can be of more value to them than a period of reduced activity of the kind that fasting affords. Instead of treating (suppressing) individual symptoms we should correct the systemic conditions that cause these symptoms. Instead of forcing an already overworked organism to do more work, we can accomplish real and lasting results by giving it less work to do. Nothing will serve this purpose better than fasting under proper conditions.

Part II

Cancer

CHAPTER IX

An Introduction To Cancer

All forms of life ranging from the simplest microscopic amoeba to the most complex living organism--the human being--are composed of cells. A cell is the smallest basic unit of life which can replicate itself. In the body, a collection or mass of cells of the same kind is called a tissue. Our body is composed of numerous tissues such as nerve tissue, muscular tissue, connective tissue, etc. An aggregation or collection of tissue constitutes an organ, such as the heart, the lungs, the liver, etc. The cells are specially adapted to carry out specialized groups of functions. Thus, the cells of the eye transmit visual impulses, the cells of the stomach perform the functions of digestion, and so on. As the body grows from infancy to adulthood, the cells divide and subdivide until no more increase of cells is required except for the normal wear and tear of the body. The rate at which an organ should grow and when it should stop growing are under the control of the body's self-regulatory mechanisms.

Cancer arises from an abnormal and uncontrolled division of cells which then form tumours that invade and destroy the surrounding tissue. Cancer cells, in other words, do not stop multiplying and continue to increase exponentially even when they are no longer required to do so. This failure of the body's self-regulatory mechanism to stop its own cells from multiplying is the hallmark of cancer. Cancerous cells multiply at the cost of the normal cells, which are slowly starved to death for lack of nutrition.

To be more precise, cancer is a disease of DNA, the master molecule that encodes the genetic script of life. One of DNA's tasks is to govern cell division, the process by which a cell makes a copy of itself and splits in two. Ordinarily, cell division is tightly regulated, but cancer cells divide uncontrollably, pushing into surrounding tissue and organs.

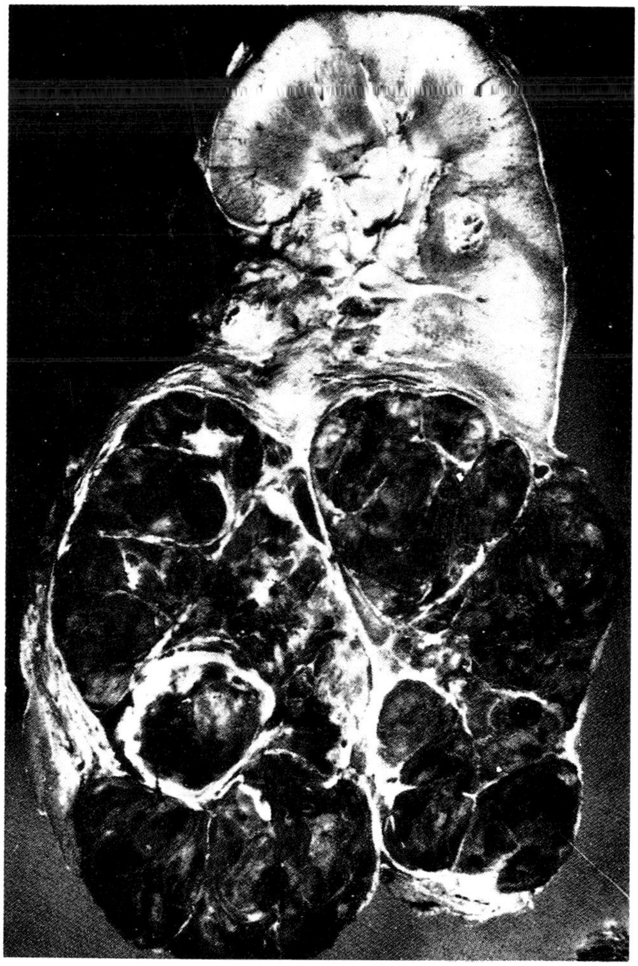

Unlike normal cells, cancer cells do not remain confined to one part of the body, but infiltrate into the adjoining tissue and dislocate its function. Sometimes, cancer cells leave their site of origin and travel by blood and lymph channels to sites distant from the original tumour and form fresh colonies. These are called metastasis or secondary growths, where they once again begin to grow at the cost of normal cells. This is how cancer destroys the well-regulated functioning of the body and brings about its end. The word cancer probably derives from the Latin for crab – to mean a disease that obstinately sticks to any part it seizes upon like a crab.

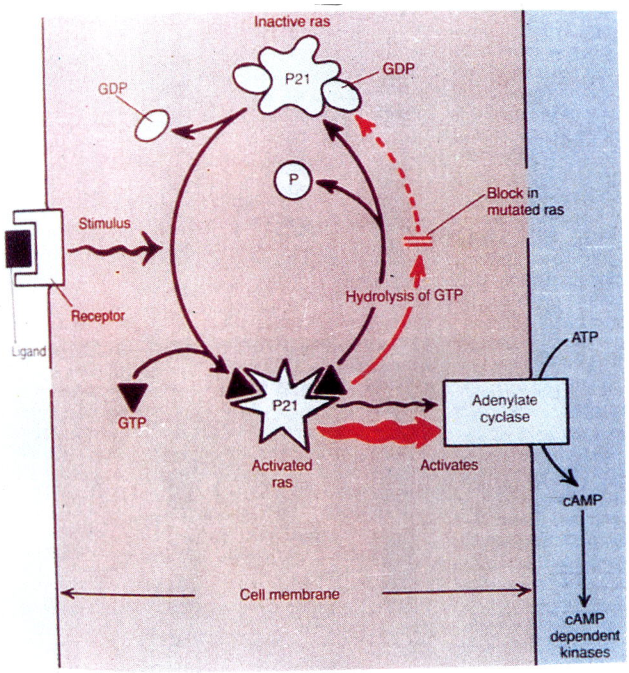

The spread of cancer occurs through any or all of the three following routes:

Local Spread. The cancer infiltrates the adjoining tissue and organs.

Lymphatic Spread. The lymph glands or nodes trap the cancer cells present in the lymph fluid and cancer grows within them. Progressive spread along lymph vessels and glands may occur and in the process quite distant glands may become involved.

Bloodstream Spread. If cancer invades the blood vessels the cancer cells may be carried to other parts and settle over there, producing secondary cancers. The veins are more readily penetrated than the arteries. The major site of spread in cases of bowel cancer is the liver. The lungs are the most common site of metastasis from other cancer sites. The spread to many other organs is also common.

The rate at which a cancer grows depends on the tissue in which it occurs and on the type of cancer. Rapidly growing cancers send metastasis in other organs, and are much more dangerous than slow-growing cancers. Sometimes the primary cancer may grow slowly, as for example, that of the stomach and remain unnoticed, while the secondaries spread rapidly in the liver, abdominal lymph glands, etc. These secondary cancers are noticed first. Whatever the factors inducing the growth of cancer, the earlier the disease is treated, the greater the chances of control and cure.

The growth of cancer cells generally leads to the formation of a nodule or tumour. Cancerous tumours are generally firm to the touch, and are fixed to the surrounding tissue. Every nodule is not a cancer. Some like warts, cysts or adenomas are benign and do not turn into cancer. A biopsy reveals the nature of the tumour. In medical jargon, a tumour is called neoplasm, to mean "new growth". The phenomenon of this growth is called neoplasia. Oncology is the study of tumours (Greek oncos=tumour; logy=study). The eminent British oncologist Sir Rupert Willis defines neoplasm as "an abnormal mass of tissue, the growth of which exceeds and is uncoordinated with that of the normal tissues and persists in the same excessive manner after cessation of the stimuli which evoked the change." This abnormal mass is purposeless, preys on the host competing with normal cells and tissues for energy supplies and nutritional substrate, and is virtually autonomous, though all neoplasms ultimately depend on the host for their nutrition and vascular supply; many forms of neoplasia require endocrine support.

It is difficult to pinpoint the exact time of the emergence of a cancerous tumour, and to establish an empirical correlation between its growth and the patient's death. This is because there is no precise code or pattern for the growth of cancer. Also, tumours artificially grown in laboratories differ considerably from those that occur naturally.

Cancer is curable, provided it is detected well in time and excised before it spreads. The treatment of cancer in its early stages is, however, difficult because it is generally discovered when it has either spread to a discernible extent in a particular part or has developed into an obvious tumour. A surgical operation can remove a cancerous tumour or tissue only when it is confined to a limited area. The good news is that remarkable progress has been made during the past two decades in the treatment of cancer by the use of surgery and radiation therapy. The discovery of a variety of anti-cancer drugs has, to a large extent, revolutionized the treatment of cancer during the past few years. Naturopathic treatment can relieve most patients of their debilitating symptoms and has succeeded in bringing about a complete remission of the disease in several forms of cancer.

Cancerous tumours may or may not be painful. A tumour may remain undetected in the body without causing pain or any other symptom even as long as fifteen years. In several instances, cancerous tumours remain painless both during the after treatment. Tumours of this nature caused death of the well known cancer researchers Dr. Mayo, Dr. Dorn and Dr. William, who carried on with their research until the last few days of their lives because their tumours caused them virtually no pain whatsoever. Their tumours were too widespread to be removed fully, and their renewed growth after surgery eventually resulted in the death of these scientists.

The fatality of cancer depends essentially on the stage at which it is detected. Cancer is more of a "whole body disease" than a localized one. Even though it originates in a specific localized region of the body, its effects are felt throughout the body. Its secondaries also generally spread from its primary site to other parts of the body--mainly to the intestines, heart, kidneys and brain. The spread of cancer is so uncertain that it cannot be forecast with any degree of accuracy. This is why cancer patients generally die after its secondaries have spread to other parts. It is therefore more logical to treat not just a single part of the body of cancer patients, but their whole body. Naturopathy believes that regardless of where the disease originates, its treatment must encompass the whole body. It is the understanding of naturopathy that the disease originates due to the assimilation of an extraordinarily high amount of toxins and other contaminations in the entire body and its treatment should therefore consist of a purification of the body. After this purification process, there is generally a considerable improvement in the local membrane of the part in which the cancer had originated.

Genetic Contribution to Cancer

A pivotal discovery in the etiology of cancer was made in 1976, when Drs. J. Michael Bishop and Harold Varmus at the University of California, San Francisco, made a startling observation. They saw that a viral gene known to cause cancer in chickens was virtually a carbon copy of the normal gene found in the bird. This finding helped lead to a general conclusion: cells become cancerous because their normal genetic machinery goes awry. The damage may be initiated by viruses, radiation, environmental poisons, defective genes inherited from parents, or a combination of all these.

Until mid-1994, researchers had found perhaps 100 cancer genes, at least three dozen of which commonly occurred in human tumours. Some, known as oncogenes, turn on cell division, whereas others, called tumour-suppressor genes, switch the process off. In their normal form, both kinds of genes work as a team, enabling the body to perform such vital tasks as replacing dead cells or repairing defective ones. But mutations in the chemical make-up of these genes, inherited or acquired, can disrupt these finely tuned checks and balances. A cell containing a faulty oncogene is often likened to a car with a stuck accelerator; and a cell with a damaged tumour suppressor gene to a car with no brakes. The malignant cell thus is not an intrinsically evil villain but an ordinary machine that has broken down in very specific, and potentially hazardous ways. Scientists who have studied the life history of a cancer cell have found errant genes at almost every step of the way, from the initial formation of a tumour to the advanced stages of metastasis, the lethal spread of the disease through the body.

Canada's McMaster University has identified a telltale enzyme which is found in cancer cell--but is conspicuously absent from most normal cells. If cancer researchers can find a way to deactivate this enzyme, known as telomerase, they may at last have the magic bullet they have long been seeking. Molecular biologists at Myriad Genetics, a biotechnology firm in Salt Lake City, Utah, have found that a majority of cancer cells lack functioning copies of the telomerase gene that serves as a circuit breaker and shuts down the abnormal cell growth that causes malignancy.

At the US National Cancer Institute, Dr. Curtis Harris, a molecular epidemiologist, has found in cancer cells mutations in a tumour-suppressor gene known as p53 (p stands for the protein the gene makes and 53 for the protein's molecular weight). Smokers who develop lung cancer, Harris has found, show tiny alterations in the p53 gene. This gene is often described as "the guardian of the gnome" because it keeps watch over DNA during cell division. When damage occurs, p53 commands other genes to bring cell division to a halt. If repairs are made, then p53 allows the cell cycle to continue. But if the damage is irreparable, p53 activates other genes that cause the cell to self-destruct. Mutations in p53, which have been detected in more than 50 per cent of all human cancers, are therefore extremely dangerous. In laboratory cultures, some cancer cells that possess mutant versions of p53 do not die when challenged by anti-tumour agents, while those that have normal p53 genes are destroyed.

Perhaps the critical stage in the life of a tumour comes after it expands to about a million cells. At this point, it is "much smaller than a BB," says Dr. Judah Folkman of Harvard Medical School. This tiny mass, known as a carcinoma in situ (lit. cancer in place), is malignant, but not yet dangerous. This is because the cells at the centre of the tumour are too far from the bloodstream to obtain essential nutrients, and are less vigorous. Like a society with zero population growth, a carcinoma in situ adds about as many new cells as it loses old ones.

Months, years, even decades may pass. Then an ominous transition occurs. Some cells in the tumour begin secreting chemicals that attract endothelial cells--the key components of blood vessels. These cells form capillaries that grow into the tumour. They also pump out molecular messengers called growth factors that stimulate the tumour to divide more quickly.

What triggers blood-vessel formation, or angiogenesis, as the process is known? A major factor, scientists believe, is a sudden drop in the cancer cell's production of thrombospondin, a protein that inhibits the growth of new blood vessels. In the normal adult, angiogenesis is not only a rare event but one that cells strive to prevent, save for special circumstances like wound healing. For blood vessels invading joints can cause arthritis, and those invading the retina of the eye can cause blindness. To prevent such damage, cells keep blood vessels at bay by pumping out thrombospondin. At a recent scientific conference, Noel Bouck, a molecular biologist from Northwestern University Medical School, stunned her colleagues by presenting preliminary data suggesting that thrombospondin production may be regulated by that ubiquitous gene, p53.

Angiogenesis is the harbinger of metastasis. The same vessels that feed the tumour also provide it with avenues of escape. Not all the myriad cells shed by tumours survive their turbulent voyage through the bloodstream, notes experimental oncologist Ann Chambers of the London Regional Cancer Centre in Ontario. But those that do, eventually slip through blood-vessel walls with ease. Using a video camera attached to a microscopic lens, Chambers has watched as melanoma and breast-cancer cells, injected into liver. Three days later, her camera resolved the spidery shapes of tiny metastatic growths. The lesson, Chambers believes, is depressingly clear. Cancer cells zip in and out of blood vessels so readily that, once angiogenesis occurs, they should be presumed to have already spread around the body.

Cancer Suppressor Genes (Anti-Oncogenes)

We have so far considered the possible involvement of cancer promoting elements in genes (oncogenes). To date, however, only 15 to 20 per cent of human tumours have been found to contain activated oncogenes. It is possible that some tumours contain oncogenes that remain to be identified. Alternatively, some cancers may arise not by activation of growth-promoting genes but by inactivation of genes that normally suppress cell proliferation. The influence of such genes would be felt only when they are absent, and hence techniques such as transfection of tumour DNA would not be expected to reveal their existence. Indeed there is accumulating evidence that loss of certain "cancer suppressor" genes may be an important mechanism underlying malignant transformation.

Like many discoveries in medicine, the cancer suppressor genes were excavated by digging among rare diseases, in this case retinoblastoma, a tumour that affects about 1 in 20,000 infants and children. Approximately 60 per cent of retinoblastomas are sporadic, and the remaining 40 per cent are familial, with the predisposition to develop the tumour being transmitted as an autosomal dominant trait. To explain the familial and sporadic occurrence of an apparently identical tumour, Knudson proposed his now famous "two hit" hypothesis of oncogenesis. He suggested that in hereditary cases one genetic change ("first hit") is inherited from an affected parent and is therefore present in all somatic cells of the body, whereas the second mutation ("second hit") occurs in one of the many retinal cells (which already carry the first mutation). In sporadic cases, however, both mutations (hits) occur somatically within a single retinal cell, whose progeny then form the tumour. Knudson's hypothesis has been amply substantiated by cytogenetic and molecular studies.

Types of Cancer

Carcinoma. Cancer that arises in epitheliums, the tissue that lines the skin and internal organs.

Sarcoma. Cancer of connective tissue. These tumours may occur in any part, as they arise in the tissue that makes up an organ rather than being restricted to a particular organ. They can arise in fibrous tissue, muscle, fat, bone, cartilage, blood and lymphatic vessels, etc.

Leukaemia. It is a cancer of the blood in which the bone marrow and other blood forming organs over-produce immature or abnormal white cells.

Lymphoma. Any malignant tumour of lymph nodes or lymph gland.

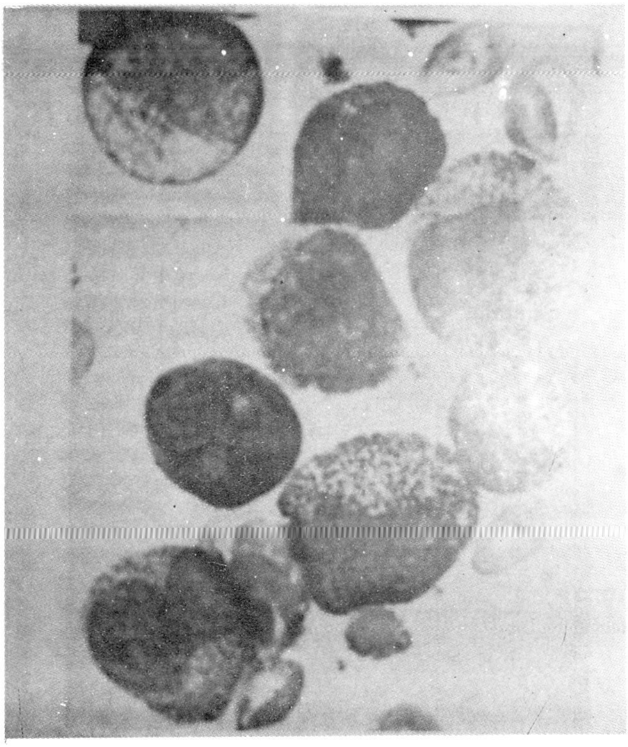

Acute promyelocytic leukemia (M3). Peripheral blood smear shows hypergraular promyelocytes. Iset (Upper left) shows a cell with promiet Auer rods. (Courtesy of Dr. Robert W. Mckenna, Southwester Medical School, Dallas, Texas)

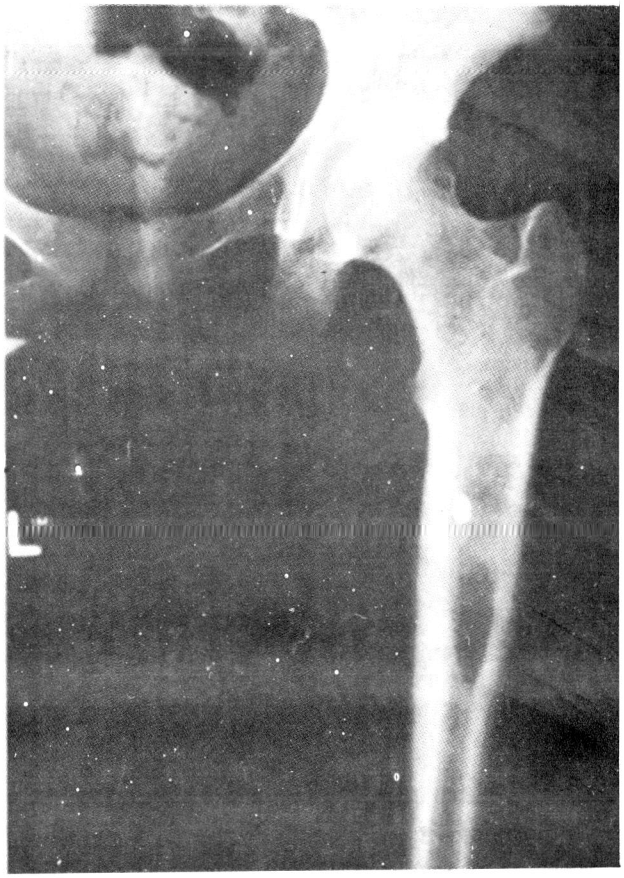

Ewing's sarcoma of the femur. The tumor has iduced a lytic lesion in the metaphyseal region accompanied by subperiosteal new bone formation with widening of the shaft. (Courtesy of Dr. Herbert Gramma, New England Deaconess Hospital).

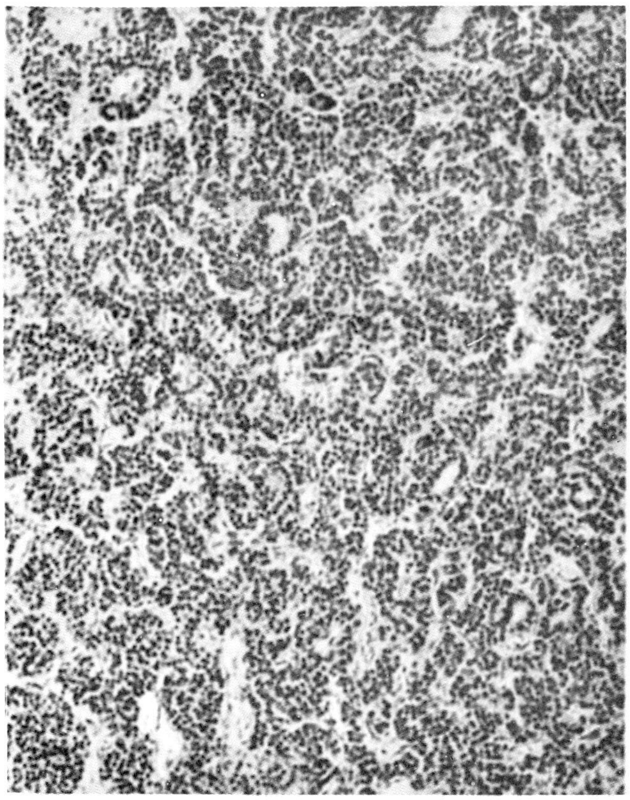

A moderately differetiated thyroid carcinoma. the tumor cells comprise disorgaized cords of cells, and only occasioal follicular spaces suggest a thyroid origin.

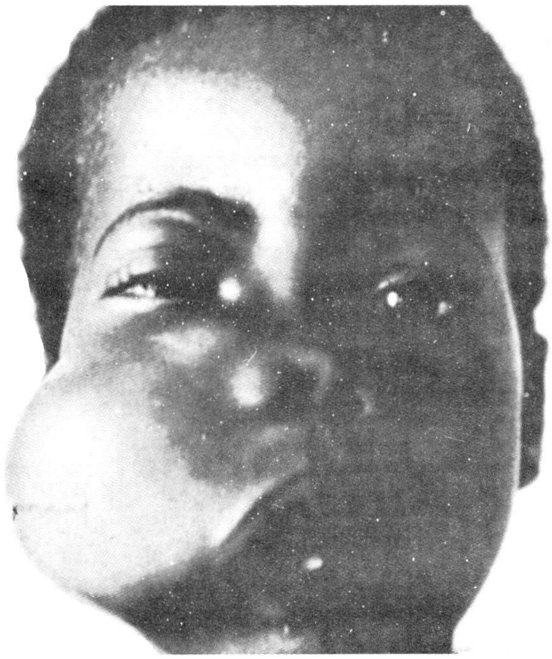

A moderately differetiated thyroid carcinoma. the tumor cells comprise disorgaized cords of cells, and only occasioal follicular spaces suggest a thyroid origin.

Incidence of Cancer

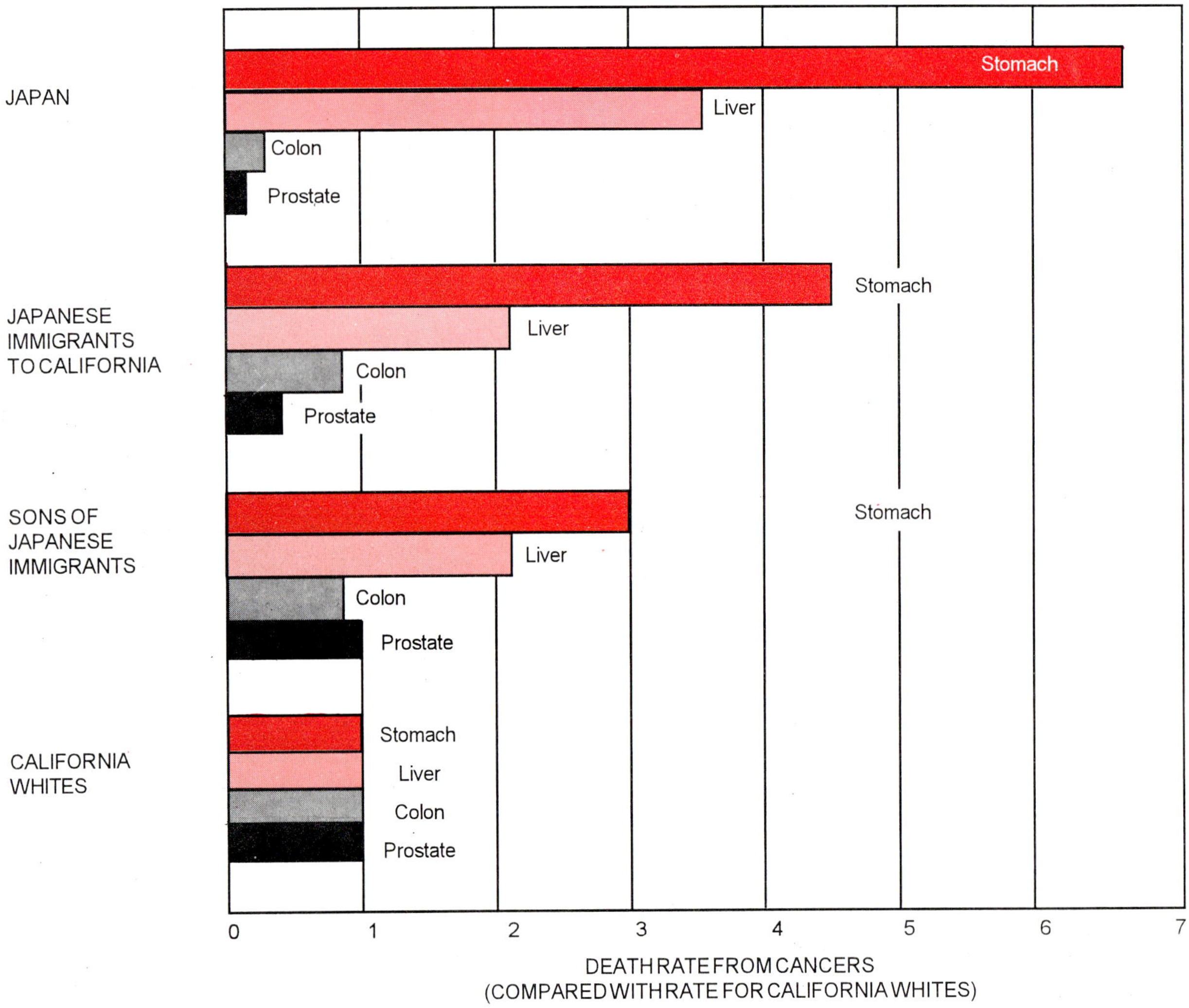

Cancer is the second common cause of death in the developed countries next to cardiovascular (heart and blood vessel) diseases. In Europe and North America, approximately one in five die of cancer. According to the WHO, out of an estimated total of 50 million deaths annually in the world, more than 5 million are attributed to cancer, and the incidence of cancer fatalities is increasing throughout the world.

Approximately 500,000 new cases of cancer occur every year in India. With the increasing life span, more cases of cancer are observed here also. Cancer is thus regarded as an emerging health problem in India. According to Dr. D.J. Jussawalla, founder Secretary of the Indian Cancer Society, "Cancer is one of the ten leading causes of death today in India, and is advancing in rank year by year." The Indian Cancer Society estimates that about 1.5 million people suffer from cancer at any point of time in India. Oral cancer and cervix cancer are in the majority.

The common cancers in India are those of the lungs, larynx, stomach, mouth, oesophagus and pharynx among men, and of uterine cervix, breast, oral cavity, pharynx and ovary among women. It has also been estimated that the life-time chance (up to the age of 64 years) of developing cancers in the metropolitan cities of India ranges between 1 out of 10 to 1 out of 16 persons.

Predisposition to Cancer

The concept that chemicals can cause cancer arose from the observations of Sir Percival Pott, who related the increased incidence of scrotal cancer in chimney sweeps to chronic exposure to soot.

In some measure, a person's likelihood of developing a cancer is expressed by national incidence and mortality rates. For example, about one in five Americans have a chance of dying of cancer. In males the overall cancer death rate has significantly increased, whereas in females it has fallen slightly. Male cancer-related fatality is mainly on account of increased incidence of lung cancer. The improvement in female cancer figures is mainly attributable to a significant decline in death rates from cancers of uterus, stomach, and liver. There is, however, alarming increase in lung cancer in both sexes. The rising slope of the curve is about the same in both sexes, and neither current-day efforts to control smoking nor "low tar" cigarettes have yet shown signs of reducing the mortality rate. In females carcinomas of the breast are about three times more frequent than those of the lung. However, because of a striking difference in the cure rates of these two cancers, bronchogenic carcinoma became the leading cause of cancer deaths in women in 1989. The decline in the number of deaths caused by uterine cancer probably relates largely to the earlier diagnosis and better cure rate. More mysterious is the downward trend in deaths from stomach and liver cancer.

Remarkable differences can be found in the incidence and death rates of specific forms of cancer around the world. For example, the death rate for stomach cancer in both males and females is seven times higher in Japan than in the United States. In contrast, the death rate from lung cancer in Scotland is nearly double that in the USA, which itself is a little more than double that in Japan. Skin cancer deaths are six times more frequent in New Zealand than in Iceland, which is probably attributable to differences in sun exposure. The age-standardized mortality rate for prostate cancer in American blacks is more than twice the rate for whites. Racial predispositions cannot therefore be ruled out, but it is generally believed that most of these geographic differences are the consequence of environmental influences. This is best brought out by comparing mortality rates for Japanese immigrants to the United Sates, and Japanese born in the United States of immigrant parents (Nisei) with those of long-term residents of both countries. This points strongly to environmental and cultural rather than genetic predisposition. Yet enigmas remain: the death rate for breast cancer in females is higher in Denmark than in Sweden, yet environmental differences between these two countries are not immediately apparent. Many hypotheses have been offered. For example, differences in number of pregnancies, age of the mother at first birth, and breast-feeding practices may be involved because they tend to reduce the uninterrupted cyclic estrogenic stimulation.

Asbestos, vinyl chloride, and 2-naphthyulamine can serve as examples of occupational hazards. Overall, mortality data indicate that persons more than 25 per cent overweight have a higher death rate from cancer than do their "trim" neighbours. Alcohol abuse alone increases the risk of throat and mouth cancer, and through the intermediation of alcoholic cirrhosis, liver cancer. Smoking, particularly of cigarettes, has been implicated in cancer of the mouth, pharynx, larynx, esophagus, pancreas, and bladder but most significantly is responsible for about 77 per cent of lung cancer among males and 43 per cent among females. Indeed, cigarette smoking has been called the single most important environmental factor contributing to premature death in the United States. Alcohol and tobacco together multiply the danger of incurring cancers in the upper aero-digestive tract.

Mortality for the Five Leading Cancer Sites for Males by Age Group, United State – 1995

All Ages **All Cancer** **246,914**	**Under 15** **All Cancer** **1,042**	**15 - 34** **All Cancer** **4,029**	**34 - 54** **All Cancer** **25,733**	**55 - 74** **All Cancer** **136,869**	**75 +** **All Cancer** **79,220**
Lung 83,854	Leukemia 418	Leukemia 679	Lung 8,926	Lung 53,756	Lung 20,996
Colon & Rectum 27,612	Brain & CNS 230	Skin 469	Colon & Rectum 2,247	Colon & Rectum 14,749	Prostate 15,132
Prostate 25,943	Non-Hodgkin's Lymphomas 66	Brain & CNS 444	Brain & CNS 1,272	Prostate 10,488	Colon & Rectum 10,422
Pancreas 11,542	Connective Tissue 50	Non-Hodgkin's Lymphomas 438	Non-Hodgkin's Lymphomas 1,214	Pancreas 6,652	Pancreas 3,672
Leukemia 9,442	Bone 33	Hodgkin's Disease 301	Skin 1,208	Stomach 4,485	Bladder 3,380

Contd.

Mortality for the Five Leading Cancer Sites for Females by Age Group, United States – 1985

All Ages All Cancer 214,649	Under 15 All Cancer 798	15 - 34 All Cancer 3,608	34 - 54 All Cancer 27,001	55 - 74 All Cancer 106,299	75 + All Cancer 76,921
Breast* 40,383	Leukemia 296	Breast 649	Breast 8,297	Lung 24,322	Colon & Rectum 14,542
Lung* 38,839	Brain & CNS 192	Leukemia 347	Lung 4,960	Breast 20,301	Breast 11,131
Colon & Rectum 28,839	Bone 41	Uterus 347	Colon & Rectum 1,911	Colon & Rectum 12,200	Lung 9,279
Pancreas 11,560	Bladder 36	Brain & CNS 321	Uterus 1,778	Ovary 6,380	Pancreas 5,211
Ovary 11,531	Non-Hodgkin's Lymphomas 36	Non-Hodgkin's Lymphomas 202	Ovary 1,666	Pancreas 5,542	Ovary 3,346

Source : Vital Statistics of the United States, 1985, From CA – A Cancer Journal for Clincians 39:7,1989.
*In 1989, lung cancer overtook breast cancer as the leading cause of cancer deaths in females (p. 263)

Evidence indicates that for a large number of types of cancer there exist not only environmental influences but also hereditary predispositions. For example, lung cancer in most instances is clearly related to cigarette smoking, yet mortality from lung cancer has been shown to be four times greater among non-smoking relatives (parents and siblings) of lung cancer patients than among nonsmoking relatives of controls. Similar data (a twofold increase) were obtained with smoking relatives. So it appears that genetic influences may contribute to the development of cancer even when there are clearly defined environmental factors. A genetic predisposition to breast cancer in females can also be shown. In general, the risk of the same neoplasm developing in close relatives of a cancer patient is about three times greater than in control populations. The best "guesstimates" suggest that about 5 per cent of all cancers are genetic. Genetic predisposition may also contribute to some proportion of so-called "environmental" and "spontaneous" cancers. The converse is equally true: Environmental factors must contribute to the initiation of many hereditary tumours.

Cancer does not, however, seem to be contagious or infectious. Experiments conducted by taking cancerous tissues and injecting or implanting them on volunteers once or twice or many times, over a period of many weeks and months, have not produced cancer in them. This shows that normal people have some defence mechanism in their bodies which does not allow the cancerous tissue to take root.

Cancer and Age Factor

Some cancers occur more often in children. Table 1 shows their percentage of occurrence in childhood.

TABLE 1. Occurrence of Cancer in Children

Type	*Per cent of Total Cancers*	
Leukaemia	3	0
Nervous system (Retinoblastoma)	1	2
Bone sarcoma	1	2
Soft tissue sarcoma	1	2
Neuroblastoma	1	0
Wilms' (Kidney) tumour		8
Lymphoma		8
Hodgkin's disease		6
Others		2

Cancer occurs more often in those above 50 or 60. In octogenarians, some characteristics of cancer have been noted during ther lifetime. Post-mortem studies of people who have died of causes other than cancers also have shown the presence of cancer symptoms.

1. Small microscopic cancer of the prostate is very common in males.
2. Lung and stomach cancer is seen in both males and females.
3. Lung cancer of the type of adenocarcinoma is found more commonly in females than males.
4. Multiple cancers are not an uncommon feature.
5. Lesions regarded as precursors to cancer are often observed in the stomach, the colon and the lungs.
6. The rate of growth of cancers in general is slow.

CHAPTER X

Causes And Prevention Of Cancer

Over the last few decades, it has been found that the environment plays a direct and indirect role in the causation of 80 to 90 per cent of all cancers. The following environmental factors have been proved to cause cancer.

Physical Reagents or Reactive Substances

In eighteenth-century England, young boys were employed as chimney sweeps. The half-dressed urchins had to crawl down chimneys to sweep them before the onset of winter. Most of them developed cancer of the scrotum when they grew up. The cause of this cancer was found to be the deposition and rubbing of soot, coal-dust and coal tar on their skin over many years. Scientists have now isolated substances such as dibenzanthracene from coal tar, which caused skin cancers in mice when it was painted daily on their skin for a few months.

Benzapyrene, a substance akin to dibenzanthracene has been found in a number of edibles and also in the atmosphere of polluted cities. Benzapyrene is a part of smoke. Rainfall brings it down to earth, where it is absorbed by vegetables and plants. Benzapyrene enters our bodies when we eat the fruits and vegetables infected with it.

Other chemical agents suspected of causing cancer include tars, dyes, aromatic ??amnesia, ??urethrae, various metals (e.g. nickel, beryllium arsenic, chromium), asbestos, synthetic hormones, and more recently aflatoxin. A number of chemicals used as medicinal compounds can also cause cancer. Diethyl stilbesterol (a female sex hormone) has been known to cross the placenta and cause vaginal cancer (adenocarcinoma) in the offspring of women who take large doses of it during pregnancy. The use of estrogens in menopausal women has also been found to be associated with a significant increase in the risk of uterine cancer. Alkylating agents and other compounds employed in the treatment of cancer have been found to be carcinogenic in animals and their potential risks and benefits must be carefully evaluated when they are used for treating human beings.

Mesothelioma, a cancer of the pleura, is a rare tumour and occurs in individuals who have been exposed to asbestos. In recent years, it has also been found that workers in asbestos factories have a significantly high probability of developing lung cancer. However, this risk is also associated with smoking, which has a dramatic synergistic effect. The asbestos worker who is also a heavy smoker has a twenty-fold increase in the risk of developing lung cancer. Cancer of urinary bladder occurs frequently in workers in aniline dye (synthetic colour) factories.

Food Additives. Some years ago, some people--scientists included--suspected that the enormous number of additives in our food supply might be a major cause of cancer. Today, most authorities believe that food additives are most likely an unimportant or even insignificant cause of cancer. One estimate, by scientists at Oxford University, exculpates food additives of responsibility for cancer with the possible exception of nitrates and nitrites added to products like smoked fish, bacon, hot dogs and liver wrust. Nitrates occur bountifully in perfectly wholesome foods, such as spinach; and even more curiously, they occur abundantly in saliva. What is more, the chemicals which react with them to form the possibly dangerous nitrosamines also occur abundantly in many foods. Perhaps foods with nitrates and nitrites ought to be consumed with foods rich in vitamin C, which largely blocks the formation of those nitrosamines. In any event, meat packers today are using less nitrite than before, and many are adding vitamin C in such form as sodium ascorbate or erythorbate to bacon, to provide a built-in blocker. The moral of all this is not that food additives are perfectly harmless, but unless you are allergic to them they are probably not worth getting paranoid over.

Tobacco

The suspicion that cancer of the mouth is associated with the use of tobacco, goes back several decades when several cases of cancer of the mouth were reported to be caused by the chewing of tobacco. A correlation between the increase of cigarette smoking and the rising incidence of lung cancer was first commented upon during the first quarter of the twentieth century in the USA, Germany and Great Britain. In the 1950s a cause-and-effect relationship was shown to exist, with a fair degree of certainty, between excessive cigarette smoking and the development of lung cancer. Innumerable studies regarding the correlation between smoking and cancer have been conducted in Great Britain, USA, West Germany, Finland, France, Japan, the Netherlands, Norway and Switzerland. The British investigations, which started in 1947 under Dr. Doll and Dr. Hill, drew the maximum attention. These investigations covered 1,465 lung cancer patients who were compared with an equally large group of carefully selected controls (those of same age and sex who did not have cancer). The analysis of the data from this and other studies conclusively revealed that smokers run a far greater risk of getting lung cancer. This risk increases with the amount of tobacco consumed. Heavy smokers (who smoke more than 25 cigarettes a day) run a much higher risk than light smokers do.

Tobacco smoke is a gaseous mixture containing finely divided solid and liquid particles. It is said to contain about a thousand chemical constituents, of which only 270 have been officially recognized till now. The most important among them are nicotine, carbon monoxide gas and a mixture of many chemicals which on deposition form a brownish tarry substance commonly called smoke tar. The active agents in the tar which lead to the production of cancers have been identified as different polycyclic aromatic hydrocarbon compounds. These are not present in the tobacco but are produced as a result of its incomplete combustion. Roughly, one cigarette ingests about 20 mg. of smoke tar into a smoker's body. A smoker of 20 cigarettes a day thus absorbs about 150 gm. of smoke tar in a year.

In a study carried out in Britain, a questionnaire was sent in 1951 to 60,000 doctors of or above the age of 35 years. Sufficient information was received from 40,000 of them to enable the investigators to classify the smokers according to their prevailing smoking habits at the time of enquiry. Upon the death of any of them details about the causes of their death were obtained and confirmed, the results of which showed that lung cancer mortality increases consistently and steeply with increased tobacco smoking. For heavy smokers (25 cigarettes or more a day), the mortality is 24 times more compared to non-smokers; for moderate smokers (15-24 cigarettes a day), it is 12 times more, and for mild smokers (1-24 cigarettes a day), it is 7 times more.

A series of studies conducted by Dr. Hammond and Dr. Morn in the USA investigated the smoking habits of 187,766 male whites between the ages of 50 and 70 years belonging not only to large and small towns but also to rural areas. Their conclusions were that those who regularly smoke up to 20 cigarettes a day are about 25 times more prone to lung cancer than non-smokers. This figure mounts to roughly 45 times for those who smoke between 20 and 40 cigarettes a day and reaches a multiple of approximately 90 for chain-smokers who smoke more than 40 cigarettes a day.

There are other interesting observations which indicate the cause-and-effect relationship between cigarette smoking and lung cancer.

1. The Icelanders smoked little until 1941. An analysis of the post-mortem examinations performed between 1932 and 1938 revealed lung carcinoma to be a rare disease. But during the war the Icelanders took to smoking because of their contacts with the American occupying troops. Today, lung cancer is one of the common cancers in Iceland.
2. In post-mortem examination of 11,365 Bantu miners in South Africa who died between 1916 and 1949, lung cancer was found only in 6 cases, while it was found in 114 of the 8,465 white miners. Bantus scarcely smoked cigarettes, while the whites did.
3. A much higher death rate from lung cancer was found among European-born Jews in Israel in 1957, than among those of Asian and African origin. Smoking was more prevalent among the whites then.
4. In the non-smoking, non-drinking community of Seventh Day Adventists in the United States, only one case of lung cancer was observed between 1952 and 1956. According to general statistics of cancer incidence in the USA there should have been at least 10 to 11 cases of lung cancer among them.

5. Lung cancer has scarcely been seen among the Sikhs whose religion forbids the use of tobacco in any form.
6. Several examinations of the lungs of smokers dying of causes other than lung cancer have revealed pre-cancerous changes in their lung cells.

There is evidence also from experiments on animals in the USA. When distilled tobacco tar was applied on the shaved skin of mice for some weeks, it was found to produce cancerous changes in the skins of only some of them in numerous experimental studies in the 1950s. Later, when smoke tar was collected under conditions that simulated human smoking, and was applied on the shaved skins of mice, and the process was continued for their natural life span, changes which were similar to those caused by lung cancer in human beings, were detected in their skin. Also when the mice were exposed to tobacco smoke in glass vessels and this process was continued for weeks on end, changes suggestive of those leading towards lung cancer were produced in many of them. Experiments have also been carried out under simulated conditions akin to human smoking. For example, a batch of 24 dogs was taught to inhale smoke by means of tubes inserted directly from their wind pipes into their lungs. Two and a half years later, after having smoked seven cigarettes a day, two of these animals developed lung cancer similar to that of human beings.

If, therefore, tobacco chewing can be controlled, the incidence of oral cancer would be substantially reduced. Oral cancer is a preventable, detectable and treatable cancer. In India , one-third of all the cancer cases are of mouth cancer, mainly because of the widely prevalent habit of chewing tobacco. In other countries, its incidence is much less--4.6 per cent in Russia, 4.7 per cent in the UK, 3.4 per cent in the USA, 2.6 per cent in Japan and 2.6 per cent in Scandinavian countries. Those who habitually chew tobacco every day run eight times the risk of developing mouth cancer than non-chewers. The risk is higher in those who have started the habit at an early age. How long the quid is kept in the mouth is also relevant. Tobacco chewers who keep tobacco in the mouth while they sleep increase the risk of getting cancer exponentially. The risk increases further if the quid is kept only on one side.

As regards lung cancer, the longer a cigarette is, the more tar and nicotine one inhales. The last half of the cigarette contains twice as much tar and nicotine as the first half. This applies to 'king-sized' cigarettes as well. No method of treating tobacco or filtering the smoke has yet been demonstrated to be completely effective in significantly reducing or eliminating the scourge of lung cancer. Giving up smoking decreases a person's susceptibility to it in proportion to the number of years that smoking has been given up for.

MALE (505,000)			FEMALE (505,000)		
Rank	**Site**	**No. Cases (%)**	**Rank**	**Site**	**No. Cases (%)**
1.	Prostate	103,000 (20.3)	1.	Breast (invasive)	142,000 (28.1)
2.	Lung	101,100 (20.0)	2.	Colorectum	78,000 (15.4)
3.	Colorectum	73,000 (14.4)	3.	Lung	54,000 (10.6)
4.	Bladder	34,500 (6.8)	4.	Endometrium	34,000 (6.7)
5.	Hodgkin's disease and lymphomas	21,000 (4.1)	5.	Hodgkin's disease and lymphomas	19,200 (3.8)
6.	Leukemia	15,200	6.	Pancreas	14,000 (2.7)
7.	Stomach	11,900 (2.3)	7.	Cervix (invasive)	13,000 (2.5)
8.	Pancreas	13,000 (2.5)	8.	Leukemia	12,100 (2.3)

Anti-tobacco Community Education

The proportion of tobacco-related cancers in India varies from 42.5 to 69.8 per cent in males as against 14.2 to 36.6 per cent in females. Based on the data obtained from the three population-based cancer registries in Mumbai, Bangalore and Chennai, it has been estimated that 6.36 lakh persons have developed cancers in 1991. Of these, 2.15 lakh had cancers attributable to tobacco usage. The corresponding figures projected for the year 2001 are 8.06 lakh due to tobacco use.

Anti-tobacco community education has been identified as a major component of India's National Cancer Control Programme. In the search for a cost-effective strategy for anti-tobacco community education, a multicentric project has been initiated for studying the feasibility of involving the health infrastructure, school children and teachers, and community volunteers. Paramedical workers were also trained in this study, in the examination of the oral cavity for early detection of cancerous and pre-cancerous lesions.

In Goa, three years intervention through schools alone resulted in reduction in the prevalence of tobacco usage by 33.5 per cent in men and 45.5 per cent in women, compared to 37.6 per cent in men and 50.4 per cent in women when intervention was carried out through schools and the health infrastructure combined (in contrast to an observed reduction of 8.5 per cent in men and 33.3 per cent in women in the control area). Based on the findings of this study, the Government of Goa has proposed to include 8 hours of teaching on tobacco hazards, as part of the curricular activities in schools for students in the fifth standard and higher classes.

The Agra centre tested the feasibility if using community volunteers to induce quitting the habit of tobacco. One year intervention by the project staff showed a tobacco quitting rate of 14.4 per cent. After one year's intervention through community volunteers 26.3 per cent men and 10.5 per cent women quit or were reported as likely quitters (i.e. tobacco use has been stopped for up to 6 months by these).

A special project under the title Radio DATE (Drug, Alcohol and Tobacco Education) was developed and implemented to assess the effect of using the radio as an instrument for bringing about a reduction in the use of drugs, alcohol and tobacco consumption in the community. The programme was broadcast in Hindi as well as regional languages. The community survey carried out in rural Karnataka showed that 31.6 per cent of the potential audience had listened to Radio DATE, and that most of them had listened to more than two episodes of the programme. The presence (or absence) of tobacco habit had no association with the probability of listening to the programme. In Goa, the programme covered 26.7 per cent of the listeners. Most of the listeners felt that such programmes, if continued, could have in due course, a positive impact on users as well as non-users. In Karnataka, nearly 6 per cent tobacco users reportedly quit the habit, 31.4 per cent reduced the frequency of use, and another 39.8 per cent had serious intention to quit the habit.

It has been estimated that the number of tobacco-related deaths in 1991 in India were at least 8 lakh. Efforts for prevention of tobacco-related diseases in the country have not been intensive, partly due to the large revenue generated by the tobacco trade. It is likely that the expenditure incurred by the Government for the treatment of tobacco-related diseases is much more that the revenue generated by tobacco. Studies carried out so far show that a patients of tobacco-related cancer spends approximately Rs. 4,881 on his illness even before the diagnosis of cancer is made and about Rs. 7,225 towards treatment, after diagnosis of cancer is established.

Many of us used to feel that pollution in general was a major cause of cancer, one even more difficult to avoid. But here the Oxford University epidemiologists we mentioned before have a word of reassurance. They estimate that pollution is probably responsible for no more than 2 per cent of all avoidable risks. A number of other studies, however, indicate that people who are exposed to relatively high amounts of air pollution over a long period of time, either at home or on the job, have a much increased rate of lung cancer if they also smoke. So, while the harmful effects of air pollution certainly cannot be ignored, the best thing that you can do about it (besides supporting clean air legislation) is not to smoke.

Radioactive Substances and Solar Radiation

During the nineteenth century, there was high incidenc of lung cancer among mine workers of the Schoenberg and Jachymov mines (now in Czech republic). It was later found out that these mines contained various cancer-causing radioactive substances. It has been experimentally proved that prolonged exposure of laboratory animals to X-rays and other radioactive substances produces cancer. Many inexperienced technicians working with X-ray machines in the past developed cancer of the skin over their hands and some even developed leukaemia. Bone cancer has been noted to occur more frequently in girls who are employed in watch factories in Asia to paint dials of watches with luminous paints which contain radioactive materials. Leukaemia and other cancers developed among many Japanese who were exposed to the atom bomb explosions of Hiroshima and Nagasaki. Solar radiation has its share in the etiology of cancer. In Australia, New Zealand and some parts of the USA, skin cancers are common among sun-bathers; this is attributed to the thinning of the ozone layer in atmosphere which prevents the harmful rays of the sun from reaching the earth.

Skin Irritation and Poor Hygiene

Chronic irritation can also cause cancer. A slight but constant injury which is repeatedly inflicted on the same part of the body over a period of many years, has been known to lead to cancer of that part. For example, a jagged edge of a broken tooth rubbing against the tongue, gall stones rubbing constantly against the lining of the gall bladder, all result in cancer. The smoking of short clay pipes by labourers in Eastern Europe leads to cancers of the tongue, lips and the gall bladder.

In the Godavari region of Andhra Pradesh, many smoke locally rolled cigars (*chutta*), with the burning end inside the mouth. Some of these people are known to develop cancer of the mouth. In Kashmir, the people keep the *kangri*, which is an earthen pot containing burning coal, underneath the garments directly in contact with the skin in order to keep warm. *Kangri*-induced cancer among the Kashmiris develops over the skin of the abdomen and thigh due to the constant irritation of the skin on the stomach by the hot *kangri*. *Dhoti* (loin cloth) induced cancer below the navel seen among Maharashtrian men has also been attributed to chronic irritation of the skin of the navel by the *dhoti*.

Cancer of the penis, fairly common among the uncircumcised, is almost unknown among the Jews and is rare among Muslims. The incidence of cervical cancer is also significantly less among females married to circumcised males. Among the Jews, circumcision is done within a week of birth, and among the Muslims between the ages of four and fourteen years. The protection that circumcision provides can also be obtained by keeping the skin over the penis hygienically clean.

Viruses

Peyton Rous first showed in 1911 that a virus caused sacrum in chickens. But it was not until the late 1950s and early 1960s, after the isolation of the marine (mice) leukaemia viruses and the discovery of the polymoa virus, that serious consideration was given to a virus etiology for human cancers and fresh expectations for its control with vaccines was generated. When cancer-related viruses enter the body they upset the normal cell functioning mutating them.

Many cancers in animals, plants and birds have been recognized to be caused by viruses. Currently, it is being convincingly stated that leukemia and Hodgkin's disease (a malignant disease of the lymphatic tissue) are associated with some kind of virus. The association of the Hepatitis-B virus with primary liver cancer is now fairly well established. The African lymphoma described by Burkitt in 1958, is suspected to be due to the Epstein-Barr virus.

Hormones

Excessive hormonal levels often cause cancer, and a reduction in their levels alleviates cancer. Cancer of the prostate in men and of the breast in women can be greatly relieved by the removal of their testes and ovaries respectively, or by the removal of adrenal glands which are a secondary source of sex hormones in both sexes. The administration of counter-hormones (estrogens in males and androgens in females) also results in a marked improvement in such cases.

Genetic and Personal Factors

The environmental factors described above do not invariably lead to the development of cancer in all those who are exposed to them. So it would appear that there is something in the body of cancer patients which predisposes them to develop cancer when they come in contact with the environmental conditions described above. The following genetic factors play a major role in the incidence of cancer.

Age. The incidence of cancer increases with age, especially after 50. Possible explanations for this enhanced vulnerability are: (a) the changes in the body due to the ageing process; (b) a long incubation period of certain types of cancer; and (c) long exposure to a carcinogens (i.e. cancer causing substances).

Sex. There are sex differences in the frequencies of certain types of cancers. For example, lung cancer and cancer of esophagus are more common in men than in women.

Race. It is difficult to empirically disentangle the influence of race from that of the environment. It has been found, however, that fair-complexioned people have an excessive incidence of skin cancers, especially those of the face and neck, as opposed to coloured races.

Marital Status. Cancer of the cervix is more common among married women with multiple pregnancies and also among those who marry at an early age. The risk factors significantly associated with cervical dysplasias are: illiteracy, deliveries conducted by untrained birth attendants, re-use of old cloth during menstruation, low age at consummation of marriage (below 18 years), and non-abstinence from sex during the post-partum period. Post-marital promiscuity has also been observed to be an important risk factor for cervial dysplasias and cancer.

Heredity. Genetic influences on cancer have been suspected for a long time. Napoleon is said to have died of cancer of the stomach. His grandfather, father, brothers and sisters all died of cancer of the stomach. Retinoblastoma (cancer of the eye) occurs commonly in siblings (i.e. in children of the same parents). Osteosarcoma (malignant cancer of the bone), cancer of the colon and thyroid cancers frequently occur in twins. Mongoloid children are more likely to develop blood cancer (leukaemia) than normal children. There are strong indications that chromosomal damage and deformity is a characteristic of some forms of cancer, but a definite cause-effect relationship has not yet been established.

Socio-economic Status. There is a definite relationship between socio-economic status and the incidence of cancer. For example, cancers of the stomach, the skin and the cervix are more common among low-income groups. Breast cancer is common among women of higher socio-economic groups, probably because of late child bearing.

Low Immunity Levels. Transformation of normal body cells into abnormal cells is not a rare event. But the body's immunological cells – lymphocytes and macrophages--at once recognize these abnormal cells and kill them before they divide and subdivide. In an immuno-deficient person, the normal surveillance provided by the defending immunological cells is weakened, so they are unable to kill the cancer cells when they grow in the body. These then multiply rapidly to set up the disease.

Preventive Measures

Cancer prevention methods attempt to eliminate the disease by protecting both the individual and the community from its etiological agents. This is called *primary prevention*. This method essentially involves the environmental monitoring of cancer-causing agents (carcinogens), the identification of high risk groups and procedures to abolish contact points between the carcinogens and the hosts (i.e. the people).

Cancer prevention also aims at correcting cancer-prone pathological states. This is called *secondary prevention*. The identification and management of such cases is made possible through mass screening techniques for detecting cases of commonly prevalent cancers like those of the cervix, lung, mouth, stomach and liver.

Education is the most important method of primary prevention. It involves the mass dissemination of knowledge and awareness about the causes of cancer. The aim of imparting this education is to make people aware of the dangers that they are likely to face when they expose themselves to cancer-causing agents.

The measures for the primary prevention of cancer are:

1. Improvement of personal hygiene in areas such as the mouth, the skin and the genitals.
2. Control of air pollution.
3. Testing all drugs, cosmetics and food additives for carcinogens.
4. Efforts to reduce the amount of radiation (including medical radiation) received by each individual without reducing its benefits.
5. Enforcement of measures to protect workers from carcinogenic agents in industries.
6. Reduction and regulation in the use of pesticides of various types such as DDT, BHC and malathion.
7. Strict enforcement of air pollution legislation in cities and for inserting a statutory warning notice on cigarette packets.
8. Necessary change in diet and life-style. Also all insecticides should be thoroughly washed off fresh fruits and vegetables before they are consumed. Artificial sweeteners like saccharin should be avoided as far as possible.
9. Statistical recording of the number of cancer patients is an important means of cancer prevention because

it provides a base for assessing the magnitude or the problem in each area of the country and for planning the necessary cancer detection and treatment services.

Study of Cancer Statistics

The National Cancer Registry Programme (NCRP), set up in 1982 continues to provide authentic information on cancer occurrence. Currently, the network has six Population-Based Cancer Registries (PBCR), at Mumbai, Bangalore, Chennai, Bhopal, Delhi and Tiruvanantapuram. The data from the PBCRs assist in the calculation of incidence rates at various sites. The study of the incidence rates according to place time and various characteristics of people has helped in the formulation of a hypothesis on the etiology of some of these malignancies.

Hospital-based Cancer Registries (HCRs) collect detailed information on cancer patients seeking specified hospitals. A comprehensive report on the five-year (1984 to 1988) data has been compiled. Epidemiological studies on cancers of the pharynx, oesophagus and stomach are being carried out. The multicentric study on stomach cancer is aimed at understanding the reason for the geographic variations in the incidence of this cancer, with special emphasis on dietary factors. A study on cancer of the oesophagus currently under way aims at defining the factors (including dietary patterns) associated with higher prevalence of this cancer in the north-eastern parts of India, while another study is testing the association of chilies and other spices and consumption of rice and jowar preparations. A case control study in search of etiological factors for pharyngeal cancer has also been completed.

Secondary Prevention

Screening for cancer comes under this category. The two important cancers that come under this head are: cancer of the uterine cervix and cancer of the breast.

Uterine Cervix Cancer. In many Western countries, deaths from cervical cancer have been reduced by up to 50 per cent in the last 20 years. During this period, there has been an increasing awareness of the importance of its early diagnosis and a concerted effort to screen for the disease using the cervical smear technique or pap test. This involves the scraping of cells from the lining of the cervix. Many of the cancers detected by this method are localized on the surface and are called *in-situ* cancers. These tests should be carried out on all women who are over 40 in symptomless cases, and even earlier in those who have abnormal vaginal bleeding or a persistent vaginal discharge. Women whose cervical smear reveals the existence of abnormal cells that are indicative of a pre-cancerous change called dyspepsia, will need to have a biopsy of the cervix to confirm the diagnosis. Cervical cancer, when caught at this stage, has a cure rate of 95 per cent.

Breast Cancer. Self-examination of the breasts should be carried out monthly. Among women who have regular periods this must be done at the same time each month as the shape and feel of the breasts changes with the menstrual cycle. The best time to examine the breasts is 7 days after the start of each period. A careful examination can easily pick up even the smallest lump. The technique of doing it can easily be learnt from a cancer specialist. Breast examination by a doctor should usually be done every six months. Briefly, the procedure for self-examination of the breasts is as follows:

1. Look at your breasts in the mirror with your arms by your side, then with them in the air and watch out for any signs of puckering.
2. Lie down, and with the left arm behind the head, examine the left breast first with the flat of the right hand and then with the fingers. Work from the upper, inner quarter into the nipple.
3. Feel around the nipple, then continue to the lower inner quarter.
4. Put your arm by your side, and then working from outside the breast, feel towards the lower outer quarter, the nipple, and lastly the upper outer quarter.
5. Check the breast tissue across the top of the breast to the armpit.
6. Feel inside the armpit.

Examine the right breast in a similar manner.

Mammography is a special X-ray of the breast and is useful for detecting cancers which are too small to be palpated. This is done in high risk patients, usually after the age of 50 years. All patients with a breast lump should be seen by a specialist so that it may be investigated further and if necessary, biopsies performed.

The majority of breast lumps that are biased do not contain cancer (i.e. they are benign), but this can only be proved by examining a transverse section of the lump tissue under a microscope. Any decision regarding whether or not to perform a biopsy can only be made by a specialist, and general practitioners should refer all patients with breast lumps to a cancer specialist immediately.

Warning Signs of Breast Cancer. (a) Unusual difference in size or shape of the breasts. (b) Alterations in the position of either nipple. (c) Retraction (turning in) of either nipple. (d) Puckering (dimple) of the skin surface over the breast. (e) Unusual rash on the breast or nipple. (f) Unusual prominence of the veins over either breast. (g) Unusual discrete lump or nodule in any part of either breast on palpation.

Summary: What To Do To Avoid Cancer

- ❑ Try not to smoke or use tobacco in any form–paan, bidis, cigarettes etc.
- ❑ Drink alcoholic beverages in moderation or avoid them altogether.
- ❑ Eat foods with a low fat content. They are the main causes of heart problems as well.
- ❑ Eat a balanced diet consisting of plenty of fresh vegetables, fruits and whole grain cereals and eat less spicy and tinned food.
- ❑ Avoid unnecessary X-rays.
- ❑ Do not expose yourself to too much sun. Wear protective clothing, caps and sunglasses, and carry an umbrella.
- ❑ Keep yourself safe while working on hazardous jobs. Use protective devices like face masks, gloves, etc., whenever necessary.
- ❑ Do not use contraceptive pills over a prolonged period of time.

CHAPTER XI

Common Symptoms Of Cancer

Early detection is vital for successful treatment of cancer. The following symptoms warrant a consultation with one's his physician or a cancer specialist immediately.

Abnormal Bleeding. Unusual bleeding after a slight injury, vomit mixed with blood, non-injury bleeding from the skin, mouth or any other bodily orifice, blood in the stools, vaginal bleeding other than menstrual one or after the sexual act, or vaginal discharge mixed with blood; phlegm containing blood; blood in the urine; continued bleeding after delivery; and bleeding from a mole or what looks like a mole.

A lump or a hard area. A lump on the abdomen which is found out to be the spleen; a lump in the arm, leg, or any other part .

A raised birthmark. A sudden growth in a mole or in a birthmark, and the formation of new moles.

A hard based chronic sore that does not heal. This is a high risk factor, particularly if it is located on the penis.

A persistent change in digestive or bowel habits, for example chronic constipation. This factor is particularly significant if it alternates with loose motions.

Loss of weight without any visible cause, especially among adults, in spite of good appetite and intake of nourishing food.

Unexplained diminished or lost appetite and aversion to food.

Feeling of tiredness without any apparent reason or accompanied by low-grade fever and increasing weakness and anemia.

Painless/painful swelling. These are different from nodular swellings or a lump. Such swellings can be often on one side of the neck or the abdomen. Cancerous swellings can be painless with a hard base in the cheek, or accompanied by discomfort or pain (sometimes severe) in the upper abdomen, or manifest in enlarged and painful testes, etc.

Difficulty in swallowing solid or semi-solid food and the vomiting of recently consumed food, sometimes mixed with blood.

A persistent cough or hoarseness in a smoker.

Unexplained low-grade fever manifesting in a variety of ways.

On external surfaces, any thickening of the tissues, formation of a nodule or tumour, persisting sores and carbuncles, can be a feature of cancer. Internal cancers may grow for some time before they cause any symptom. But weight loss, anaemia and low-grade fever in older people even without symptom, should arouse suspicion.

Cancer-related symptoms may be categorized as: (a) those which are common to any cancer; (2) those that depend upon the site of cancer and the type of cancer; and (c) those in which symptoms are caused by cancer treatment like chemotherapy and radiation. The common symptoms of cancer and their usual methods of alleviation are--

Loss of appetite and weight. Loss of appetite and weight are the commonest symptoms of cancer. These may be a result of: (a) a poor appetite, which results in reduced intake of food; (b) the presence of cancer tissue which burns up the excessive energy of the body; (c) vomiting and diarrhoea which do not allow food to be absorbed.

To increase the appetite, appetizing foods are normally given. Appetizers like mild alcoholic drinks may also be prescribed. Sometimes steroids prove helpful when other measures fail.

Nausea and vomiting. These are common symptoms after chemotherapy or radiation. When severe, they may be difficult to tolerate. Anti-vomiting anti-hysteric tablets are normally prescribed for mild or moderate cases.

Diarrhoea. This is generally the effect of chemotherapy treatment, but sometimes may be due to the cancer itself. Anti-diarrhoeal drugs are helpful in alleviating these symptoms.

Constipation. This may be due to diminished appetite or loss of appetite, inactivity, change in diet, or even due to pain relieving drugs. Stool softeners such as liquid paraffin are helpful in such cases.

Insomnia. Many symptoms of cancer, or the depression and anxiety associated with it can make patients lose sleep. Proper treatment of these symptoms with sedatives and hypnotics can provide patients with the much needed relief. Depression can also be helped by tricycle drugs.

Pain. As many as half the cancers, even at an advanced stage, do not cause any pain. But where pain is present, it may be continuous and can gradually increase in intensity which can sometimes become difficult to bear. Pain-relieving drugs are prescribed for regular intake. The choice of the drug depends upon the severity of the pain.

Shortness of breath. Shortness of breath, often with cough, is not uncommon in advanced cancers. It is commonly caused by cancer in the lung in which there is a collection of fluid in the pleural cavity around the lung, scarring and fibrosis of the lungs and infections in the lung such as pneumonia. The treatment of this symptom depends upon its cause. Lung cancer patients, for example, will need either surgery, radiation or chemotherapy to alleviate this symptom.

Cough. Coughs can only be treated after finding out their cause. Coughs caused by infection in lung cancer are treated by giving appropriate antibiotics. Irritant coughs without much phlegm can be suppressed by cough mixtures containing codeine or related compounds.

Urinary incontinence. Cancers in the which the pelvis irritates or presses upon the bladder can cause increased frequency or incontinence. Radiation and/or chemotherapy may help. If incontinence continues, a catheter is passed through the urethra which drains the bladder into a container without soiling the patient's bed. Care is necessary to see that no infection enters the urethra and the urinary bladder while inserting the catheter.

Bowel obstruction. Obstruction or blockage of the bowels is most often caused by cancer of the large bowel. It usually starts slowly with an occasional attack just like a colic pain in the abdomen. The pain is often accompanied by loud bowel sounds and swelling of the abdomen. The symptoms of bowel obstruction are usually colicky abdominal pain, nausea and vomiting. Sometimes, the constipation may become so complete that the patient cannot even pass any wind.

The following measures are suggested as part of the treatment of this symptom: (a) no food or drinks are taken by mouth; (b) fluids are given intravenously; (c) in cases of severe vomiting, a tube is passed through the nose into the patient's stomach in order to drain out excess fluids; (c) in some cases, the obstruction may settle down with this treatment. If it does not, surgical intervention becomes necessary.

Collection of fluid in the abdomen (Ascites). Sometimes cancer in the abdomen causes the accumulation of fluid. This can lead to uncomfortable swelling and also difficulty in breathing. A wide-bored needle or a plastic tube is generally passed through the skin of the abdomen and the fluid is drawn up into a syringe to alleviate this symptom.

Sore mouth. This may be due a to drug reaction, a vitamin deficiency, aphthous or small ulcers, fungal infections or bacterial infections. Careful cleaning of the mouth is very important. For fungal infections, anti-fungal lozenges are helpful. Miconazole is used also to rinse the mouth at least four times a day. Ketoconazole can also be used. In the case of anti-cancer drugs which produce sores in the mouth, the basic treatment is to keep the mouth hygienically clean.

Difficulty in swallowing. Cancer in or near the oesophagus (the food pipe) can cause difficulty in swallowing (dysphagia). Some cancers respond to treatment but many do not. In such cases, surgery is performed to insert a tube from the upper end of the oesophagus through the cancerous segment, to its lower end.

Cachexia

Cancer frequently leads to a syndrome known as cachexia. It manifests in weakness, loss of weight and appetite anorexia. The patient appears ill and emaciated. The fat content of muscle cells of patients with cachexia is generally around half that of healthy people. There is also an increased breakdown in the proteins of their muscles.

There has been an increasing awareness of cachexia as a cause of death in cancer patients. In one autopsy series, more than 22 per cent of the patients died not of their cancer, but of the systemic effects of cachexia.

The cause of anorexia remains complex and unclear, but there are some contributing factors such as the following:

1. Cancers at specific sites like the oesophagus produce mechanical obstructions to the passage of food.
2. It has been postulated that metabolic demands are increased in cancer patients due to competition by cancer cells for nutrition. Various studies have demonstrated increased nutrient-consumption ratios in patients with widespread sarcomas.
3. Other mechanisms like abnormalities of smell and taste, deranged nervous system control and the presence of cancer cell secretions in the blood, all lead to the development of cachexia.
4. The cancer treatment itself can also influence the development of cachexia. Chemotherapy and radiation therapy can lead to malnutrition by causing mucositis, enteritis and vomiting, while the stress of surgery produces a hyper-catabolic state. The nutritional consequences of cancer chemotherapy are secondary to its side-effects such as nausea, vomiting, oral pain, diarrhoea and fever.

In cachexia cases, adequate nutritional support in necessary. It is likely that by offering such nutritional support before, during and after the treatment, a patient's clinical responses may improve along with his tolerance to therapy.

When voluntary oral intake is unsatisfactory and the gastro-intestinal tract is not functional, feeding via a gastric tube is indicated. In more serious cases, total intravenous nutrition may become essential. Total intravenous support is a newer and more effective method of nutritional support through which carbohydrates, fats and other nutritional requirements are given. This is a useful treatment both before and after radiation and chemotherapy. However, it involves close monitoring of metabolic needs and a careful adjustment of the mineral and trace metal levels in the body.

Dental Problems

Oral symptoms are among the earliest symptoms of leukaemias, and patients with undiagnosed leukaemias may first seek dental care. Fever and septicaemia predispose the onset of serious bleeding. In these cases, serious bleeding from the gums is directly related to low platelet count, and platelet transfusions have proved effective in checking bleeding.

Oral perblems can also be treatment induced, and can start with a reddening of the inside of the mouth. They are generally observed after a week of treatment. By the middle of the second week, white patches appear on the lining (mucosa) of the lips, cheeks and tongue. The irritation becomes progressively more severe. A sloughing of the mucosa occurs by the third week, and by the fourth and fifth week, the lips and corners of the mouth generally have an ulcerated appearance. The mucosa may become very painful and the oral discomfort may become so severe that the patient avoids all chewing and swallowing. An alkaline mouthwash, to which a large spoonful of milk of magnesia is added, gives some relief. Rinsing of the mouth with topical xylocaine before meals may help the patient to eat.

A side effect of radiation therapy is the severe depression of salivary secretion leading to a marked, persistent and irreversible sensation of dryness of the mouth.

CHAPTER XII

Diagnosis And Treatment

Every passing year the approach to laboratory diagnosis of cancer becomes more complex, more sophisticated, and more specialized. For virtually every tumour, a number of subcategories have been characterized by experts.

The laboratory diagnosis of cancer is, in most instances, not difficult. The two ends of the benign-malignant spectrum pose no problems; however, in the middle lies a ''no man's land'' where wise men tread cautiously.

Occasionally what can, at the time of the first non-invasive examination seem to be caner may turn out to be a non-malignant condition. Various diagnostic investigations are necessary to confirm the diagnosis of cancer. Diagnosis may be done by study of cells (cytology) or of tissue (histology). If a cancer is found, a series of X-rays, blood tests and other special tests are normally carried out to ascertain whether there are any signs that the tumour has spread.

Cytological Methods

Cancer Markers in the Blood. Cancer cells differ from normal cells. The bio-chemicals that they produce and pour into the blood are also different. The presence of cancer tissues in the body can be detected by the presence of these biochemical products known as cancer- or tumour-markers in the blood. These are normal metabolic constituents that are found in either abnormal amounts or at an inappropriate time of life, like for example, foetal proteins being re-expressed in adult life. Tumour-markers of this type are useful in the diagnosis of some forms of cancer. The presence of tumour-markers can also be of clinical value in monitoring the progress of patients as their quantity reduces with recovery from cancer.

Cytologic (Papanicolaou) smears provide yet another method for the detection of cancer. This approach is widely used for suspected cancer of the cervix, and also for many other forms of suspected malignancy, such as endometrial carcinoma, lung, bladder, prostate and gastric cancers; for the identification of tumour cells in abdominal, pleural, joint, and cerebrospinal fluids; and, less commonly, with other forms of tumours.

Cytologic interpretation requires a great deal of expertise but can yield with cervical smears nearly 100 per cent correct positive diagnosis. Smears for other types of tumours (e.g. lung, stomach, prostate) are more difficult to evaluate. With all, a positive finding almost always provides strong evidence of the existence of a cancer but a negative report does not exclude the presence of a malignancy.

Fine needle aspiration. The procedure involves aspirating cells and attendant fluid with a small-bore needle followed by cytologic examination of the stained smear. This method is employed most commonly for the pre-operative assessment of readily palpable lesions in sites such as the breast, thyroid, lymph nodes, and, with the aid of a special needle, the prostate. Modern imaging techniques enable the method to be extended to lesions in deep-seated structures such as pelvic lymph nodes. Fine needle aspiration is less invasive and more rapidly performed than are needle biopsies. In experienced hands it is an extremely reliable, rapid, and useful technique.

Immunocytochemistry depends for its analysis on the presence of specific monoclonal antibodies in the cells. *DNA probe analyses* and *DNA flow cytometry* are some other cytological diagnostic methods which are more recent introductions.

Examination of Ascetic Fluid. If the patient has a swollen abdomen and physical examination reveals the presence of fluid in it, then this fluid is removed either for diagnostic or for therapeutic purposes in order to relieve him of the discomfort. The withdrawn fluid is then sent for cytological and bacteriological examination and chemical analysis.

Histological Methods

Barium Meal. A contrast meal such as barium compound which is opaque to X-rays is given to the patient to swallow. This makes the part in which the barium flows, opaque to X-rays in contrast to the rest of the body. Any abnormality in the organs through which it passes can then be noticed on an X-ray. Stomach cancer shows up on X-rays as a filling defect in the barium-filled organ. The whole examination requires 6 to 24 hours to complete. The patient is asked to take a light meal the previous night and fast until the X-ray examination is over.

Biopsy involves examining tumour tissue taken from the body under a microscope. It often involves relatively minor surgery and may be done using a local anaesthetic. Many patients need only spend the day in hospital.

Before a patient undergoes any test, it is always worthwhile for him to find out everything about them and just how they are done. Medical tests and operations often seem much more frightening when one doesn't know what one is facing.

Some suggested questions to ask at the outset of cancer investigations are:

* Why is the test being done?
* Just how is it done?
* Is any special preparation needed?
* How long does it take?
* Can I go home immediately and do I need someone to accompany me?
* How long will I be in Hospital?
* Will I need to convalesce?
* How long will I be off work?
* Are there any special do's and dont's before and after the operation?
* Will there be any immediate side-effects?
* Are there any long-term side-effects?

Your surgeon may not be able to give a clear-cut answer to all your questions as some answers may depend on what he finds during the operation. When you are discharged from hospital you will come back into the care of your family doctor, so it is useful to also discuss your problems with him.

CONVENTIONAL METHODS OF TREATING CANCER

1. Radiotherapy

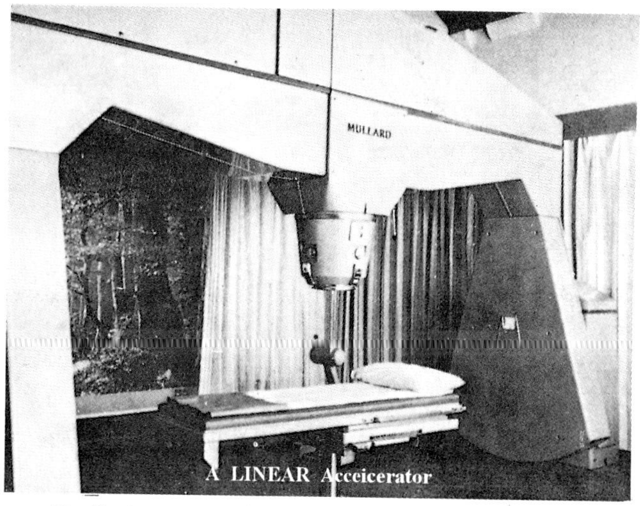

A LINEAR Acceicerator

Radiotherapy is the use of energy rays to kill cancer cells. It is also variously called deep X-ray therapy, cobalt therapy, or radium treatment depending upon the different types of radiation given. Radiotherapy can cure some malignant tumours and can be used to control the symptoms and slow their growth in case of others.

In the past, radiotherapy often had a rather unfortunate reputation. This was partly because it was used to control symptoms in terminal cases. Very often, because the situation had not been fully explained to the relatives, the patients' subsequent death was blamed on the treatment. A further factor was the higher risk of side-effects with the old fashioned treatments. Modern radiotherapy is able to deliver a precise dose of radiation to a tumour deep in the body.

Before the treatment starts, the radiotherapist (the doctor in charge of this treatment) normally spends some time planning the treatment. During this time, the area to be treated is marked out on the body (often with a purple dye). This should not be washed off as these marks are used to place patient in the correct position for each treatment. The total dose of radiation is usually delivered in a series of short treatments (called fractions) over several days or weeks. Most treatments are given four times a week for three to four weeks. The radiographer (the person who delivers the treatment) does not stay with the patient during a fraction, but can see and talk to him all the time through a microphone.

The side-effects of radiotherapy vary somewhat, depending on which part is being treated. In general, the following side-effects are common to most types of treatment: (a) tiredness and lack of energy; (b) nausea and possible vomiting, especially if the abdomen is being treated; (c) mild reddening of the skin at the site of treatment.

Before undertaking radiotherapy it is worth asking the doctor whether there are any other troublesome side-effects. Other possible questions include:

* Will I have a low energy level and tire easily?
* Can it cure my cancer?
* Are there any alternative treatments?
* Which part of my body will be treated?
* How often is treatment given, and how long is each treatment?
* How long will the full course of treatment be?
* Can I drive myself to hospital or do I need transport?
* Should I take any special precautions during treatment?
* Are there any particular side-effects?

Chemotherapy

Chemotherapy is the general term used to describe the drugs that treat cancer. The main advantage with chemotherapy is that it can treat a tumour anywhere in the body, in contrast to surgery or radiotherapy which are local treatments. The first anti-cancer drugs were developed about forty years ago and currently over thirty drugs are commonly used. Each drug has its own pattern of activity against cancer and its own side-effects.

Because the media often paints a somewhat lurid picture of chemotherapy, most of us have the impression that all patients who are administered chemotherapy have dreadful side-effects. Some anti-cancer drugs cause little or no side-effects, through others can cause a lot of them. Though some of these drugs can be taken by mouth as tablets or capsules, most of them need to be injected into the body.

Most anti-cancer drugs work by poisoning cells that are actively dividing and growing. Because of this, they often affect some of the normal cells in the body which are also busy dividing. This is why many chemotherapeutic drugs cause side-effects, though as mentioned above, there is a wide variation in toxicity from drug to drug. Anti-cancer drugs are often used in combinations of three or four drugs. This is done in an attempt to reduce the chance of cancer cells becoming resistant to treatment. Although it is likely that some of the cancer cells will become resistant to a single drug, it is much less probable that they will become resistant to all three or four of the drugs being used. As these combinations of drugs can cause quite severe side-effects, it is usual to allow gaps of about three weeks between each treatment to give the body time to recover and get back to normal.

While some malignant tumours are very sensitive to anti-cancer drugs, other respond poorly. Because of this and the side-effects that the drugs produce, it is important to make sure that chemotherapy is administered in a planned and balanced manner.

Some of the less common cancers are very sensitive to anti-cancer chemotherapy and, provided the patient is reasonably fit, intensive dose therapy is used. This almost invariably means that the patient will suffer some, possibly severe, side-effects. Since the goal is cure, however, side-effects are usually acceptable if the patient is getting better. Anyone who saw the film or read the book about the jockey Bonn Champion will know that this treatment can be very rigorous, though the end result certainly justified the means in his case. If you are about to embark on a course of chemotherapy, ask about possible side-effects and problems that you may face. Much can often be done to reduce the side-effects of treatment and it is best to know what to expect.

Quite a few of the common cancers do not respond well to chemotherapy. Since most chemotherapy causes side-effects, it is often best not given or, at most, relatively simple, non-toxic treatment is administered on patients with these cancers.

Often, the cancers that do respond well to chemotherapy are rarely cured by it. Here it is important to make sure that the correct balance is kept between the benefits gained from shrinking the tumour and the side-effects of the treatment.

The side-effects of chemotherapy vary from drug to drug, and from patient to patient, so it is important for each patient to ask what he should expect from his particular treatment regime. The common side-effects of chemotherapy include: Nausea and possibly vomiting; hair loss; tiredness and malaise; loss of appetite and change in taste; changes in the blood, reduction in white blood cells leading to an increased risk of infections and a reduction in the clotting cells (platelets) which can lead to bursting or bleeding. Some drugs reduce fertility, especially in men. Some drugs may also have specific effects on the kidneys, liver, lungs, heart, and nerves. Nearly all side-effects from anti-cancer chemotherapy are reversible, but their effects on fertility may be permanent. So, a patient should ask about his treatment, find out if hair loss does occur or if nausea is a problem. If this is the case a wig can be provided before hair loss occurs, and good anti-sickness treatment can be given to reduce any nausea.

Some suggested questions to ask prior to chemotherapy are:

* Why is chemotherapy necessary?
* Is there any alternative?
* What are the goals of treatment?
* How is the treatment given, and how often?
* Exactly what are the side-effects, particularly on fertility?
* Do I need to take any special precaution during chemotherapy?

Interferon–A Panacea ?

The interferon story began in 1957, when Alick Isaacs and Jean Lindermann, working at the National Institute for Medical Research in England, isolated a substance which seemed to prevent virus infections. They had infected the membrane of an egg with certain viruses and were trying to discover why it was impossible to infect the same cells later with other kinds of viruses. They found that an extract from the infected cells added to a separate group of completely healthy cells caused the second group to become resistant to a wide range of virus infections. The active ingredient in the extract was a protein, and because it seemed to interfere with a virus's ability to infect cells, was named interferon.

Viruses work by invading a cell, taking over the genetic control of its biochemical systems, and using those systems to produce identical copies of themselves. The infected cells, disturbed in their normal functioning, rapidly disintegrate, releasing the newly manufactured viruses into the bloodstream and lymphatic system which transports them all over the body to infect the healthy cells.

One of the last actions of the dying cell, however, is to release a minute quantity of interferon into the surrounding tissue, the lymphatic system fluid and the bloodstream. Molecules of interferon then attach themselves to special receptor sites on the surfaces of healthy cells, causing the production of enzymes which in turn hopefully protect these cells from virus attack.

From a clinical point of view, it is significant that once the body has been altered by interferon, its cells become resistant to a wide variety of virus and not just to the particular infection which sparked off the reaction. The earliest samples of human interferon confirmed that the substance could indeed help to control viral infections. A single nasal spray containing interferon gave protection for up to two weeks against the common flue virus, and doctors at Moorfields Eye Hospital in the U.K. showed that it could protect victims of shingles against blindness.

The discovery of a substance that was potentially a cure for all virus-caused diseases was greeted with enthusiasm, and many laboratories began experimenting with interferon. It soon became clear, however, that there were obstacles to its immediate use.

For a start, scientists found that the chemical structure of the substance varied critically from species to species, and as a result, interferon from animals simply would not work in human beings. Obtaining human interferon proved a daunting task partly because interferon is present only in extremely small concentrations, and partly because it is far from easy to purify.

Hoping to demonstrate that interferon would also work against a cancer causing virus in mice, the American scientist Ion Gressor injected mice with mouse interferon. He expected the interferon to prevent the further spread of the tumours, but to his astonishment, the tumours gradually shrank and in some cases disappeared altogether.

Funds for further research became rapidly available. Soon it was shown that in animals, large doses of interferon appeared to have a twofold effect against cancer. In the first place, it activated the scavenging white cells in the blood stream which normally destroy all foreign material in the body. Second, the surface coating of tumour cells which have become exposed to interferon undergo a slight change. The effect of the change is that cancer cells become very recognizable to the body's natural immune system as foreign material, and this encourages their destruction.

In the mid-1970s, in a series of experiments at the Karolinska Hospital in Sweden, thirty-five patients with a rare form of bone cancer were treated thrice a week for eighteen months. More than twice the expected number of patients showed long-term recovery but the number of people treated was too small to enable the drawing of any general conclusions of real worth from this treatment. Many doctors were sceptical and saw interferon as another 'wonder drug' that failed to live up to its initial promise. So the American Cancer Society funded a much more detailed programme costing millions of dollars, and using up almost the whole world's supply of interferon. The programme involved 150 patients. But, even these trials have proved inconclusive. Some cancers improved, while others did not.

The main block to interferon research is the lack of an adequate method of its production. Future hope lies in finding a large-scale, cheaper source of the drug. The aim is to. produce interferon artificially in quantities which are not restricted by the need for human material. So far, three different approaches to the problem look promising. The method which is furthest advanced is to culture human white blood cells that have lost their normal growth control function and therefore multiply readily. One problem is that the best way of making the blood cells multiply is to expose them to a special virus which has been implicated in certain types of human cancer. It is thus vital that the interferon produced is contaminated with an agent that will cause the very disease that the drug is designed to cure. There will also be difficulties in scaling up production for large scale commercial cultures.

A variation of this approach is to dispense with white cells and use fibroblast cells instead. These cells, which can easily be obtained from human foreskins removed during circumcision, will multiply in culture without being treated with dangerous viruses. While the interferon produced by this method is slightly different form white-cell interferon, it seems to work just as well. Indeed, some researchers claim that a mixture of both types is most effective.

A quite different artificial method of producing interferon in large quantities has become possible as a result of recent advances in genetic engineering. A section of DNA (representing the gene coding for human interferon) has been successfully inserted into the DNA of a bacterium called "Scheerchia coli", which then produces interferon as it grows and divides. The major problem concerns the extraction and purification of the interferon so produced. Chemical synthesis is also being tried out, for which the precise sequence of the 150 or so amino acids that comprise the interferon protein must be known. This, in turn, depends on having extremely pure samples of human interferon, and materials of this quality have only recently become available.

But a serious obstacle remains in the way of both the direct synthetic production of interferon and the use of bacterial chemical factories to achieve the same result. Interferon is not simply a protein, it also contains residues that are not required by the gene for producing interferon. Hence the chemical constitution of the interferon molecule is partly affected by the type of cell that makes it. It is possible that interferon from bacteria which have undergone genetic engineering and that from straightforward chemical synthesis will both be chemically different from natural human interferon. Whether this difference significantly reduces the power of artificial interferon to help destroy cancer is not known. It may be responsible for the inability of interferon from one species to act properly in the body of another. At the moment, therefore, interferon seems unlikely to be a cure-all for cancer.

Surgery

Because there are no specific medicines for cancer, one of the best ways of eradicating a malignant tumour is to remove it surgically. Only if the surgeon removes all the cancer cells, will such an operation result in a cure. Surgery was the first successful treatment for cancer and still remains the most important of all the treatments available. Cancer surgery may involve just a biopsy or a major surgical operation. Biopsy may be–

Excisional Biopsy. Cutting out the whole tumour, if it is relatively small.

Incisional Biopsy. Cutting away a part of the tumour if it is too large to remove easily in one piece.

Needle Biopsy. Taking away a thin core of tissue and its cells by inserting a sharp needle into the lump.

Endoscopic Biopsy. If the suspected tumour is inside the body, an instrument is passed into the body to the tumour. For instance, a thin tube called gastroscope can be swallowed for inspection of a tumour in the stomach. The gastroscope allows the doctor to see the tumour and take a biopsy. Endoscopy is the medical term that is used to describe this procedure.

Staging Operation. Very rarely, surgery is necessary to see if there has been an internal spread of a cancerous tumour. This is known as a staging operation. It is most commonly done in Hodgkin's disease where the doctor has to decide whether the disease is limited enough to be controlled by treatment with radiotherapy or if it needs drug treatment (chemotherapy).

If there is no evidence that the tumour is spreading, a cure may be possible if all the visible cancer is removed surgically. Examples of this type of operation are, a removal of a part of the bowel in colon cancer, or part or all the breast in breast cancer.

Sometimes, even when a cancer is too advanced for there to be a chance of a cure, surgery is done to control a patient's symptoms or to prevent problems from developing. For instance, a tumour in the bowel may be removed to prevent an obstruction developing even when it is clear that the cancer has already spread to other parts. Provided care is taken to ensure that the benefits of surgery outweigh its discomforts, these operations can improve a patient's quality of life and sometimes even prolong it.

There is another purpose of surgery as well. Some benign growths may become cancerous if left in the body. Such growths are generally removed surgically. The most common example is the removal of a polyp from the colon. Sometimes, even a major operation may be done to remove an organ which has a great risk of developing cancer. This is most commonly done when there are hundreds of polyps in the colon (familial polyphonies), or where there is chronic ulcerative colitis. Removal of the large bowel in these cases is a drastic thing to do, but the risk of cancer is so high that this is often the only chance a patient may have for survival.

Management of the Terminal Phase of Cancer

A difficult part of the management of a cancer patient is when it becomes apparent that active measures to arrest the further growth of the cancer are no longer proving effective. When to tell a patient that he/she has a terminal illness is a matter of experience and judgment that cannot be easily mastered. Avoiding such discussions can only enhance the patient's sense of loneliness and isolation. It is not always appropriate to present all the facts to a patient, especially on a single occasion, and time must be spent to determine the patient's awareness of his situation. Noncommittal, even ambiguous statements about the future may be appropriate but the patient should never be told what is known to be untrue.

The most important principle of managing a terminal illness is to provide adequate time for talking with the patient. The doctor must learn to develop the ability to listen to the patient and to learn from him how best to provide him with psychological support. The help of an appropriate religious person or social worker is very useful in such a situation. At this stage psychological support is most important aspect, supplemented with positive measures to relieve pain, to ensure adequate and appropriate nutrition levels and to treat specific symptoms such as cough, nausea, vomiting, pain, etc.

A patient's reaction to the inevitability of death from a fatal disease depends on a host of interrelated variables including his or her cultural and religious background, age, education, reaction of family and dependants, etc. A period of initial disbelief and denial is often replaced by resentment and anger. This, in turn, is followed by a period of depression. Many patients, with or without medical intervention, enter the final phase of cancer peacefully, accepting the inevitability of death.

The Naturopathic View of Cancer

Cancer is a disease which affects the whole body and not just a part of it. Therefore, localized treatment alone will not eradicate it from the body. Surgical operations of X-ray treatment of the affected part can hardly be of any help in eradicating its roots. Panch Karma is the only effective remedy in purifying all damaged parts.

Naturopathy has an elaborate system of dietary control for all diseases including cancer. No other system of medicine cures ailments through diet. Though the roots of cancer and other chronic diseases pervade the whole body, their influence is most evident in the delicate organs. Naturopathy emphatically prohibits surgery on the delicate organs.

Heat treatment is used extensively by naturopaths in the West to treat cancer. Indian naturopaths are more circumspect in prescribing this treatment; for the wrong application of heat can lead to more harm than good. The following considerations should be borne in mind before prescribing heat treatment for cancer: the season; the patient's age; proportion of action (i.e. the extent of heat); the location of the disease in the body. Also, heat is merely a system of surface treatment, and will only be effective if combined with dietary methods.

In naturopathic treatment, the doctor would need the following information from his patients: level of vitality; age; the effect of the seasons on his disease; geographical area from where he comes; body parts affected by cancer; duration of illness; form of cancer.

SITES	SEX	1950-52	1980-82	PERCENT CHANGES	COMMENTS
All Sites	Male	169.8	216.0	+ 27	Steady increase mainly due to cancer
	Female	146.7	135.4	– 8	Slight Decrease
Bladder	Male	7.2	6.5	*	Slight fluctuations ; overall no change
	Female	3.1	1.9	– 39	Some Fluctuations, notceable decrease
Brain	Male	3.5	4.7	+ 34	Steady slight increase in both sexes,
	Female	2.3	3.2	+ 39	reasons unknown.
Breast	Male	0.3	0.2	*	Constant rate,
	Female	25.8	25.3	+ 3	Slight fluctuations, overall no change
Colon and rectum	Male	25.8	25.3	*	Slight fluctuations; overall no change
	Female	24.9	18.0	– 28	Slight fluctuations; noticeable decrease.
Esophagus	Male	25.8	25.3	*	Some fluctuations ; slight increase
	Female	1.2	1.5	*	Slight fluctuations ; overall no change in female
Kidney	Male	3.3	4.8	+ 45	Steady slight increase.
	Female	2.0	2.2	*	Slight fluctuations; overall no change.
Leukemia	Male	7.7	8.7	+ 13	Early increase, latter leveing off and decrease.
	Female	5.3	5.1	*	Slight early increase, later leviling off.
Liver	Male	6.7	4.7	– 30	Some fluctuations, Steady decrease in both
	Female	7.7	3.5	*	Slight early increase, later leveiling off.
Lung	Male	23.7	72.1	+ 204	Steady increase in both sexes due to
	Female	4.9	29.9	+ 510	cigrette smoking
Oral	Male	6.1	5.5	*	Slight fluctuations; overall no change in both
	Female	1.5	2.3	*	sexes
Ovary	Female	8.1	7.9	– 2	Steady increase, later leviling off and decrease.
Pancreas	Male	8.4	10.5	+ 25	Steady increase in both sexes, then leviling off
	Female	5.5	7.0	+ 27	reasons unknown.
Prostate	Male	20.7	22.8	+ 10	Fluctuations throughout; overall slight increase
Skin	Male	3.2	2.7	*	Slight fluctuations, overall slight increase
	Female	2.0	1.4	*	both sexes.
Stomach	Male	23.6	8.1	– 66	Steady decrease in both sexes ; reasons
	Female	12.8	3.8	– 70	unknown.
Uterus	Female	20.7	7.6	– 63	Steady decrease

Chapter XIII

Some Common Cancers

LEUKAEMIA

Childhood leukemia is different from leukaemia that occurs among adults.

Childhood Leukemia

Symptoms. (a) Tiredness without any apparent cause; (b) bleeding from gums or other places after slight injury; (c) frequent fever; (d) enlargement of lymph glands; (e) discomfort or pain over bones; (f) anaemia.

Prognosis. About half of all children with acute lymphatic leukaemia can be cured with the current methods of treatment. The risk of relapse is the greatest in the first two years of treatment, and becomes progressively less.

Treatment. Bone marrow transplant gets good results for leukaemia patients in the younger age group, provided a suitable donor of bone marrow is available. A sibling donor is preferable. The transplant essentially involves talking cells from a normal marrow and giving them intravenously to a patient who has been specially prepared. Thereafter, cells begin to produce enough white and red blood cells and platelets. It takes longer (months or years), for the normal bone marrow to stabilize.

Leukemia in Adults

Symptoms. (a) Tiredness; (b) loss of weight; (c) loss of appetite; (d) fever; (e) pain or discomfort in abdomen due to enlarged spleen or a mass in the upper left abdomen; (f) anaemia; (g) occasional bleeding from any source.

Prognosis. Control of the disease and symptomatic improvement for a number of years is achieved in most patients, but ultimately an aggressive, untreatable stage develops in most cases.

LYMPHOMAS

Lymphoma (Hodgkin's disease) is thought to arise in one region of the body and spread from there. It has four clinical stages. It is important to establish the stage of the disease because staging largely determines treatment. The four stages of lymphoma are: *Stage I*. Only one group of glands is involved anywhere in the body. *Stage II*. More than one group of glands is involved, but only on one side of the body. *Stage III*. More than one group of glands is involved, on both sides of the body. *Stage IV*. Besides the glands, there is involvement of the lungs, liver and bones.

Symptoms. (a) Lymph node enlargement is usually painless unless it has developed very quickly; (b) painless swelling in a group of glands, more often on one side of the neck; (c) tiredness and lassitude; (d) loss of weight; (e) loss of appetite; (f) fever with sweating, which comes on and abates frequently.

Symptoms also depend on the site of the lymphoma. If it is located in the chest, there may be breathlessness and coughing; if in the abdomen, there may be enlargement of the abdomen, discomfort, pain, obstruction in the intestinal tract or jaundice.

Prognosis. The patient may live for over ten years. Also, recent advances in chemotherapy have increased life expectancy.

CANCER OF THE BRAIN

Brain cancers are amongst the commonest childhood cancers, after the leukaemias, lymphomas and the kidney cancers. Approximately 15 to 20 per cent of all brain cancers occur below the age of 15 years.

Brain cancers occur either primarily in the brain itself or spread to the brain from other sites such as the lungs, breasts, etc. The latter is more common than primary cancer in the brain. Both primary and secondary cancer of the brain produce identical symptoms.

Brain cancer can arise from any of the different cells that constitute the brain substance. Each cell type may behave differently with regard to symptoms and treatment. The important types of brain cancers are: (a) medulloblastoma and (b) glioma. The latter is the commonest cancer of the brain, occurring in the young as well as the old.

In a study reported from the All India Institute of Medical Sciences, New Delhi, 419 cases of cancer of the brain in children below 16 years were seen between the years 1968-1980. There were 7 patients below 2 years of age. The highest incidence was between 10 and 15 years. There was a distinct male preponderance--the male-to-female ratio being 1.9:1. The male sex predominance was even more marked in cases of ependymoma and medulloblastoma where the ratio reached 3:1.

Symptoms. Since the skull provides no scope for expansion, when the cancer mass grows, it causes pressure symptoms on other parts of the brain. The symptoms of brain cancer also depend on the area involved and the severity of pressure produced by the cancer mass on other parts of the brain. Common symptoms are: (a) constant and increasing headache; (b) nausea and vomiting; (c) epileptic fits; and (d) loss of function of some body part.

Diagnosis. An X-ray of the skull may reveal the location and spread of cancer. An electro-encephalogram (EEG) can indicate the site of the lesion, but not its nature. A cat-scan is one of the most precise methods of diagnosing brain cancer. It involves the injection of condensed radioactive material into the blood and following its progress with a gamma camera. The cancer tissue shows up in the photographs as an inactive area. A cat-scan of the brain is generally used to indicate the site and size of the cancer. A careful examination of its density in the scan may indicate the type of the cancer.

The exact nature of the cancer, in the majority of the cases, can only be determined by examining the tissue. The treatment given depends upon the cell-type of the cancer. Both radiotherapy and chemotherapy are generally given.

Radiation. High dose radiation is given at the site of the cancer mass, and low dosages of radiation are given all over the rest of the brain and the spinal cord for about six to eight weeks.

Chemotherapy. The drug is given intravenously and/or through injection into the cerebro-spinal fluid by piercing the covering (theca) of the spinal cord.

As a result of the combined effect of surgery, radiation and chemotherapy, more than half the children live for five years or more.

CANCER OF THE MUSCLES (RHABDOMYOSARCOMA)

Cancer of the muscles can occur anywhere in the body. It is easy to diagnose because it is present in the superficial surfaces of the body, such as the extremities and the abdomen. It is not a common cancer. Its causes are unknown.

Symptoms depend on the site of the cancer. A lump may appear in muscles of the arm, leg or neck. This lump does not appear after an injury and gradually increases in size.

Prognosis depends upon the site of the cancer. If it is superficial and detected at an early stage, its remission rate is more than 50 per cent. Younger children have better chance of survival than adults.

CANCER OF THE SKIN

The two main types of cancers of the skin are malignant melanoma and neuroblastoma.

Malignant Melanoma

This type of cancer is fast growing and also spreads locally into the regional lymph glands.

Causes. Prolonged exposure to the sun is the most common cause. It also occurs in parts not exposed to the sun.

Symptoms. (a) A skin ulcer that does not heal, but infiltrates into the surrounding area; (b) sudden growth in a mole or birthmark; (c) bleeding from a mole or what looks like a mole; (d) formation of new moles around an old one.

Prognosis. Detected and treated early, over 90 per cent of this type of cancer is curable.

Neuroblastoma

This is a common cancer of childhood, forming 10 per cent of all cancers in this age group. It arises from the cells of the sympathetic nerves and in the adrenal glands which are spread over all parts of the body, but occurs more commonly on the skin of the abdomen. It spreads rapidly across the body through the blood vessels as well as through the lymphatic system. These cancer cells produce a substance called catecholamine which raises the blood pressure.

Symptoms. (a) Lump in the abdomen; (b) weight loss; (c) diminished appetite; (d) swelling in the neck; (e) protrusion of the eyeball due to the proliferation of cancer cells behind the eyeball.

Prognosis. The younger the age, say 1 to 2 years, the better the chances of cure.

CANCER OF THE BREAST

Breast cancer is one of the most common cancers. It usually occurs in women over the age of 40 years, though it has been seen to occur in younger women as well. The incidence of breast cancer in India is reported to be 20 per 100,00 women. It occurs a decade earlier in Indian women than in white women-the mean age of its occurrence is about 42 years among Indian women as compared to 53 years among white women.

However, the incidence of breast cancer is higher in Western countries than it is in India. Different studies have shown the incidence per 1,00,000 women in western countries to be as follows:

USA	71.4
Denmark	49.1
Switzerland	70.6
England	48.0
Israel	55.5
Yugoslavia	28.3

In Japan, the incidence of this cancer is less than it is in India, viz.. 13.0 per 100,000 women.

Etiology. The major known determinants of risk for breast cancer are delayed age at first pregnancy, family history of breast cancer, giving of estrogens, firbrocystic breast disease, and exposure to ionizing radiation.

Symptoms. (a) A lump or a nodule in the breast; (b) as this lump grows, it gets attached to the skin of the breast; (c) lymph nodes become enlarged and palpable in the axilla closest to the site of the disease.

Treatment. If the cancer mass is of moderate size, then besides surgery, radio-therapy is given to patients in order to kill any remaining cancer cell. Radiation is given four to five times a week for four to six weeks. The main side-effect of radiation is soreness or discomfort to the exposed area. Radiation is also given in cases of recurrence of the disease.

Prognosis. If the breast cancer recurs after any or all modes of treatment, the chances of cure are not bright. But even such patients can live for several years. An older patient can generally live up to her normal life span.

CANCER OF THE LUNG

Cancer of the lungs is categorized depending upon the type of cells involved. The two categories are: small-cell cancer and non small cell cancer.

Small-cell cancer accounts for about one-fourth of all lung cancers. It is also called oat-cell cancer because under the microscope its cells look like oat grains. A quickly growing cancer, it is seldom associated with smoking.

Non-small-cell cancer has three varieties: squamous or epidermoid (associated with tobacco smoking); adenocarcinoma; large-cell cancer. All these varieties grow less rapidly than the small-cell cancer and hence their treatment is more or less on similar lines.

Lung cancer accounts for more than 50 per cent of all male deaths from cancer in the Western countries. Small-cell carcinoma accounts for 25 per cent of deaths from lung cancer, squamous for 50 per cent, large cell for 10 per cent and adenocarcinoma for 10 per cent.

Lung cancer arises from bronchial epitheliums or mucous glands and at an early stage may include the bronchial lumen. When the cancer mass obstructs a major bronchus, it causes a collapse of the lung. However a tumour arising from a peripheral bronchus may attain a very large size without producing a significant degree of lung collapse.

Lung cancer may involve the pleura either directly or by lymphatic spread, causing a pleural effusion which is often blood-stained. It may also extend into the chest wall and cause severe pain. The cancer or its lymph node metastasis may extended into the mediastinum, the space between the two lungs in the chest. The incidence of lung cancer in India is about 4 per cent of all cancers.

Etiology. After World War II, the incidence of lung cancer has sharply increased in developed countries. In England and Wales, the lung cancer-related death rate is continuously increasing and had reached a level of 37.5

deaths in males and 5.8 deaths in females per 100,000 population in 1975. Cancer of the lung, particularly of the squamous cell type, has increased in incidence all over the world where tobacco is smoked, particularly tobacco in the form of cigarettes.

Symptoms. (a) Cough, sometimes with blood in the phlegm; (b) fever; (c) loss of appetite; (d) loss of weight; (e) hoarseness of voice (only sometimes); (f) pain in the chest; (g) breathlessness; (h) clubbing of the finger nails.

Metastasis to the brain are commonly produced by lung cancer resulting in a variety of other symptoms.

Diagnosis. An X-ray, followed by a biopsy is the normal method of diagnosis. Additionally, in cases where there is suspicion of the presence of cancer secondaries in other organs such as the liver, bones or brain, an ultra-sound examination of the liver, or CT scan of the other organs can confirm their diagnosis.

Treatment. *Chemotherapy* is done in small-cell type of cancer. *Radiation* is generally given over the parts of the body that have both large and small-cell type lung cancers, but this is primarily to treat the symptoms and not for curing the cancer.

While these modes of treatment may decrease the symptoms for some time, the side-effects that they produce such as nausea, vomiting, hair loss and risk of increased infection, are major hazards. Also, they generally reduce these symptoms for some time, but do not generally result in the cure.

Prognosis. Since most cases of lung cancer present themselves when the cancer has spread from the lungs to the glands or other parts of the body, its cure is difficult.

Secondary Tumours of the Lung

Blood-borne metastatic deposits in the lungs my be derived from a primary cancer almost anywhere in the body. The secondary deposits are usually multiple and bilateral.

CANCERS OF GASTRO-INTESTINAL TRACT

The main functions of the gastro-intestinal system along with its associated organs such as pancreas, gall-bladder and liver are the digestion and absorption of food. Gastro-intestinal tract cancers begin in the mouth and end at the anus. In between, they spread from the mouth into the pharynx, oesophagus, stomach and small and large intestines.

Cancer of the Mouth, Cheek and Tongue (Oral Cancer)

In the Western countries, cancers of the tongue, mouth and pharynx account for only 3 to 5 per cent of all cancers. These are much more common in India, Bangladesh, Sri Lanka, Thailand and Indonesia, accounting for as much as 30 to 50 per cent of all cancers in India.

Cancer of the tongue involves the back of the tongue and grows unnoticed for months. It then involves lymph glands in the neck which become enlarged and it is generally for this reason that patients seek medical advice. This kind of cancer is generally seen more often in men than in women.

Causes. (a) Approximately 90 per cent of oral cancers in India can be attributed to tobacco chewing and smoking. These cancers almost always occur on the side of the mouth where the tobacco quid is kept, and the risk of cancer rises drastically for those who keep the tobacco quid overnight in their mouths. A link also seems to exist between HSV infection (Herpes simplex virus) and oral cancer.

(b) Cancer of the lower lip is generally caused by the habit of keeping *khaini* (a mixture of tobacco and lime) under the lower lip from where it is chewed slowly. This type of cancer is seen in eastern Utter Pradesh and Bihar.

(c) Cancer of the cheek appears as a hard thickening which is painless. Sometimes an ulcer forms over it. If a painless swelling or an ulcer with hard base forms and does not heal in about two weeks, one must consult a competent doctor to rule out cancer.

(d) Chewing or smoking tobacco and the chronic irritation caused by irregular teeth are suspected to lead to cancer of the cheek.

Symptoms. The onset of mouth cancer is usually preceded by a white patch on the inner lining of the lip on which a hard mass slowly develops, the top of which sometimes becomes an ulcer.

Treatment. These cancers are treated with radiotherapy when there is a suspicion of their spread is present and if the lymph nodes are involved.

Cancer of Oesophagus

In India, the oesophagus is the commonest site of gastro-intestinal cancer, after oral cancers. The oesophagus is a part of the gastro-intestinal tract that connects the pharynx of the mouth with the stomach. The lower end of the oesophagus which connects with the stomach normally remains partially closed so as not to allow the acid content of the stomach to come out and injure the oesophagus.

Causes. Cancer of the oesophagus is more common in Kashmir. Kashmiris consume large amounts of very hot, saltish tea (noon chai), have a high intake of spices such as chilis and animal fats, and are fond of smoking. These factors, along with an attendant vitamin deficiency combine to injure the oesophageal lining, leading to the high incidence of oesophageal inflammation.

Symptoms. (a) Difficulty in swallowing solid or semi-solid food and, in later stages even liquid food; (b) pain in the middle of the chest and also in the back; (c) loss of weight; (d) vomiting of freshly consumed food, sometimes mixed with blood.

Prognosis. Oesophagal cancer has a grim prognosis, as it does not produce clear symptoms early enough. Vague discomfort during swallowing and heaviness or uneasiness underneath the sternum are usually ignored by the patient, causing delayed detection.

Cancer of the Stomach

The stomach is the first part of the gastro-intestinal tract where food is broken down and digested. If the food contains any carcinogenic substance, the stomach is the first to be affected.

Etiology. The basic cause of this cancer is not known. Heavy alcohol drinkers are more prone to stomach cancer than non-drinkers. It generally occurs in the older age group of people between 50-70 years. Its incidence is the highest in Japan.

Symptoms. The symptoms of stomach cancer are very vague to begin with. Generally, the only symptom is a diminished appetite and a feeling of being unwell. This is a very misleading symptom which seldom makes doctors realize that their patient has cancer until it is too late. Some of the other symptoms are: (a) loss of weight; (b) discomfort and pain in the abdomen; (c) vomit containing blood.

Cancer of the Colon and the Rectum

The large bowel forms the lower 1.5 metre part of the gastro-intestinal tract which goes up from the right abdomen as the ascending colon, then horizontally as the transverse colon, then comes down on the left side as the descending colon and then becomes the rectum and ends at the anus. Cancers of the colon and rectum are one of the most common sites of cancer in the USA, Denmark and some other European countries. In the USA nearly 45,000 people die of this cancer.

Etiology. Those who pass stools once or even twice a day because they have more roughage in the diet, do not generally get cancer of the large bowel. Those who pass stools less frequently because their diet contains little or no roughage, have a higher predisposition to development of colon cancer. This might be either due to the increased length of time that the cancer-causing wastes stay in their intestines, or due to the production of bacteria due to putrefaction of faecal matter which can eventually become carcinogenic.

Symptoms. (a) Constipation alternating with diarrhoea; (b) pain in the lower abdomen; (c) blood in the stool; (d) early fatigue; (e) loss of weight.

CANCER OF THE LIVER

The liver is situated on the right side of the upper part of the abdomen, just under the diaphragm. Its main function is to convert the digested food into integral special cells which have the capacity to regenerate themselves. In India, the commonest disease of the liver is infectious hepatitis or common jaundice.

Cancers of the liver may either be primary, i.e. arising from the liver itself or secondary, i.e. arising from another organ (metastasis) which then spread to the liver. The incidence of the primary cancer of the liver shows greats geographical variations. It is common in Africa, South East Asia and India, and less common in western countries. It occurs predominantly in males and in 80 per cent of the cases, the patient already has cirrhosis of the liver.

Primary Cancer of the Liver

A liver which has developed cirrhosis because of an earlier attack of infectious hepatitis caused by the Hepatitis-A virus or due to an excessive intake of alcohol is more liable to develop primary liver cancer. The presence of some chemical substances in the food such as aflatoxin, which occurs particularly in groundnuts infected with a fungus called *aspergillus famigatus*, is also known to cause liver cancer. In most cases, however, the cause of this form of cancer cannot be pinpointed.

Symptoms. (a) Loss of appetite; (b) weakness; (c) discomfort or pain, sometimes very severe, in the upper abdomen; (d) swollen abdomen due to rapid enlargement of the liver and/or the presence of fluid in the abdomen, a condition called ascites.

Diagnosis. Special liver function tests always show an impairment of the liver. Liver ultrasounds and CT scans show the outline of the liver and its consistency, and therefore indicate the nature of the disease. A liver biopsy taken through a fine needle indicates the exact nature of liver cells and therefore gives a precise diagnosis.

Treatment. *Radiation* only helps in relieving some symptoms such as pain, but only for some time. *Chemotherapy* rarely helps.

Prognosis. Patients of liver cancer generally die within a year.

Secondary Cancer in Liver

The spread of cancer secondaries to the liver after the initial occurrence of primary cancer in other parts of the body is a very common occurrence. Secondaries in the liver usually originate from cancers in the bronchus, breast, abdomen or pelvis. They may be single or multiple. About 30 to 50 per cent of patients who have advanced cancers generally have secondaries in liver. The average survival of such patients ranges between two and six months. Surgery and radiation are unhelpful, but in isolated cases a positive response may be obtained by chemotherapeutic drugs.

CANCER OF THE GALL-BLADDER

Diseases of the gall-bladder are commoner among females. Gall-bladder cancer occurs in older age-groups.

Etiology. The precise etiology of this form of cancer is not known. A diseased gall-bladder that has gall-stones which irritate its walls may make it more liable to develop cancer.

Symptoms. The initial symptoms of gall-bladder cancer are vague and generally consist of abdominal discomfort or pain in the upper abdomen or under the right rib. The other symptoms that often manifest themselves are: (a) indigestion; (b) loss of appetite; (c) jaundice in the later stages; (d) loss of weight.

CANCER OF THE PANCREAS

The pancreas is situated between the lower border of the stomach and the upper border of the duodenum, in the first part of the small intestine. It produces digestive enzymes which pass into the duodenum by a duct to digest the food. The pancreas produce insulin which maintains the balance of sugar in the blood. Cancer of the pancreas generally occurs in older people of both sexes.

Etiology. The etiology of this form of cancer is not known.

Symptoms. (a) Pain in the upper abdomen, and also sometimes in the back; (b) loss of weight; (c) loss of appetite; (d) jaundice in the latter stages. There may be no symptoms at all, till the cancer has spread into the adjoining tissues which then produces secondary symptoms.

Treatment. *Radiation* can only work to the extent of reducing the size of the cancer or any obstruction, if present. *Chemotherapy* has only a limited role. Most patients do not respond favourably to any form of chemotherapy.

Prognosis. A cure is rarely possible because this form of cancer is usually detected very late.

CANCER OF THE BONE

Cancer of the bone occurs both in all ages and in both sexes. Its most common types are: osteogenic sarcoma; Ewing's sarcoma; and multiple myeloma.

Osteogenic Myeloma

This cancer occurs predominantly in males between the ages of 10 to 25 years. Any bone may be involved. Its causes are not known.

Symptoms. (a) Pain and tender swelling of the bones and the tissues around it; (b) loss of weight; (c) fatigue; (d) the involved bone may break without much of an injury.

Prognosis. If detected when localized, the chances of cure after surgery are above 50 per cent. In some osteogenic sarcomas which are slow-growing, the chances of success are as high as 70 to 80 per cent.

Ewing's Sarcoma

This is a tumour of the bones which generally occurs in children, more among boys between the ages of 5 and 15 years. It may involve any bone. Its etiology is not known.

Symptoms. (a) Continuous and increasing pain over a bone; (b) swelling of a bone.

Prognosis. Until two decades ago, Ewing's Sarcoma was described as the most lethal primary cancer of the bone. Its reported five-year survival was 0 to 12 per cent. The availability of new chemotherapeutic agents has, however, changed the picture and today, with couch chemotherapy, five-year survivals are now reported to be around 70 per cent.

Treatment. Radiation and chemotherapy together can effect a cure in cases where the cancer is localized and has not spread in other parts. In cases where the cancer has spread, this treatment prolongs life and lessens suffering.

Multiple Myeloma

This is a cancer of the plasma cells of the bone marrow and occasionally of the soft tissue. Plasma cells normally produce antibodies. When these cells become cancerous, they cannot produce antibodies, with the result that the patient is very susceptible to even the smallest of infections.

This cancer is uncommon under the age of 30 years. Its occurrence becomes increasingly frequent thereafter, with its peak incidence occurring between 60 and 70 years. Males are affected more frequently than females. There is a long pre-clinical phase, in some instances up to 25 years and the disorder is generally discovered only incidentally by laboratory tests during this phase. The patient my thereafter be under observation for years before any symptoms develop. The etiology of this form of cancer is not known.

Symptoms. (a) Anaemia; (b) fatigue; (c) loss of weight; (d) fever; (e) recurrent infections; (f) bone fractures. Most of the symptoms usually reflect some degree of bone involvement, impairment of the immune function, kidney damage and anaemia. The first intimation of trouble may be the sudden onset of acute localized pain due to a pathological fracture. These symptoms arise mainly in the weight-bearing bones. The vertebrae, pelvis and femur are particularly susceptible. The collapse of a vertebra is common and produces severe nerve root pain. Weight lifting may also cause pain in arms. Patients are often severely crippled. The progressive impairment of the immune function due to deficiencies of normal immunoglobulins and the excess of abnormal immunoglobulins, renders these patients susceptible to infection, particularly of the respiratory tract. Pneumonia is quite frequently the presiding illness and is often the cause of death.

Prognosis. After chemotherapy, most patients live longer and comfortably for may years. When chemotherapy becomes ineffective, a patient is treated only for the relief of symptoms.

CANCER OF THE GENITO-URINARY SYSTEM

These two separate systems of the body have been grouped together here for the convenience of the description. Genito pertains to reproduction and urinary to the formation and excretion of urine.

Cancer of the female genitals, particularly the uterus and the cervix is one of the most prevalent cancers of females in India.

Cancer of the Uterine Cervix

The cervix is the last part of the uterus which protrudes slightly into the vagina. Cancer of the uterine cervix accounts for 25 to 50 per cent of all cancer cases in women seen in hospitals in different parts of India. The following figures published in 1980 give an indication of its incidence: Guntur (Andhra Pradesh), for 61.5 per cent; Visakhapatnam 71.8 per cent; Vellore (Tamil Nadu) 54.5 per cent; Calcutta 23.3 per cent. Cancer of the cervix is also widely present in South East Asian countries. The incidence of and mortality from cervical cancer has declined considerably in Western countries in recent decades. Hygienic measures, early detection by cervical cytology and effective treatment have contributed significantly to this decline.

Causes. Cervical cancer has multiple causes. The important risk factors of this cancer include poor genital hygiene, early marriage, early coitus, multiple sexual contact and repeated childbirth. This cancer is rare in nuns; in contrast, prostitutes have a very high incidence. Also, cancer of the cervix is more common in the lower socio-economic groups, reflecting the importance of poor genital hygiene.

Symptoms. (a) Vaginal discharge mixed with blood; (b) bleeding in between periods of after the sexual act.

Prognosis. If this cancer is detected and removed surgically in the earliest stages, it can be cured.

Prevention. An annual PAP test in all women going to a gynecologist.

Cancer of the Uterus

The uterus, located in the lower part of the abdomen, is the organ where the foetus grows during pregnancy. The uterus is prone to developing hard, roundish masses in its well, which also protrude into the cavity of the uterus, and cause excessive bleeding. They may be present more than one at a time. There are called fibroids and they are not cancerous. Cancer of the uterus is quite common in India. In Bombay, Dr. Jussawalla (1973) found its incidence to be 25.1 per 100,000 females.

Symptoms. (a) Bleeding from the vagina at times other than the menstruation; (b) vaginal discharges.

Prevention. There is mounting evidence of a steady rise in the incidence of uterine cancer in India. It was supposed to be confined to the post-menopausal age group, but lately, it is also being seen with increasing frequency in the middle-age and early-age groups. The diagnosis of the form of cancer in its pre-invasive stage is clearly the key to its control.

Cancer of the Ovary

The ovaries are the organs of reproduction in females and·are located in the abdomen. Cancer of the ovaries occurs in the older age groups of women. Cancer of the ovary is the most fatal female cancer. Its late detection contributes to its lethality. No definite causes of this cancer are known.

Symptoms. (a) Discomfort of the abdomen, due to the spread of the cancer and presence of fluid; (b) loss of weight.

Choricarcinoma or Cancer of the Placenta

This is a rare form of cancer. The placenta is the tissue that links the foetus with the uterus of the mother during pregnancy.

Etiology. This cancer develops from an abnormality of the placenta called a hydatiform mole. It spreads very quickly to other parts and may show itself in the mother after an abortion or miscarriage or even after the completion of the pregnancy.

Symptoms. (a) Continued vaginal bleeding after delivery; (b) abdominal pain; (c) cough due to spread of the cancer to the lungs; (d) multiple symptoms due to its spread in different parts of the nervous system.

Cancer of the Testes

Enlarged testes are the most common manifestation of this cancer, but not all enlargements of the testes are cancerous. Most often they are due to either epididymytis, i.e. inflammation of the tube leading to and from the testes, or hydrocele, which is presence of fluid in the pouch around the testes. Cancer of the testes occurs in younger men between the age of 15 and 40.

Cancer of the testes is mainly of two types: seminoma and teratoma.

Etiology. The failure of the testes to descend completely from the abdomen where they are situated in the foetus, to the scrotum, is one of its known causes. The remaining causes of this cancer are not known.

Symptoms. The main symptom is malignant tumour of the testes, which generally appears as a painless swelling in the scrotum. The other symptoms are enlarged and painful testes. The secondaries of this kind of cancer generally spread into the lungs.

Prognosis. If detected early, the cure rate is high.

Cancer of the Prostate

The prostate is a chestnut-shaped gland in males which encircles the uppermost part of the urethra which connects it to the urinary bladder. Prostate cancer accounts for 16 per cent of all cancers in males. It is uncommon among men under forty, but it is the third highest causes of male cancer deaths in men over fifty-five and the leading cause of cancers among men over seventy-five. The etiology of cancer of the prostate is not known.

Symptoms. Prostate cancer has to be differentiated from benign prostatic enlargement which is quite common in the same lower age group and causes almost the same sort of symptoms. It usual symptoms are: (a) hesitancy at the start of passing urine; (b) increased frequency of passing urine; (c) getting up at night also to pass urine; (d) retention of urine.

Men who get cancer of the prostate carry the disease with them for many years without suffering any noticeable symptoms. As many as 90 per cent of the cases are not detected until the cancer has metastasized beyond the prostate gland. Indeed, the condition is often not even discovered until an autopsy is performed after death from some other cause. An estimated 15 to 20 per cent of men over fifty may unknowingly be suffering from prostate cancer.

Diagnosis. Prostate cancer may first reveal itself in the bones as metastasis or secondaries. An X-ray of the bones can reveal this condition. Thereafter, an isotope-scan of the suspicious bones can be used to confirm the diagnosis.

Prognosis. The chances of a cure are the highest when the cancer is confined to the prostate and is removed surgically.

Cancer of the Penis

Cancer of the penis is a frequently reported cancer among uncircumcised males of all races. Its incidence is highly variable. It accounts for less for than one per cent of male cancers in the United States. Poor hygiene of the inside of the skin that covers the glans penis seems to be one of the major causes.

Symptoms. A hard-base chronic sore that does not heal and infiltrates the area around as it grows is the main symptom.

Cancer of the Urinary Bladder

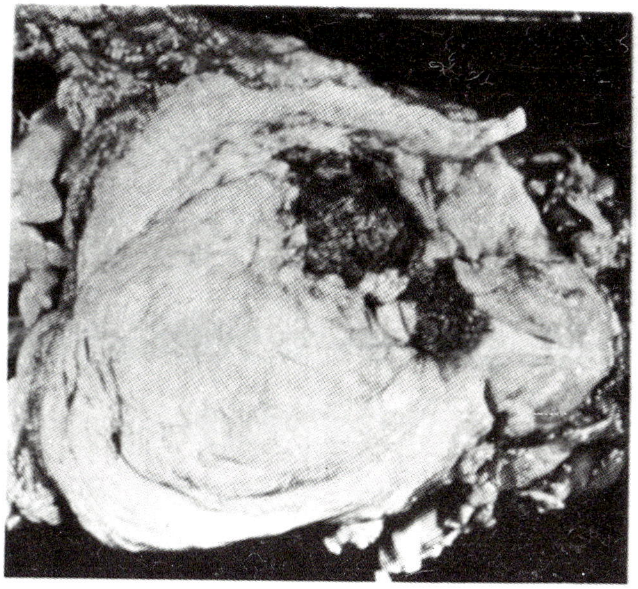

Cancer of the urinary bladder occurs mostly in older people of both sexes. It is easy to detect and difficult to cure. The causes of this type of cancer are not known. Aniline dyes and other industrial chemicals are often known to cause cancer at this site.

Symptoms. (a) Increased frequency in passing urine; (b) blood (haematuria) in the urine; (c) pain on passing urine; (d) pain in the lower abdomen when the cancer has spread.

Diagnosis. A biopsy is generally carried out to diagnose primary cancer of the urinary bladder. Bone scans and liver ultrasound are then done to see if cancer secondaries have spread to other organs.

Prognosis. The chances of survival depend very much on the extent of the spread of this cancer and the stage at which the patient begins treatment.

Cancer of the Kidney

The two kidneys which are located on either side of the abdomen, cleanse the blood of various harmful metabolic products such as urea and creatinine, and maintain the balance of water and other electrolytes in the body. Cancers of the kidney are of two types: hypermephroma and Wilm's tumour. Hypermephroma is found in adults and older age-group people, while Wilm's tumour occurs more frequently in children.

Hypermephroma

The causes of this type of cancer are not known. Smokers suffer from kidney cancer five times more than non-smokers. Some industrial chemicals can also cause it. It occurs most often in males above the age of 50 years.

Symptoms. (a) General ill health in the early stages; (b) loss of weight; (c) loss of appetite; (d) blood in urine; (e) fever of unexplained origin; (f) pain in the abdomen.

Diagnosis. A biopsy of the kidney tissue is carried out to diagnose primary cancer of the kidney. Bone scans and lung X-rays are then carried out to see if the secondaries have spread to other parts.

Prognosis. The prognosis is variable. Sometimes, spontaneous remissions may occur. At other times, the patient may not live very long.

Wilm's Tumour

This is a cancer of the kidneys which generally occurs among children between the ages of 1 and 5 years. Its etiology is not known. Children who suffer from this cancer often have partial or complete absence of the iris of the eyeballs and have abnormalities of the urinary system, i.e. in kidneys, urethra or the bladder.

Symptoms. (a) A firm, irregular, non-tender lump in the abdomen; (b) abdominal discomfort; (c) blood in the urine (generally occurring in the latter stages of the disease); (d) fever; (e) loss of appetite and weight.

Prognosis. The chances of cure are the best in children under 2 years of age, when the cancer is generally still confined to the kidney. Up to 80 per cent of the patients get cured after chemotherapy.

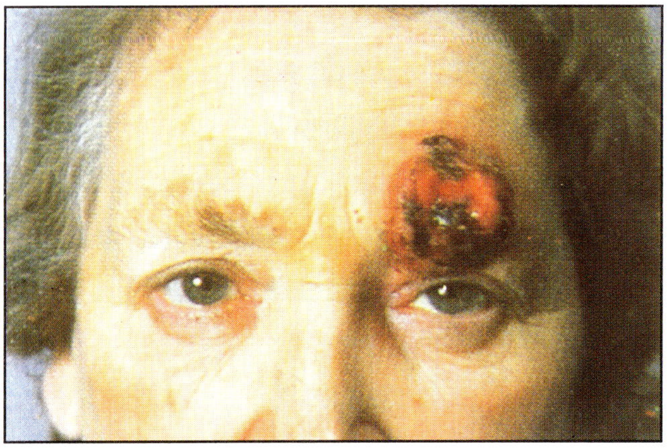

Saugmous cell carcinoma showing a tendency to Keratin formation in some Areas

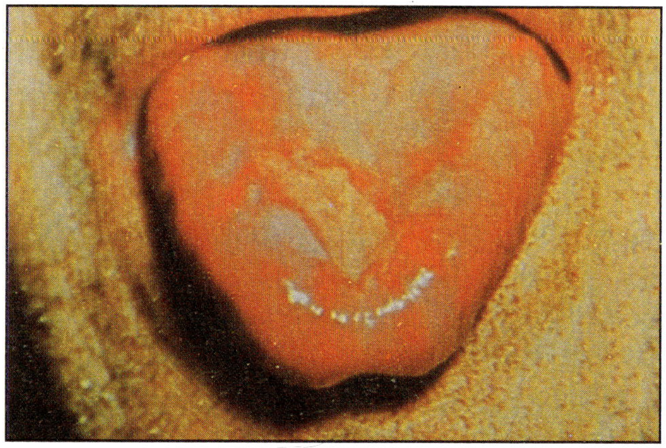

Gumma of Tongue

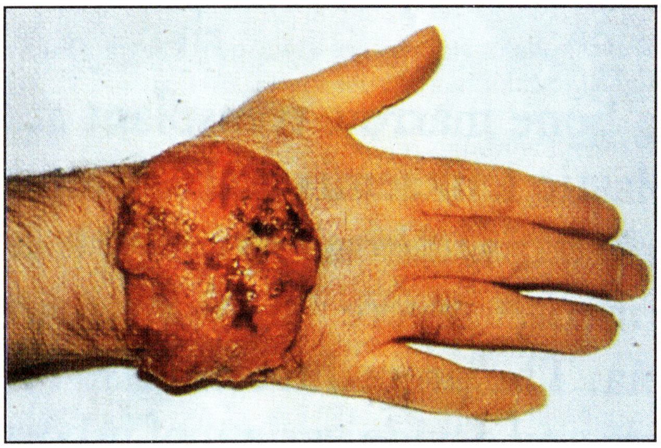

Squamous Celled Carcinoma on the back of the hand of a Tar worker

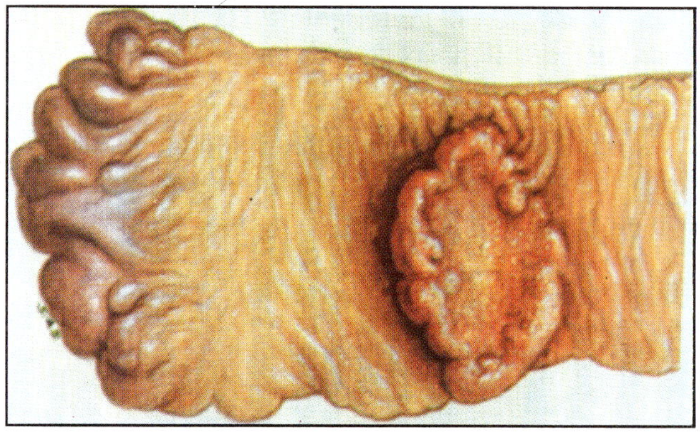

Carcinoma of the rectum A not infrequent diagnostic Pit fall.

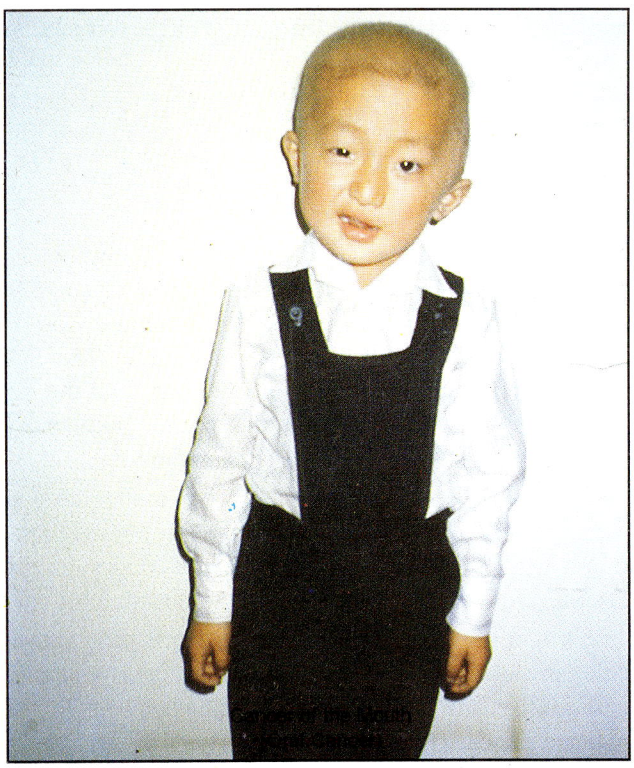

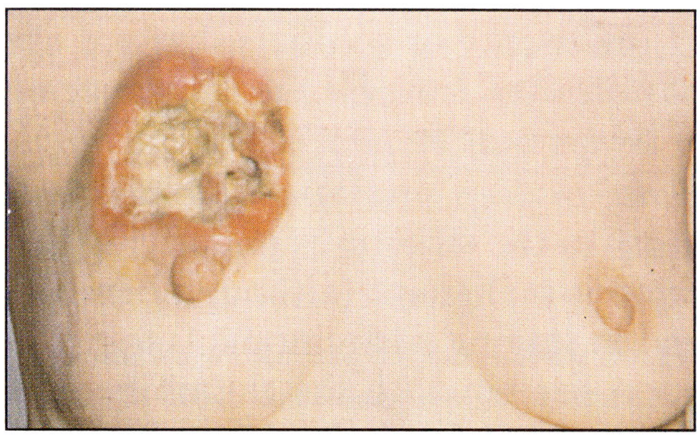

Cancer of Brest

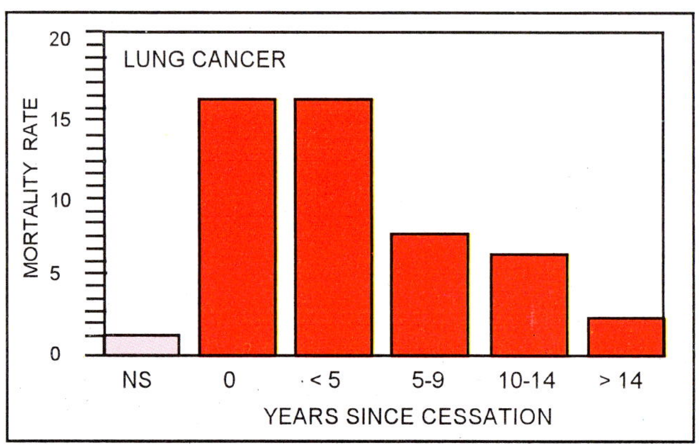

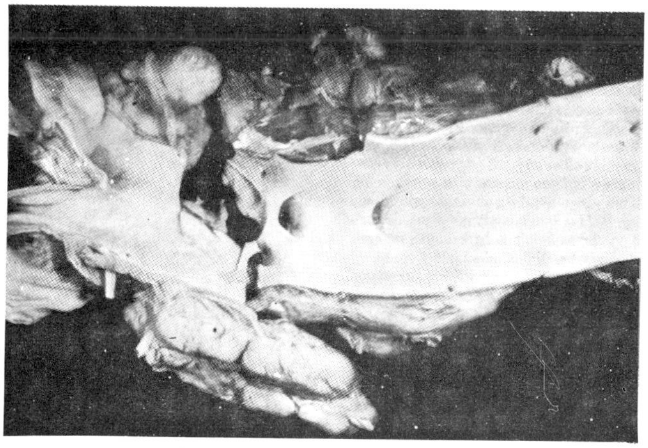

Periaorict Lymph Node Enlargment in Chronic Lymphocxtic Leukemia

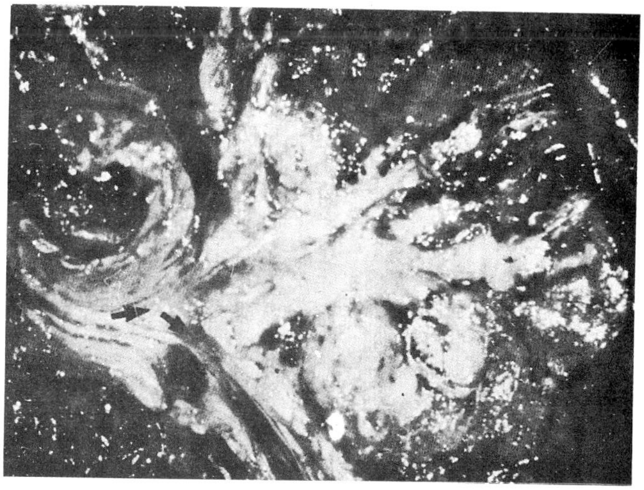

Bronchogenic Carcinoma infiltrating Peribronchial Lung Substance.

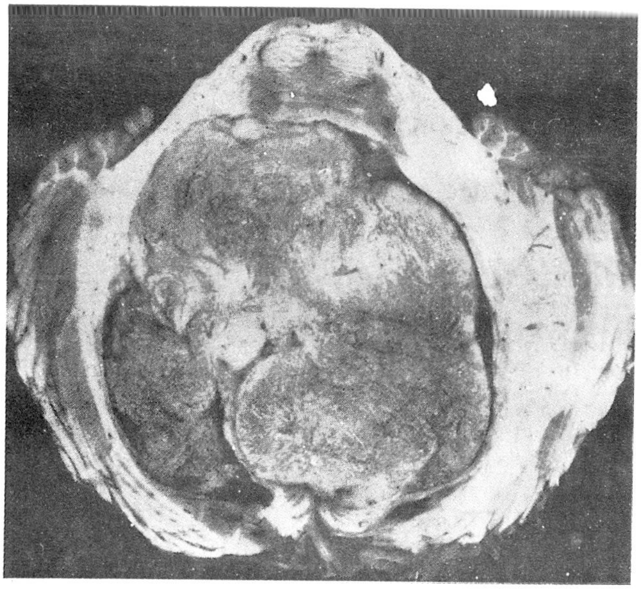

A Medulloblastoma Growing in to Fourth Ventricle, Distorting, Compressing surrounding Structures

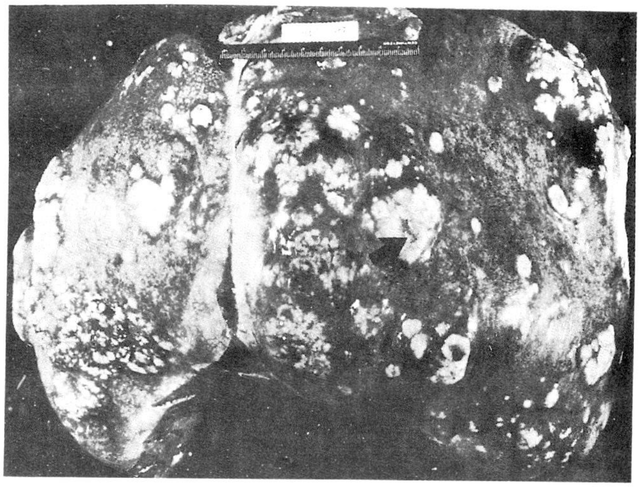

Carcinoma metastatic of liver

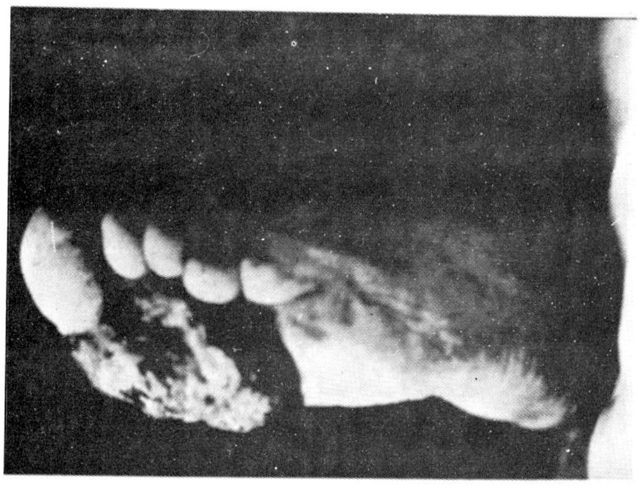

Melanoma

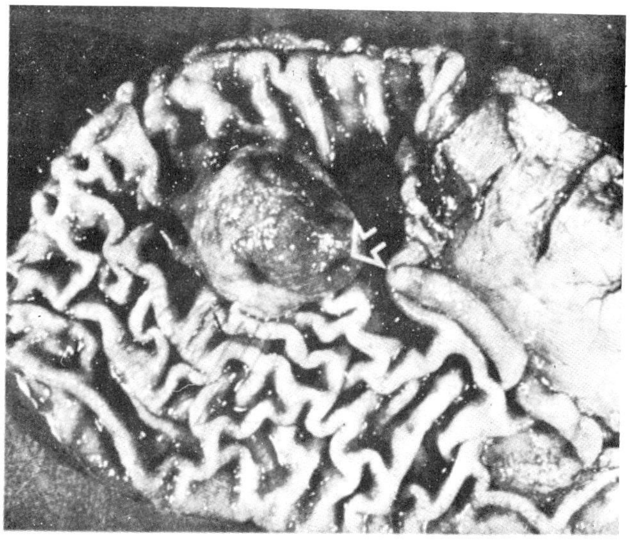

Adenomatous Palyp of stomach

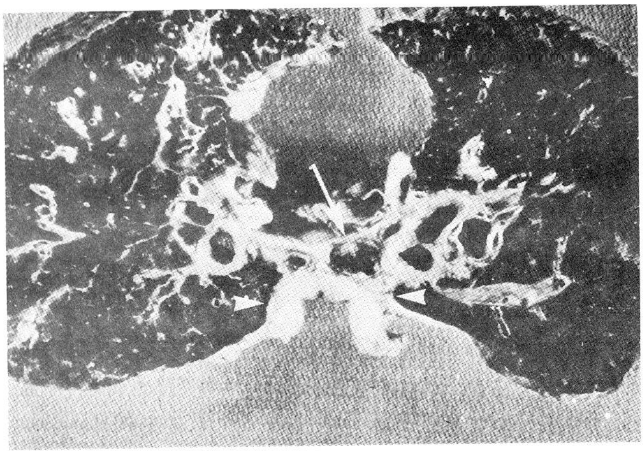

Esophageal Carinoma on transverse sectioning of esophagus

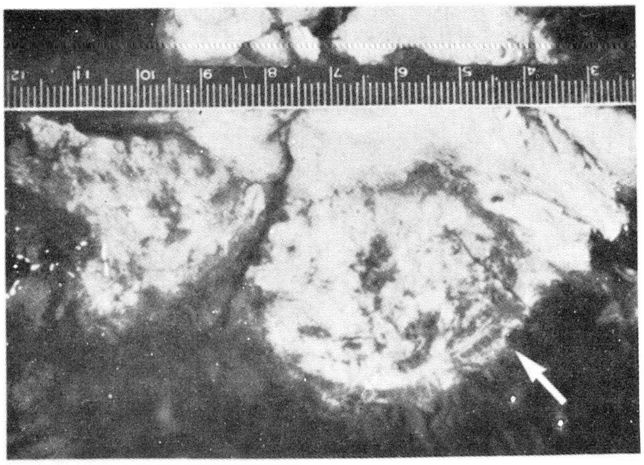

Carcinoma of Head of fancreas

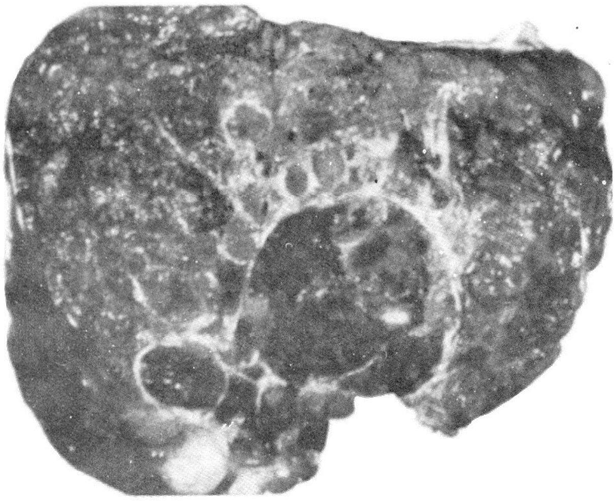

Hepatocellular Carcinoma extensively replacing the Liver subs tance
In Area, the neoplasm is Hemonhagic and necrotic.

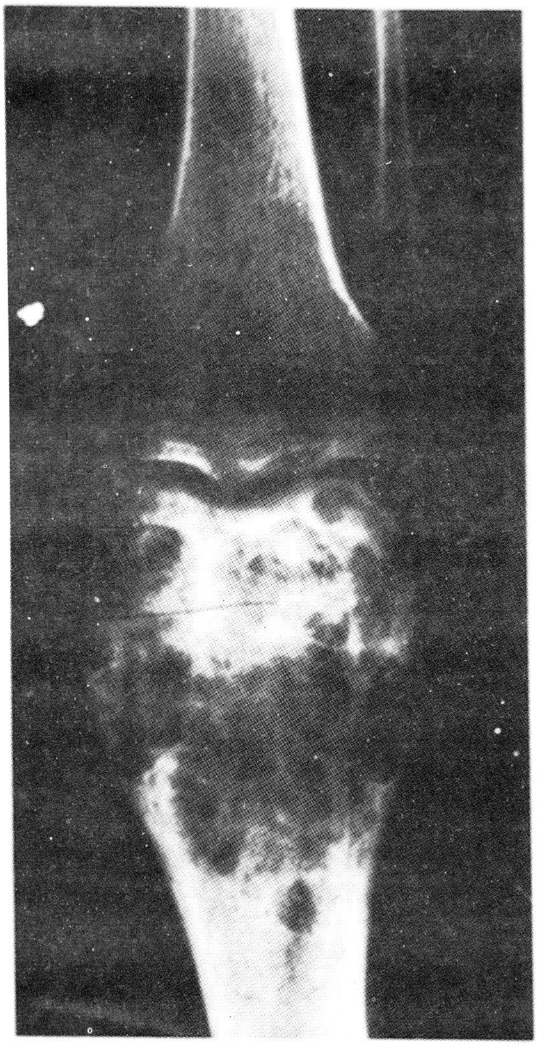

Giant Cell tumor end of the femur and
abuts on the Articular Cartilage.

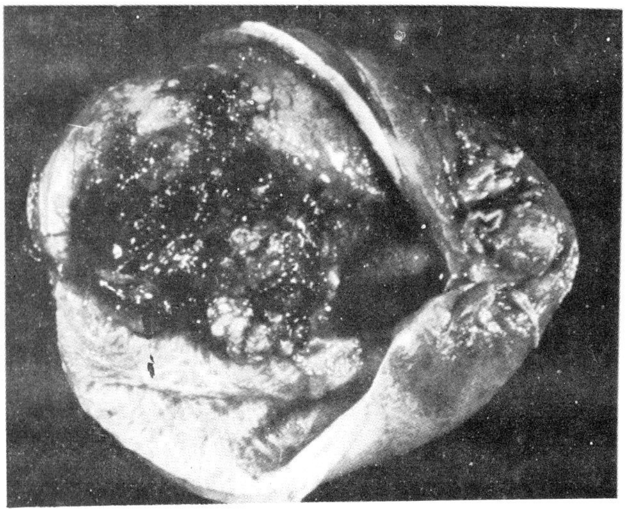

Carcinoma of Gallbladder as seen with the opened fundus

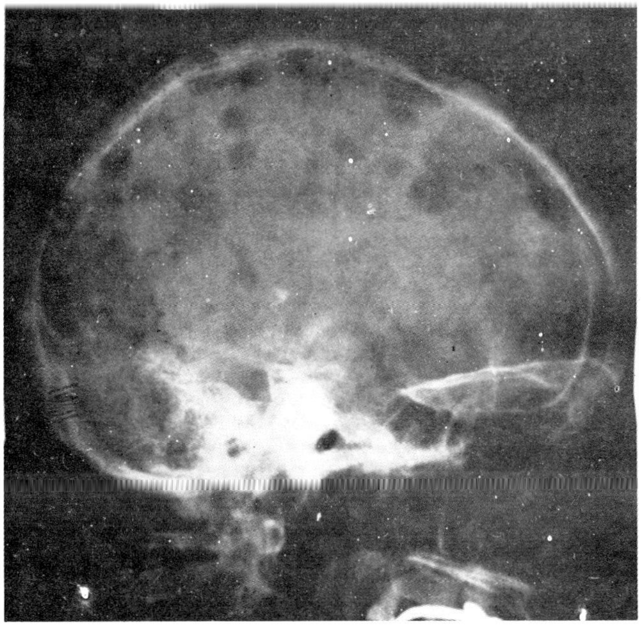

Radiograph of Skull extensively involved by focal, sharply punched out lesions of plasma cell myeloma

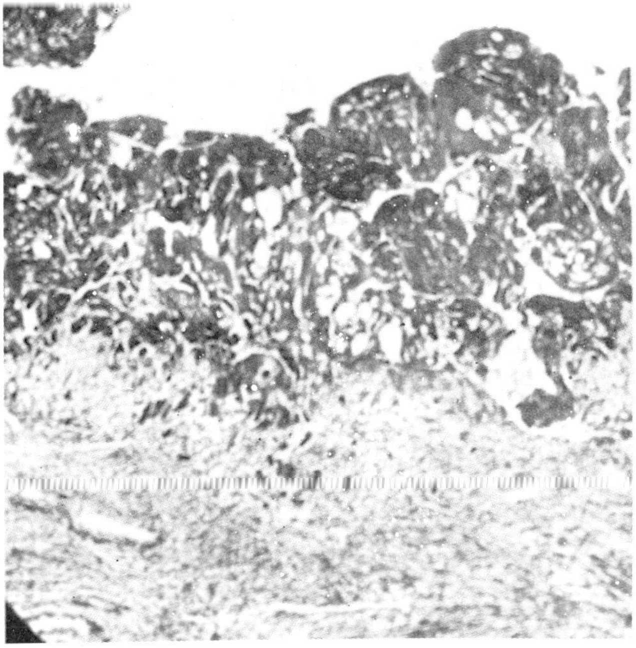

Low Power Choriocarcinoma of uterine wall showing invasion of underlyings myometrium

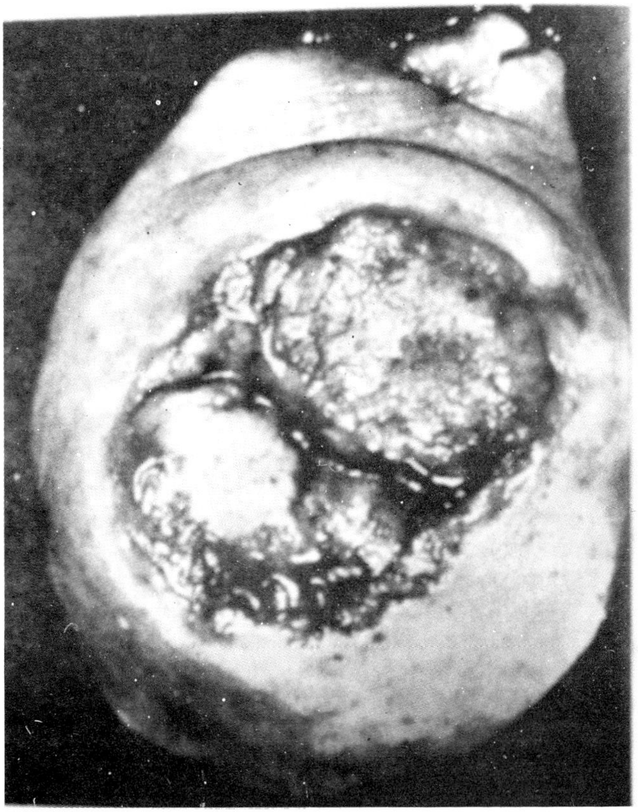

Carcinoma of Cervix well Advanced

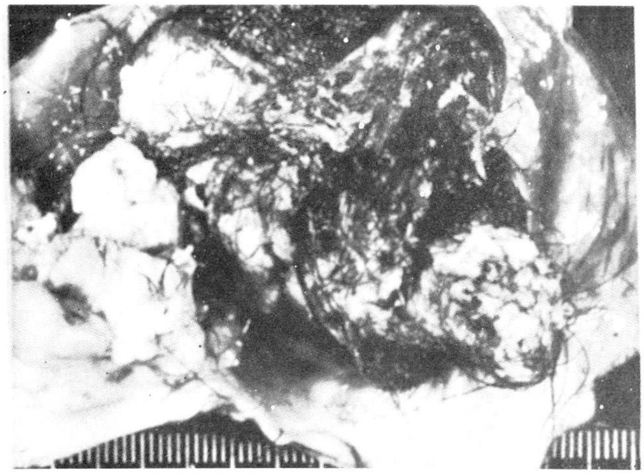

Opend dermoid cyst of Overy. Abudant hair and sebaceous material is evident

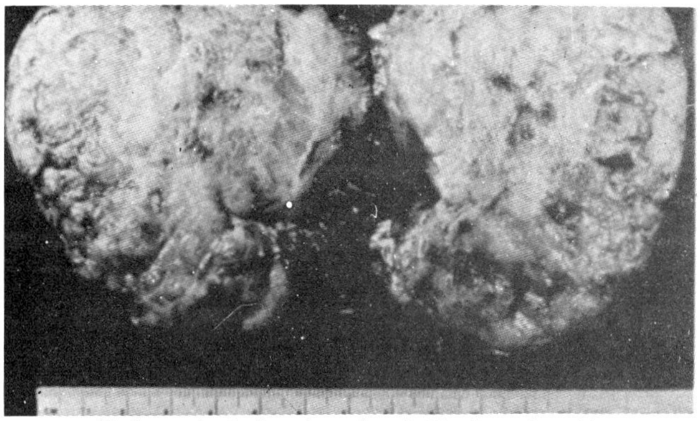

Siminoma testis is enlarged and virtually replaced by Labulated Homogenous, gray-white tumor tissue

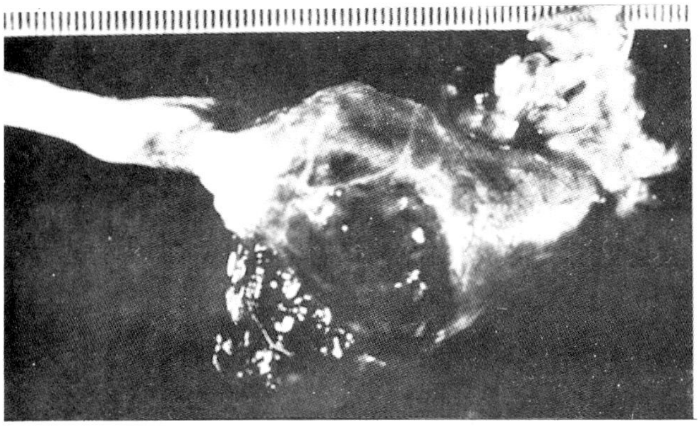

Tubal Pregancy with marked dilatation and cupture of distal end of

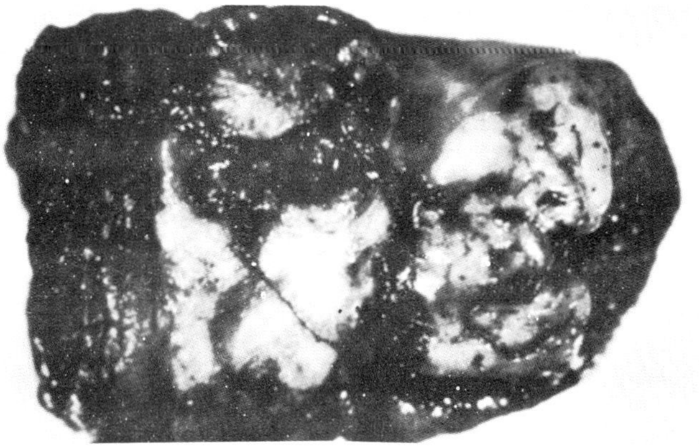

Cell Carcinoma of Penis

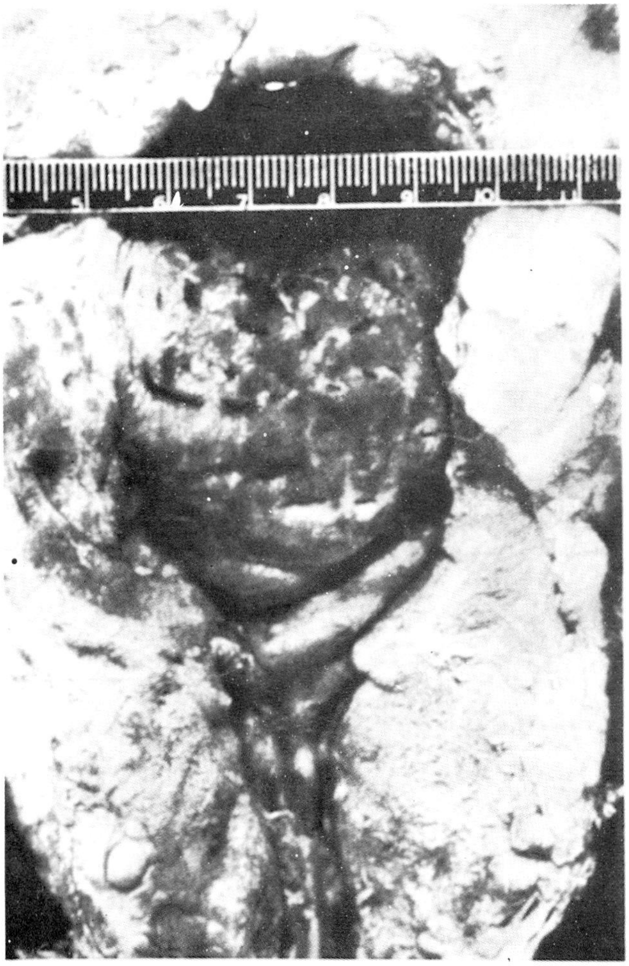

Carcinoma of Prostate

Pipillary Transitional Cell Carcinoma of Bladder

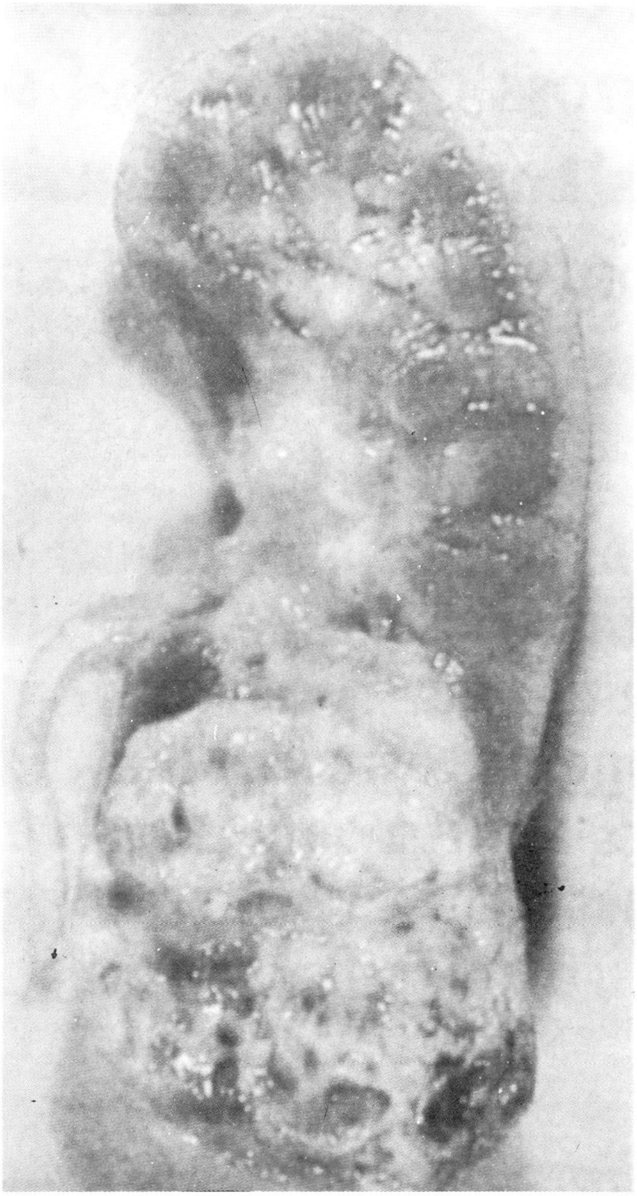

Adenocarcinoma of the KIDNEY

CHAPTER XIV

Diet And Cancer

It used to be believed that abstaining from smoking was the single most effective means to avoid cancer. New research findings have, however, led many in the scientific community to believe that nutrition plays an even more important role.

If this news has not made its due impact, it is because of two reasons. There is a big investment in the idea that the answer to cancer is to be found in a cure **and** not in prevention. Also, the idea that a disease is something that needs to be cured rather than prevented in the first place, seems to have a greater appeal to the human mind. Even if you don't have any ego investment in playing down the importance of nutrition, or in playing up the magnificence of drugs and surgery, you may still doubt the assertion that food can cause or prevent cancer. This is because foods identified as "cancer promoters" do their work not directly but in a very indirect way, altering body chemistry or processes in such a way as to encourage still other changes, which in turn, somewhere down the line, lower the body's ability to perform naturally. Such changes do not become truly dangerous unless they persist over many years. It is not a question of a few meals but the food habits you follow year after year. Likewise, foods believed to be protective against cancer may also probably work indirectly, by stimulating the body's natural resistance factors, or by diluting or buffering certain substances that may provoke cancer after a long and close contact with certain organs.

A few recent news headlines from scientific journals reflect this truth: "Diet Is Prime Factor in Triggering Cancer: High Plant Consumption Recommended", "Disordered Nutrition Blamed for Half of U.S. Cancer Deaths", "Cancer Is Not Inevitable: National Research Council Panel Recommends Changes in Diet To Reduce the Risk of Cancer". Under the headline, "Massive Data on Cancer Risk Factors Compiled", *Chemical & Engineering News* described a major study suggesting that of all avoidable cancer risks, unwise nutrition is the foremost. While the range of acceptable estimates for the relative importance of nutrition is wide, going from 10 to 70 per cent, the "best estimate" of scientists is that diet accounts for 35 per cent of all avoidable risks. Tobacco is estimated to account for 30 per cent of all cancer risks. By eating more wisely and avoiding tobacco, therefore, it might be possible to reduce our risk of cancer by two-thirds.

The High Cancer Risk Diet

Take a typical office-goer in the West, where the incidence of cancer is high. For breakfast, he has a couple of fried eggs, a few slivers of bacon, buttered toast and a cup of coffee--the first of the seven or eight cups he will have that day. A few hours later, he'll have a doughnut for a snack. For lunch today, it may be a corned beef sandwich with coleslaw and Russian dressing on rye, with a handful of potato chips. For dinner, a generous portion of roast beef ringed with dark, crunchy fat, buttered string beans and mashed potatoes mixed with butter and decorated with drippings from the roast. Later, there will be a slice of leftover apple pie topped with ice cream.

Beginning with breakfast, this diet is swimming in fat. The eggs are fried in butter, the bacon is loaded with fat, and the toast is covered with it. There is a good shot of fat in the doughnut, and lots in the corned beef sandwich–about 30 per cent by weight--not to mention all the fat in the mayonnaise used in his coleslaw and Russian dressing. Then there are his potato chips. At dinner, he gets another big dose of fat from his roast beef, from the butter and drippings on his mashed potatoes, the butter on his string beans, and finally, a big bedtime dollop from the apple pie and ice cream.

You probably thought that fat is bad if you have a weight problem or if you're worried about your circulation.

But cancer? Yes, says all the new research. Of all nutritional factors considered in a recent large-scale survey of the scientific literature by the National Research Council, the investigating committee "*found the strongest evidence for a connection between cancer and consumption of fats*". Both epidemiological and laboratory studies have shown higher rates of cancer of the breast, large bowel and prostate in populations that eat foods containing large amount of both saturated and unsaturated fats. These studies have also shown that eating less fat is associated with lower incidence of these cancers. Significantly, the cancers most clearly associated with high-fat intake--involving the colon, prostate and breasts--are among the most common fatal cancers.

Cancer of the breast, which is both the most common and most often fatal cancer in women, seems to have an especially close relationship with a high-fat diet. Countries such as Thailand and El Salvador, with very low averages of dietary fat consumption, have extremely low rates of breast cancer. Countries like Poland and Hungary, with fat intake in the middle range, have a middle-range incidence of breast cancer. In countries like the United States, New Zealand and the Netherlands, with relatively high fat consumption, breast cancer rates reach their highest levels.

A revealing comparison can be made between the United States and Japan, both of them fully industrialized nations. An American woman consumes, on the average, about 3.5 times as much fat as a Japanese woman and is just about four times more likely to develop breast cancer. When Japanese women move to the United States, their children's chances of developing breast cancer quickly increase. Even within Japan, in cities where there is a high intake of fat--mainly animal fat--there is also a higher rate of breast cancer, and *vice versa*. (Breast cancer rates have been increasing in Japan rather rapidly in recent years, which is linked to the greater consumption of fat as their diet becomes increasingly westernized.)

Further confirmation of the fat-cancer link comes from the laboratory, where many research studies have shown that when animals are challenged with cancer-causing chemicals, a high-fat diet increases the number of tumours and the speed at which they will then develop.

A substantial amount of the fat comes from meat, bacon, corned beef, roast beef. Such heavy meat eating is now considered to be a probable risk factor for cancer. And that risk may be independent of and additional to the fat content of the meat. Several studies have even pinpointed heavy consumption of beef as a special risk factor for cancer of the colon. Credibility was added to the idea of heavy meat consumption being a risk factor when a study published in the *New England Journal of Medicine* (December 16, 1992) revealed that vegetarian women tend to have significantly lower levels of circulating estrogen hormones. Women in Western countries, where the risk of breast cancer is high, are known to have higher levels of these hormones. It thus appears as though a vegetarian diet may be protective; **and** regular meat eating leads to a hormone profile that in some manner promotes cancer. It was found that besides not eating meat, the vegetarian women studied ate about 25 per cent less fat than average and also consumed more fibre. Perhaps those factors, rather than their abstinence from meat, were behind their more healthful hormone levels.

Anyone who eats meat three times a day would be hard pressed to keep his fat intake low or his fibre level high·(Meat has no fibre whatsoever.) There is no fibre also in eggs, butter, bacon, corned beef, Russian dressing, roast beef or ice cream. Toast and doughnut and rye bread, being made with mostly white flour, contain only very small amounts of fibre. Mashed potatoes, string beans and the apples in the pie give a little more fibre, but hardly enough.

Meat cooked at very high temperatures or charred (very crisp bacon and roast beef burned around the edges) constitutes yet another risk factor, since it is believed that potentially carcinogenic compounds may be formed in the process.

Two of the three servings of meat in our example--the bacon and the corned beef--were cured with sodium nitrate. Many scientists believe that these nitrate compounds, when they hit the stomach, can undergo reactions yielding new compounds, called nitrosamines, considered cancer-causing agents. High heat encourages this transformation.

The seven or eight cups of coffee consumed a day may be yet another risk factor, at least when taken along with a high-fat diet. The effect might be even worse for a person who smokes or is exposed to heavy doses of toxic chemicals. A few cups of coffee a day, you may be relieved to hear, is not so far considered to be a risk factor.

Are there any negative habits in our example that have a redeeming value? Yes, two. He's not a heavy drinker, so his risk of developing a number of cancers--

primarily in the mouth and throat area--is reduced. (He doesn't smoke, either, a habit that seems to worsen the effects of alcohol, as well as promoting cancer in numerous organs, notably the lungs.) And, although his diet is rich in fat, he isn't a big snacker, so his weight is normal. And that puts him on the good side of the obesity factor, which is also regarded as a significant risk.

The Low-Cancer-Risk Diet

All those negative nutritional factors, even when followed for many years, probably do not provoke cancer directly. They only worsen the odds against you.

A protective diet is one consisting largely of whole grains, fresh fruits and vegetables, and perhaps moderate amounts of fish and seafood. It is not exotic or expensive food. The protectors are all familiar friends, foods that you are used to. By eating more of them (and less of the negative foods), resistance to cancer may be increased.

One nutrient that now appears to be of supreme importance in helping to protect us against cancer is vitamin A. It does not follow, however, that taking huge supplemental amounts of this vitamin braces you up like a Titan. In fact, taking more than 25,000 I.U. of vitamin A every day may get you in trouble. The point is not how much vitamin A you can cram into your diet but rather to make sure that your intake isn't dangerously low. A better diet, perhaps with moderate-level supplements not exceeding 10,000 to 25,000 I.U. a day, can easily put you in the safety zone without over-dosage. We shall spend some time with this nutrient.

Of all forms of cancer, none is so lethal as lung cancer. Fully 34 per cent of all cancer deaths in men are from lung cancer, and 16 per cent in women (second only to breast cancer, which claims 9 per cent). Even when caught in its early stages, survival times are shorter for lung cancer than for any other common cancer. Anything, therefore, that decreases the risk of developing lung cancer is of utmost importance. Enter vitamin A.

One way to get some idea of whether or not vitamin A might be protective against lung cancer is to follow a large group of people over a period of time and determine if there is a relationship between habitual intake of this nutrient and the occurrence of lung cancer. Such studies have been carried out in Norway, Japan, Singapore, the United States and England, and they have all shown a tendency for people who have a low intake of vitamin A to have a relatively higher risk of developing lung cancer.

There are two major forms of vitamin A. One, called retinal, occurs naturally only in certain foods of animal origin, particularly liver, milk, cheese, butter and egg yolk. The second form of vitamin A is found only in plant foods. Known as beta-carotene, it is transformed into active vitamin A by the body to the extent needed. Because some scientists suspect that beta-carotene, but not necessarily animal-source vitamin A, is the true protective factor against lung caner, one recent major study of lung cancer risk paid special attention to this distinction. Over nineteen years, a research team headed by Richard B. Shekelle, of the Rush-Presbyterian-St. Luke's Medical Center in Chicago, monitored the dietary habits of nearly 2,000 middle-aged men employed at the Western Electric Company in the Chicago area. Then they sorted out the links between the workers' dietary patterns and cancer. When they examined the specific data on carotene intake, they discovered that among the 488 men who had the lowest level of carotene consumption, there were fourteen cases of lung cancer. But in the group of the same size that ate the most carotene, there were only two cases. What's more, even long-term cigarette smokers seemed to be protected by beta-carotene, though to a lesser degree (*Lancet*, November 28, 1981). No other nutritional difference seemed significant.

Plants rich in beta-carotene are carrots, sweet potatoes, pumpkins, winter squash, spinach, kale, broccoli and sweet red peppers. Apricots, peaches, oranges and tomatoes also are good sources.

It is possible that vitamin A protects against more than just lung cancer. A ten-year study of over 100,000 Japanese men aged 40 and over revealed a substantially lower death rate from prostate cancer among men who ate green and yellow vegetables each day (ICRDB *Cancer-Gram*, January 1979). Japanese scientists theorized that it was the vitamin A in these vegetables that might be responsible for their cancer preventing effects. Interestingly, the incidence of prostate cancer is lower and the consumption of vegetables higher among the Japanese than the Americans. Also, the prostate cancer rate is lower for American vegetarians than for meat eaters.

Any good news on the ability of vitamin A to help treat cancer once it has been diagnosed? Exciting news along these lines was presented at the First International Conference on the Modulation and Mediation of Cancer by Vitamins held in February of 1982 at the University of Arizona Cancer Center in Tucson. The emphasis is not on using vitamin A alone to treat cancer, but rather on vitamin A as part of total therapy. In one experiment with animals, for instance, a group of mice was injected with cancer cells and then given radiation treatment. Although their tumours shrank following radiation, they later regrew, and all the mice died. Another group of animals, instead of receiving radiation treatment once their tumours had become established, was given supplements of vitamin A. They survived about 50 per cent longer than the animals that had received radiation. When radiation therapy and vitamin A therapy were given to animals infected with cancer, the results were remarkably better than giving either radiation or vitamin A alone. Whereas all the mice that had been treated with a single therapy survived, on the average, no more than about two months, all the combination-therapy mice were still alive after ten months, and only 4 out of 48 animals showed any signs of having tumours (Study by Rettura and colleagues from the Albert Einstein College of Medicine).

At this writing few studies have been published showing the results of supplemental vitamin A given to cancer patients. Such research is probably under way. One glimmer of what we might expect from such work is seen in a study reported at the Tucson conference by a group of doctors representing two different cancer treatment centres. Some 213 patients with a variety of cancers who came to these institutions were extensively studied prior to treatment to ascertain their nutritional status. After treatment, the patients were re-examined to see if there was any relationship between nutritional status and the outcome of treatment. And indeed there was, with vitamin A stepping to the front.

The doctors worked out the average vitamin A content among people without cancer. Among patients with serum vitamin A levels less than average, cancer tended to worsen even following chemotherapy. Only 7 per cent responded positively to treatment, while 15 per cent remained about the same. But among patients with serum vitamin A levels equal to or greater than the average, 56 per cent responded well to chemotherapy. Cancer progressed in only 18 per cent (versus 78 per cent in the low vitamin A group). In another 26 per cent, the condition remained stable.

Were the patients who had low levels of vitamin A more ill than the others? The researchers state that was probably not the case. If it were, the patients probably would have had low levels of all vitamins, but they didn't. Only their vitamin A levels were particularly low compared to the patients who responded better (Study by Soukop and colleagues at the Medical Oncology Unit, Royal Infirmary, Glasgow, Scotland, and the Wisconsin Clinical Cancer Center, University of Wisconsin, Madison, Wisconsin).

Completing the Family of Cancer Protectors

Vitamin C. To save space, we shall treat the remaining protective nutrients more briefly. The first is vitamin C. The literature on vitamin C as a protector is not nearly as impressive as for vitamin A, but its possible importance can't be denied. While vitamin C probably helps protect against cancer in many parts of the body, the chief benefactor of its powers may be the stomach. John H. Weisburger, of the American Health Foundation in Valhalla, New York, believes that the declining rate of stomach cancer in the United States is largely the result of the Americans' greater intake of fruits and vegetables rich in vitamin C (thanks to rapid transportation and refrigeration). Work at the American Health Foundation and elsewhere has also shown that vitamin C, when eaten with a meal containing nitrite, blocks the production of nitrosamine compounds believed to cause cancer. In Japan, nitrite-treated fish and pickled foods are widely eaten, which is considered a major cause of the very high rate of stomach cancer in that country. But now that the Japanese are eating more fresh fruits and vegetables, endless nitrite-treated fish and pickled foods, their rate of stomach cancer seems to be tending downward. "If all this information is correct", Dr. Weisburger told a scientific conference, "we should be able to prevent gastric cancer from childhood onward by insuring that we have adequate vitamin C with each meal."

The possibility that vitamin C helps prevent cancer is an additional reason why we should make sure that we are getting enough of this key nutrient. All citrus fruits and melons are excellent sources; so are broccoli, brussels sprouts, cabbage, cauliflower, fruits in general, tomatoes and dark green leafy vegetables.

Selenium. Among the dietary requirements of humans are a surprisingly large number of minerals that are needed in extremely small amounts. Yet, no matter how small the requirement, if it isn't met, the results can be serious. In the case of selenium, the result may be cancer. Several studies have shown that selenium possesses definite anti-cancer characteristics. Some suspect that among other things, selenium helps out by slowing down cancer at its very earliest stages, permitting cells to heal themselves before they are taken over by the cancer process. Several highly respected researchers have repeatedly shown that when laboratory animals are injected with cancer cells, supplementing their diet with a little extra selenium substantially lowers the subsequent tumour rate.

Selenium may have a special role in protecting against breast cancer. Gerhard N. Schrauzer of the University of California at San Diego discovered that as levels of selenium in blood rise, breast cancer rates fall. Analysing data from seventeen countries, Schrauzer discovered that selenium levels in blood from blood banks in Japan, Taiwan, Thailand, the Philippines, Puerto Rico and Costa Rica were over three times as high as the samples from European countries and the United States. And the breast cancer mortality rate in Europe and the United States is correspondingly two to five times higher than in Asia and Latin America. Other researchers have found that breast cancer patients have ''significantly less selenium in their blood than do healthy women'' (*Journal of Surgical Oncology*).

Selenium, like vitamin A, can become toxic at high doses--even more so than vitamin A. But there is no danger in increasing your selenium consumption by emphasizing seafood and whole grains in your diet. A selenium supplement of from 100 to 200 micrograms a day is also judged to be safe.

Vitamin E may have certain anti-cancer properties, but not very strong. Nevertheless, vitamin E may well have the ability to give the prospective power of selenium a big boost. A study at the Roswell Park Memorial Institute in Buffalo, New York, showed that by itself, vitamin E had no effect on cancer. On the other hand, while selenium alone had a protective effect against three chemicals known to cause breast cancer in laboratory animals, vitamin E greatly enhanced this effect (Proceedings of the American Association of Cancer Research, March 1982).

Cabbage Family. While many vegetables are valued for their high content of vitamin A or vitamin C or their fibre (they are just about all very low in fat), there is one group of vegetables that has these items in abundance and appear to have unique anti-cancer properties. Belonging to the cabbage or cruciferous family, these vegetables (cabbage, broccoli, cauliflower, brussels sprouts) have been repeatedly shown to contain something that seems to help prevent cancer. The effect may be especially important in the colon and rectum. Put them down as best bets.

Highlights of Anti-Cancer Diet

The following features of the presumed anti-cancer diet may be noted.

* It looks remarkably similar to the diet currently believed to protect your heart and circulatory system–low in fat, meat and calories, and high in grains and vegetables.
* It is also remarkably similar to the diet eaten by millions who might consider themselves ''semi-vegetarians''.
* It is remarkably similar to the diet now followed by many joggers and athletes involved in endurance sports.
* It is the kind of diet prescribed at progressive spas to people who want to keep their weight down.
* It is the kind of diet many follow simply because of its rich vitamin and mineral content.
* Most remarkably, it is similar to the diet our forebears ate long before the birth of civilization.

Is it possible that what we are talking about is a diet for which the body is naturally designed? Which would go a long way toward explaining why keeping to it would maximize health, and deviating from it invite not only cancer, but other problems as well.

One of the nice parts about it all is that gradually modifying your diet to include more and more of the protective factors and fewer of the negative factors is not terribly difficult. You don't have to shop at special places or pay special prices. In fact, your food bill should go down, not up.

Elements of a Cancer-Protective Diet

Tomatoes. One of the compounds in tomatoes that is though to reduce the risk of cancer is lycopene, the pigment that makes tomatoes red. Lycopene, an antioxidant that is also found in watermelons and apricots, quenches certain cancer-triggering oxygen-free radicals. Having a low lycopene level in the blood is associated with a higher risk of pancreatic cancer, according to a Johns Hopkins University study. The study also showed that people with pancreatic cancer had lower levels of lycopene compared with healthy individuals. Lycopene is present in tomato paste and even in ketchup.

Green Vegetables. A recent Italian study showed that dark-green leafy vegetables lower the risk of many cancers. Spinach, broccoli, kale (a variety of cabbage) and dark-green lettuces are chock-full of anti-oxidants, including beta-carotene, folate and lutein. A good rule of thumb: the darker the vegetable, the more anti-oxidants it has.

Pungent Preventives. A whole host of chemicals thought to have cancer-inhibiting properties have been identified in root vegetables, which include garlic and onions. Animal studies show that many of these chemicals block the spread of carcinogens that have been linked to colon, stomach, lung and liver cancer. A study at Pennsylvania State University found that feeding rats with various garlic extracts and preparations reduced mammary tumours by as much as 71 per cent. Studies on humans suggest that those who eat more onions and garlic are less prone gastro-intestinal cancer. Research suggests that garlic compounds may even interfere with cancer progression. A recent German study found that ajoene, a garlic compound, is toxic to malignant cells. Garlic may also antagonize existing cancer by boosting immune functions, according to American researchers. Their study, done on mice, found that garlic's sulphur compounds increased the activity of macrophages and T-lymphocytes, two of the components of the immune system that destroy cancer tumour cells.

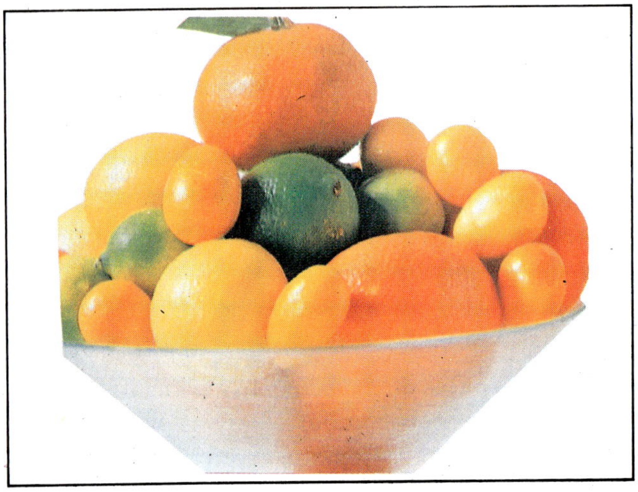

Citrus Fruit. "Eat oranges, grapefruits, lemons and limes as often as possible", says American toxicologist Herbert Pierson. He calls citrus fruits an all-around cancer package because they possess every class of natural substances (carotenoids, flavonoids and others) that have individually neutralized powerful chemical carcinogens. Citrus fruits, if consumed daily, reduce the risk of pancreatic cancer by one-half to more than two-thirds, as compared with eating citrus fruits less than once a week.

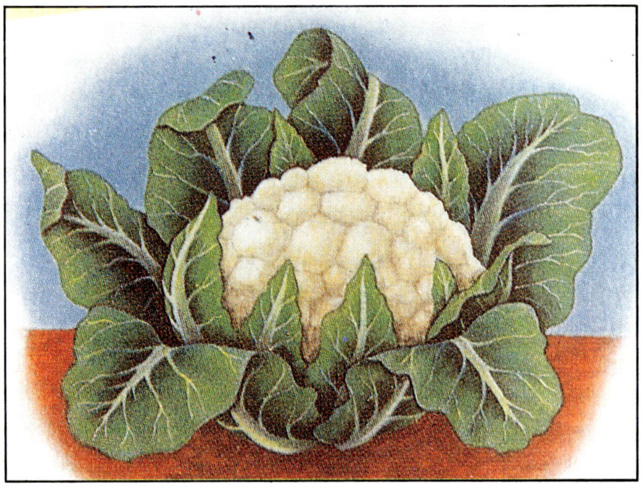

Cruciferous Vegetables. Cruciferous vegetables such as cabbage, cauliflower, brussels sprouts, broccoli, kale, mustard greens and turnips may reduce the risk of breast cancer. In fact, one research team found that feeding animals with cabbage and collard greens (also a cruciferous vegetable), along with a low-fat diet, reduced the incidence of mammary cancers. Cruciferous vegetables should be eaten either raw or lightly cooked. Over-cooking may destroy the cancer-protective compounds found in theses vegetables. Cruciferous vegetables may also work to head off stomach and colon cancer. Research has revealed that men who ate the most cruciferous vegetables had a 70 per cent lower risk of colon cancer than those who ate the least of such vegetables.

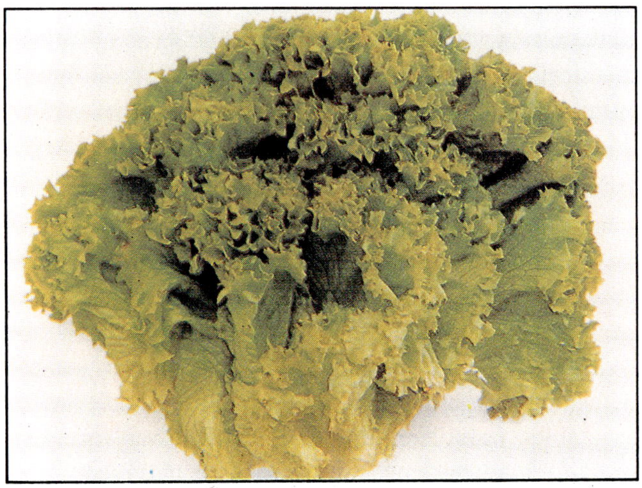

Broccoli. There is new evidence that broccoli may help ward off cancer. Scientists at Johns Hopkins

University have tested a compound isolated from broccoli and found it protects rats against breast cancer. They have also found that the compound, sulforaphane, fights cancer in laboratory animals. Now they have published a report in Proceedings of the National Academy of Sciences, on a study of 137 rats. The substance of the study was: (a) reduced tumour incidence from 68 per cent in untreated rats to 39 per cent in all the other treated animals; (b) cut in the number of tumours; (c) decreased tumor size; (d) delayed onset of cancer. ''Although how it works isn't known'', says study leader Dr. Paul Talafay, he believes that sulforaphane energizes an enzyme that breaks down cancer-causing substances.

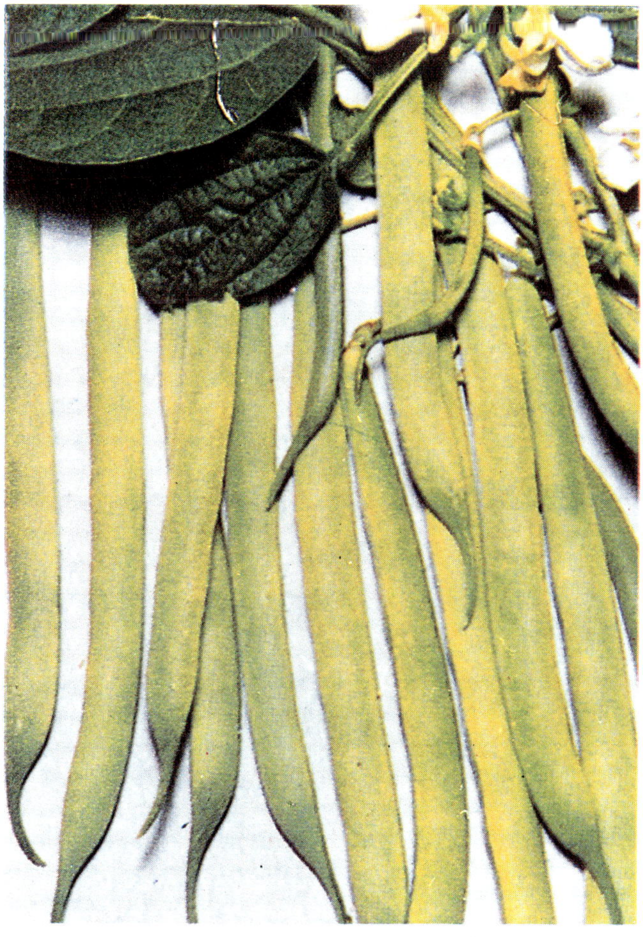

Soybeans. Soybeans contain at least five compounds believed to inhibit cancer. In fact, one of the compounds that they contain is chemically similar to the drug tamoxifen, which is routinely used to treat estrogen-dependent breast cancer and is under test to see if it can prevent the disease altogether.

Dried and Canned Beans, including chick-peas, lentils, kidney, black and white beans, contain possible anti-cancer agents as well. One California study showed that those who ate these beans weekly were 40 per cent less likely to die from pancreatic cancer than those who ate them less than once a week.

Wheat Bran. Wheat bran may lower the risk of colon cancer. A study of patients at the New York Hospital-Cornell Medical Centre found that two 30 gram servings of wheat bran cereal a day caused malignant colon polyps to shrink within six months. It Most remarkable that such a small amount of food could have such an impact. This illustrate that dietary intervention may work even after cancerous warning signs have appeared.

Low-fat Milk. While the saturated fat in milk seems to promote certain cancers, another substance in milk may deter them. Researchers at a cancer institute discovered, not surprisingly, that drinkers of whole cream milk had higher odds than non-drinkers did, of developing cancers of the oral cavity, stomach, colon, rectum, lung, bladder, breast, and cervix. But they also found that milk drinkers were less likely than non-milk-drinkers to develop cancers of the oral cavity, stomach, rectum and cervix. Scientists suspect that elements such as calcium, riboflavin may be the do-gooders.

Conclusion

To sum up, dietary factors--estimated to account for 35 per cent of all avoidable cancer risks--are of much greater importance than food additives and pollution combined--estimated to amount to about 6 per cent of the avoidable risk. Since smoking is estimated to account for 30 per cent of all avoidable cancer deaths, and excessive alcohol another 3 per cent, we can see that by focusing on these three factors--a better diet, not smoking and very light use of alcohol--all of which are under our control, we may able to achieve a surprisingly high degree of cancer protection.

Cancer develops over a long time, which means that a person has years, or typically decades, in which to hinder or promote it. Researchers are finding that what we eat may interfere with cancer growth at various stages. For example, certain foods can block the chemicals that initiate cancer. Anti-oxidants, present in some vitamins and minerals, can snuff out oxygen-free radicals--substances that are thought to make cells more susceptible to cancer, and they can even repair some cellular damage.

A recent review of 170 studies from seventeen nations reveals that people who eat the most fruits and vegetables have about half the cancer rates of those who eat the least. This includes cancers of the lung, colon, breast, cervix, stomach, bladder, pancreas and ovary. In fact, some research suggests that a high consumption of fruits and vegetables can cut the risk of lung cancer even in smokers. "It is almost mind-boggling", says Tim Byers, an epidemiologist with the US Center for Disease Control and Prevention, "that ordinary fruits and vegetables can be so effective against such a potent carcinogen as cigarette smoke."

Table of representative values of funds for nutrients.
Amounts given per 100 gms of edible portion.

Food	Water ml	calories	proteins	Fat gm	carbohydrates	Fiber mg	Calcium mg	Iron mg	Vit. A i.u.	B1	B2	Nicotinamide	VitC
1	2	3	4	5	6	7	8	9	10	11	12	13	14
Maize Whole	12	363	10	4.5	71	2	12	2.5	-	.35	.13	2	-
Rice, lightly milted	12	354	8	1.5	77	.5	10	2	-	.35	.13	2	-
Sorghum Jawar	12	353	10	2.5	73	1.5	20	4	-	.4	.1	3	-
Wheat Whole	13	344	11.5	2	70	2	30	3.5	-	.4	.1	5	-
Wheat Flour	13	341	10	1	75	-	16	1.5	-	.08	.05	.8	-
Whole Wheat sprouted	13	397	29.2	7.4	53.3	1.4	40	6	-	1.4	.54	.29	-
Bajra millet	13	361	11.6	.5	67.5	1.2	42	5	-	.33	.25	2.3	-
Barley	13336	22.5	1.3	62.6	3.9	26	8	-	.47	.20	5.4	-	-
Maash (black kidney bean)	11	329	24	1	56	4.5	150	9	40	.4	.2	2	-
Gram, Whole	10	338	22	.5	61	5.3	280	8	.4	.15	2.5	-	-
Mung bean (Green)	12	324	22	1	57	4.7	100	8	40	.45	.2	-	-
Dried Pea	10	337	25	1	57	4.5	70	5	100	.8	.2	-	-
Lubia bean	12	323	24.1	1	54.5	3.8	77	5.9	60	.51	.2	1.3	-
Red Kidney bean	12	346	22.9	1.3	60.6	4.5	260	5.8	60	-	-	-	-
Soybean	8	382	35	18	20	4.5	200	7-11	-	1.1	.3	2	-
Almond	5	657	20	59	12	1.7	150	3.5	-	.3	.6	4.5	5
Cashewnut	5	590	20	45	26	103	50	5	-	.3	.6	4.5	5
Pistachio	6	626	20	54	15	2	140	14	100	7	.5	1.5	-
Coconut Kernel	20	375	4	35	11	4	10	2	-	.05	.02	.6	-
Walnut	3	697	15	65	13	2.1	80	2	-	.4	.1	.7	-
Groundnut	6	579	27	45	17	3	50	2.5	-	.9	.15	17	-
Melon seeds without cover	6	581	25	45	19	2	50	8	-	.1	.15	1.5	-
Pumpkin seeds without cover	4	610	30	50	10	2	40	10	30	.2	.2	2	-
Spinach	85	48	5	.7	5	1.5	250	10.9	3000	.1	.3	1.5	1
Lettuce	94	19	1.4	-	3	.5	35	2.4	300	.1	.1	.4	1
Bathua leaves	90	30	3.7	.4	2.9	.8	150	4.2	-	.01	.14	.6	3
Methi leaves	85	49	4.4	.9	6	1.1	395	16.5	-	.04	.31	.8	52

Food	Water ml	calories	proteins	Fat gm	carbohydrates	Fiber mg	Calcium mg	Iron mg	Vit. A i.u.	B1	B2	Nicotinamide	VitC
1	2	3	4	5	6	7	8	9	10	11	12	13	14
mustard leaves	85	34	4	.6	3.2	.8	155	16.3	-	.03	-	-	3 3
Fresh beans & peas	70	104	7	-	19	2.5	40	2	15-500	.3	.15	1.5	2 5
Beet root	87	45	1.8	-	10	.7	15	1	-	.02	.03	.3	5
Cauliflower	90	33	3	.2	5	1	30	1	20	.1	.1	.7	-
Cucumber	96	12	.6	-	2	.5	15	.3	-	.04	.02	.2	1 0
Egg plant (brinjal)	93	22	1	-	4	1	10	1	-	.05	.03	.8	5
Gourd	92	28	.7	-	6	.3	20	.6	-	.04	.03	.6	1
Green spring onion	90	36	1.8	.5	6	1	40	3	500	.05	.1	.5	5 0
Green pepper	90	37	2	.5	6	1	20	1	130-800	.03	.03	.3	1 5 0
Redish	94	18	1	-	4	.7	30	1	-	.03	.03	.3	2 5
Tomato	94	20	1	-	4	.6	5	.4	250	.06	.04	.7	2 5
Turnip	90	34	1	-	8	.7	30	.4	-	.06	.04	.7	2 5
Potato	80	75	2	-	17	.4	10	.7	-	.1	.03	1.5	1 5
Sweet potato	70	114	1.5	.3	26	1	25	1	100	.1	.04	.7	3 0
Yarm	73	104	2	.2	24	.5	10	1.2	20	.1	.03	.4	1 0
Carrot	90	33	1	-	7	.8	40	.7	3000	.05	.05	.5	
Fresh mushroom	91	13	2.5	.3	-	1	20	1	-	.12	.5	5.8	6 3
Apple	84	61	.3	.4	14	1	4	1	20	.02	.04	.2	5
Apricot	90	36	1	-	8	.4	15	1	2000	.03	.05	.5	5
Lemon, lime grape fruit & other citrus fruits	90	37	.6	-	8.5	.4	21	.5	.04	-	.2	4	0
Orange, Malta	86	53	.8	-	13	.3	30	.5	30	.5	30	.2	45
Banana	70	116	1	.3	27	.3	7	.5	100	.1	.08	.8	30
Custard apple	75	93	1	-	22	1	25	.5	-	.1	.08	.8	30
Dried dates	20	303	2	-	74	2.4	70	2	50	.07	.05	.4	2
Fig-fresh	85	49	1-3	-	11	2	50	1	80	.05	.05	.4	2
Fig-dried	20	269	4	-	63	11	200	4	100	.1	.08	1.7	-
Grape	80	76	1	-	18	.5	20	.3	50	.04	.02	.3	5
Guava	80	58	1	.4	13	5.5	15	1	200	.05	.04	1	200
Lichi	82	71	.9	.5	16	.3	5	.5	-	.04	.04	.3	50
Mango	83	63	.5	-	15	.8	10	.5	600	.03	.04	.3	30

Food	Water ml	calories	proteins	Fat gm	carbohydrates	Fiber mg	Calcium mg	Iron mg	Vit. A i.u.	B1	B2	Nicotinamide	VitC
1	2	3	4	5	6	7	8	9	10	11	12	13	14
Musk-Melon	93	26	.5	-	6	.4	10	.4	500	.03	.03	5	30
Papya	89	39	.8	-	9	.7	20	.5	1000	.03	.03	.2	50
Peach	85	56	.8	-	13	.5	8	.5	300	.02	.03	.3	10
Pear	84	59	.3	-	15	.9	7	.4	-	.02	.02	.2	4
Pineapple	85	57	.4	-	14	.5	20	.5	100	.08	.03	.1	30
Plum	88	456	.7	-	11	.4	10	.4	30	.02	.03	.3	5
Pomegranate	80	77	1	-	18	.2	3	.7	-	.02	.02	.2	8
Butter	16	545	.5	82.5	-	-	15	.2	3000	-	-	-	-
Butter oil pure	8	828	-	92	-	-	-	-	2000	-	-	-	-
Animal fat	1	891	-	99	-	-	-	-	-	-	-	-	-
1	2	3	4	5	6	7	8	9	10	11	12	13	14
Hydrogenated oil	-	900	-	100	-	-	-	-	-	-	-	-	-
Cow milk-fresh	88	64	3.3	3.6	4.7	-	120	.1	150	.04	.15	.1	1
Cow milk skimmed	91	34	3.4	.1	4	-	120	.1	-	.05	.15	.1	1
Cow milk condensed	29	317	7.3	8	53.9	-	270	.2	350	.09	.33	.2	3.8
Mother's milk	87	75	1.3	4.6	7	-	30	.2	160	.02	.04	.2	4
Cheese from whole milk (cow) hard	39	384	24	32	-	-	800	.5	1400	.04	.5	.1	-
Cheese from skimmed milk, soft	77	87	19.5	.5	1	-	90	.4	20	.02	.02	.3	1
Fish, fresh water	787 8	95	18	2.5	-	-	50	1	-	.03	.05	1.5	-
fish dried	20	309	63	6.3	-	-	3000	8.5	-	1.	.2	6	-
Sardine canned in oil	50	309	20	2.5	-	-	50	1	-	0.5	.03	0.5	1.5-
Beef lean	66	206	19	14	-	-	10	10	1000	-	.1	.2	5
Kidney	75	127	16	7	-	-	10	10	10000	.3	2	7	12
mabmb meat	73	139	19	7	-	-	15	1.5	-	.1	.15	9	-
Pork	34	535	10	55	-	-	15	1.5	-	.5	.15	3	-
poultry mant	73	139	19	7	-	-	15	1.5	-	.1	.15	9	-
Honey	23	286	4	-	76	-	5	.4	-	-	.05	.2	-
Sugar whitle	-	400	-	-	100	-	-	-	-	-	-	-	-
Brown Khandsari	1	389	.2	-	97	-	30	2	-	0.2	.1	.3	-
Cane Juice	81	73	.3	-	18	-	6	2	-	.02	.02	.1	10
Jam	29	260	.4	-	69	.6	12	.3	-	-	-	-	10
Garlic	63	139	6	-	29	.8	13	1.3	-	.25	.08	.4	10
Tamarind	20	304	2	-	74	2	50	3	50	.4	.15	1.5	10
Black pepper	13	347	.12	7	59	4.9	130	10	-	.04	.2	1	-
Red pepper	13	347	.12	7	59	4.9	130	10	-	.04	.2	1	-
Cinnamon	12	229	12	7.8	28	35	440	17	-	.1	.4	2.4	-
Cardamon dried	20	228	10	2	43	20	113	5	-	-	-	-	-
Cumin seed	12	356	19	15	36	12	1080	31	300	-	-	2.6	-
Clove	23	293	5	9	48	10	740	5	-	.1	.2	2	-

Natural food:

Food produced on fertile land without the use of chemical fertilizers, or other chemicals is known as natural food. Pasteurized milk does not remain a natural food, nor is white wheat flour (maida). The whole wheat flour has very good proteins, natural oil, minerals, other elements and vitamins B and E in good quantities but in the production of white wheat flour most of them are lost.

Fresh fruits and vegetables are not only good to taste but also have nutritive elements in large quantities. If fresh vegetables are left in an open room for one day, almost half of their vitamin C is lost. Many people cut vegetables long before cooking. By doing this they provide greater outer surface for some of their nutritive elements to evaporate. Fruits and vegetables which are frozen in the deep freeze lose most of their vitamin B1 and B2. All the enzymes of milk are destroyed in pasteurization.

Food on which pesticides have been sprinkled, should be thoroughly washed before use. Wash them before cutting. These days some of the pesticides and chemicals sprayed are such as would not be washed away with cold water. Therefore use luke warm water for washing such foods.

Those of you who have your own land for agriculture, should grow your vegetables on that land which has been fertilized with natural compost only and where no pesticides chemicals have been used. And pluck such vegetables or fruits just a little before use. Those are best natural food.

In USSR they do not permit chemical additives to their food. Their canning process is done by heat alone and the preventing proceess by sugar and by freezing! Food with additives cannot be considered natural food.

Proteins:

The word protein comes from a greek word meaning "first in importance". Proteins are formed by a combination of oxygen, nitrogen, carbon, phosphorus and sulpher etc. Proteins are extremely important for body development. If proteins are in short supply, your body "eats" its own muscles in order to keep vital organs working.

Proteins provide the building blocks needed for growth, repair and maintenance of body tissues and organs. They are composed of more than seventy amino acids. For assimilation of proteins, body release enzymes into intestinal tract. Enzymes break the protein down into amino acid. These acids are absorbed into your bloodstream. About ten amino acids are essential for good nutrition. Proteins which have a fair balance of these essential amino acids are know as high quality proteins. Proteins of milk, almonds, nuts, coconut, soybean, eggs, and meat are of high quality. Cereals, pulses, peas and seeds have some of the essential amino acids in short supply. Their proteins are, nevertheless, of good quality. Mixing some of these foods gives the same results as a high quality protein. Deficiency in the proteins of cereals is made-up by the proteins of the pulses. It is consequently appropriate to take pulses with cereals.

Muscles, skin, enzymes and hormones are all made of amino acids. Their needs are continuous so your need for proteins is also constant. Due to shortage of proteins you feel weak and tired. If proteins are taken excess, the blood gets vitiated and rotting start inside the intestines.

Need for proteins depends upon the body weight. For every kilogram of body weight, one gram of proteins required per day. According to one school of thought if you are taking sufficient calories in you food, there will not be any shortage of proteins because ntaure has kept appropriate proportions of these two essential requirements of the body in various food items. You, have however, to pay attention to the quality of protein in the food items. You have, however, to pay attention to the quality of protein in the food you take. The quantity of protein in various food items is given Table VI.

Carbohydrates:

Chemically, Carbohydrates are compounds of carbon, hydogen and oxygen. This element in food provides us both the heat and energy. Commonest carbohydrates in human food are starch and sugar. Both of these are found in green plants. Starch causes fat to accumulate on the body. Digestion of starch puts a great strain on the liver. Shortage of carbohydrates produces listlessness and weakness. Its excess produces obesity. Reserves of carbohydrates are found in the form of glycogen in your liver and in your muscles. These reserves are handy during fasting periods.

An ordinary person requires 160 to 240 gms of carbohydrates per day.

The quantity of carbohydrates in various food items is given in Table VI.

Fats:

Many plants store oil as a reserve food material used of starch. Animal store a similar substance. Coconut, groundnut, soybean, palm and olives contain a high percentage of oil. Some nuts also have lot of oil. Meat of all animals, egg yolk and milk provide animal fat.

Both carbohydrates and fats are burnt or oxidised and in that process they free energy is transformed into muscular work and into body heat. Fats produce nearly twice as much heat as the weight of carbohydrates.

All oils and fat have two kinds of acids, one saturated fatty acid which increase blood cholesterol and hardens the blood arteries and second the poly unsaturated fatty acid, the linolink of which even helps in the reduction on blood cholesterol. Various fats have these two acids in the following proportions:

Table I

Name of the fate.	Percentage of the saturated fatty acid.	Percentage of poly unsaturated fatty acid.
Pure ghee (butter oil)	65	almost nil.
Mustard oil	6	18
Sunflower oil	16	50
Corn oil	12	58
Soya oil	14	50
Ground nut (peanut) oil	17	30
Til (Sesamum) oil	12	38

Vitamins:

Vitamins are chemical substances required in very small quantities by our bodies for promoting certain chemical, processes. Vitamins help in processing proteins, carbohydrates and fats etc. So that those elements in our food could perform their functions. Vitamins are generally, not produced by the body itself (exception vitamin K). Vitamins are contained in food. Vitamins help our body in processing food so that it creates energy, builds and help in prevention of disease. Vitamins are protective foods and promote good health.

Vit. A Promotes good eye sight, healthy skin, good teeth, general growth and vitality. Builds resistance to infection and necessary during pregnancy and lactation. Deficiency results in night in night blindness, retarded growth, retarded growth, lack of appetite. Natural sources are all coloured fruits and vegetables, milk and milk products, egg yolk, liver & liver oil. Carrots are very rich in Vit. A. Daily requirements 5000 iu. For pregnant and lactating mothers 8000 iu.

Vit. B1 (Thiamine) : Essential for normal functioning of the nervous system, heart and muscles, aids digestion and promotes carbohydrates utilization. Deficiency results in nervous irritation, mental depression, loss of weight and tickling sensation in the soles of feet. Natural sources are whole wheat, rice husk, brewer's yeast, pea-nuts, oat meal, most vegetables, milk, legumes, pork, liver, and meat. Daily requirement 1.25 mg.

Vit. B2 (Riboflavin) : Promotes generally health and growth, good for skin and healthy eyes, assists cell to use oxygen for the releae of energy from food. Deficiency may result in burning of eyes and in itching and cracking of the corners of the lips. Natural sources are whole grains and their products, milk and milk products, liver and meat foods which have Vit. B1. Daily requirement 1.50 mg.

Vit. B6 (pyridoxine) : Aids in assimilation of fat's and proteins and in blood building. Essential for normal functioning of the nervous system, brain and muscles. A very important vitamin. Deficiency may result in nervous system disorders skin eruption, loss of hair, and ultimately loss of muscular control. Natural sources are wheat germ, brain, brewer's yeast, milk, banana. Pea nuts, raisins, cabbage, blackdrop molasses, liver, kidney, eggs, fresh and meat. Daily requirement 2.0 mg.

Vit. (Cobalamin) : Helps in the formatting and regeneration of red blood cells and nerve tissue, help in utilization of fats, Proteins and carbohydrates. Promotes growth of children and a general tonic for adults. Deficiency may lead to anemia, fatigue and lack of growth, sometimes of inflated tongue. Natural sources are milk products, meat, eggs, liver. Daily requirement 6.0 micrograms.

Niacin (Nicotinamide Vit. B family) : Helps normal functioning of gastro-intestinal tract and maintaining normal skin condition, Health of nervous system including good memory and absence of insomnia etc. Deficiency may results in gastro intestinal & skin lesions and dysfunction of nervous system, low of weight, insomnia a general weakness. Natural sources are whole wheat, green vegetables, pulses and beans, pea-nuts, brewer's yeast, meat and liver. Daily requirement 20 mg.

Biotin and Folic Acid (Vit, B family) : Function as part of a coenzymes metabolism. Natural sources : fresh vegetables legumes, milk, egg etc. Daily requirement 0.3 mg each

Pantothenic Acid (Vit. B5) : Necessary for synthesis of antibodies, normal digestive and nervous systems, deficiency through rare may result skin and digestive disturbances and dizzy spells. Natural sources : whole wheat, brain, peas, brewer's yeast, molasses, liver and kidney. Daily requirement 10 mg.

Vit. C (Ascorbic Acid) : Holds body cells together, hastens healing and increases resistance to infection. Necessary for healthy teeth, gums and bones, one of the most important factors for good health and vigour, helps in resisting colds and cough. Deficiency may result in bleeding gums, general weakness, anemia. Natural sources : citrus fruits, papers, papaya, mango, tomatoes, potatoes, spinach, peppers, others fruits and vegetables. It is easily destroyed in storage and cooking. Normal requirement 60 mg.

Scientist like twice Nobel prize winner Dr. Linus Pauling strongly recommended heavy special supplements of Vit. C and Vit. E for good health. Both these vitamins are anti oxidants and take care of the incomplete molecular fragments produced in the process of oxidation. These vitamins, according to this school of thought, are remedies for aging.

Vit. D (Coliferon) : Essential for utilization of calcium and phosphorus and formation of good teeth and bones. Deficiency may result in rickets in the children. Natural sources : ultraviolet rays of the sun convert the cholesterol present in the skin to Vit. D, also in milk products and fresh liver oil, excess of it may cause toxic effects. Daily requirement 400 i.u.

Vit. E. (Tocopherol) : Works as anti oxident protecting vitamins A and C and to prevent fats becoming rancid, Vit. E prevents formation of unwanted blood clots. It promotes better circulation and promotes the formation of new skin wounds. Vit. E and oxygen are important to on another and thus Vit. E becomes the most important vitamin along with vitamin C. Deficiency may lead to early aging, loss of reproductive powers and also to muscular dis-orders. Natural sources are whole grain products, wheat germ, green and leafy vegetables, vegetable oil, margarine, butter, eggs, liver. Daily requirement 30 i.u. but could be taken upto 400 i.u. Vitamin E supplements are extremely necessary when Lecithin supplements are extremely necessary when Lecithin supplements are taken.

Vit. F : It promotes growth. Specially necessary for healthy glands, skin and hair. Helps in a assimilation of calcium and also in lowering of cholesterol levels. Deficiency may lead to skin disorders. Natural sources : vegetables oils, eg. sunflower oil, corn oil, soybean oil etc.

Vit. K (Menadione) : Helps maintenance of blood's clotting system. A person may bleed to death from even a small cut if there is deficiency of this vitamin. It is important to the healthy working of liver. It is present in whole grains, Wheat germs Wheat bran, potatoes, tomatoes, cabbage, spinach, egg yolk and liver. This vitamin is produced by bacteria in the human intestines. No necessary to taken as a supplement.

Vitamin P (Bioflavonoid) : Strengthen walls of capillaries, good for high blood pressure patients and builds resistance to colds and infection. Its deficiency may results in weakness of the capillaries and appearance of spots on the skin. Natural sources : peels and pulp of citrus fruits, especially lemon.

Vit. B15 : It makes up the deficiency of oxygen in live tissues. Its natural source is whole wheat, brewer's yeast, unpolished rice, rice polish, pumpkin seeds and sunflower seeds.

Minerals :

It is not generally realised that basic minerals and trace elements found in food are just as essential to health as protective foods, as are the vitamins. Iron for both the blood and calcium for the bones are sometimes very important in supplement form during pregnancies. Deficiency of iodine leads to goiter and low magnesium to cancer. There seems to be relationship between manganese and chromium is needed to maintain normal blood sugar levels and deficiency of zinc in the system may lead to baldness, loss of appetite and sexual dysfunction.

Calcium, phosphorus, sodium, potassium and magnesium are the five important gross or basic minerals for the body. Important trace elements consist of iron, zinc, copper, chromium, manganese, and iodine. Besides the above, nickle, cobalt, fluorine and oxygen, carbon, hydrogen and nitrogen also play a part in our physical well being.

Mineral contents of an average person of 70 kilograms body weight and the average daily intake requirement of such a person are estimated as follows:

TABLE - II Daily requirements of minerals and trace elements.

Minerals and trace elements	Contents of the body of an average	Daily requirements. person in gms.
Calcium	1250	adults 400-500 children 500-800 exp. and lacting mothers 1000-1400
Phosphorus	680	1000
Sodium	75	400 to 1500
Potassium	275	1000 to 1500
Magnesium	45	200 to 400
Iron	7	12 to 15
Copper	.1	2
Chromium	.002	.1 to .2
Manganese	.01	5
Iodine	.01	0.1 to 0.2

Minerals deficiency arises due to lack of minerals in the diet, lack of absorption in the system because of disease, protein deficiency, wrong form of supplementation and also because of perspiration or defective kidneys.

Let us now discuss the functions of individual minerals:

Calcium : It builds and maintains bones and teeth, helps blood to clot, aids vitality and endurance's and regulates heart rhythm and chloesterol level, is good for the nerves, good for muscle cramps and good for menstrual pain. Vitamin D is required specifically for absorption of calcium. Vitamin C also improves calcium absorption. Rickets in children are symptoms of calcium deficiency. Calcium contents of various food is given in table VI. Milk products, pulses, soybeans, green leafy vegetables, citrus fruits and sardines are significant sources of this mineral. If there is not enough calcium in our diet, It is taken from our bones.

Phosphorus : It is needed form the normal bone and tooth structure, inter-related with action of calcium and vitamin D. It is also needed by certain enzymes which help change food into energy. It is also involved in many varied chemical reaction in the body. Its deficiency results in general weakness, bone pain and decreased appetite. Its excess could hinder uptake of calcium. Whole grain bread, cereals, beans, pulses, milk and milk products, eggs, fish, poultry and meat are significant sources of this mineral.

Sodium : It helps maintain water balance inside and outside body cells. It is deficiency can cause muscle cramps, edema but its excess has harmful results like high blood pressure, kidney disease, cirrhosis of the liver and congestive heart diseases. Its main sources is processed food and meat besides common salt.

Potassium : It is necessary for the normal toning of the muscles, nerves, heart action and enzymes reactions. It also helps regulate body fluid balance. Its deficiency can cause weakness or muscles, irregular heart beat and irritability. Its excess can cause cardiac irregularities. Its main source are bananas, dried fruits, orange juice, potatoes and peanuts.

Magnesium : It is necessary for handling of calcium and vitamin C within the body and also necessary for proper functioning of nerves and muscles. It also activates enzymes. Its deficiency can cause cancer and twitching of muscles. Upsetting of calcium-magnesium balance can impair the nervous system. In France low magnesium content of soil is associated with greater incidence of cancer. Its significant sources are nuts and leafy green vegetables.

Iron : It helps to carry oxygen in the blood. It is required in production of hemoglobin And myoglobin which stores oxygen in muscles. Iron deficiency cause anemia, breathlessness, fatigue, weakness etc. Its excess can cause toxic build up. Its significant cereals, whole grain bread, liver, egg yolk, and meat products, Iron content of various foods, is given in table VI.

Zinc : It helps normal tissue functioning and is necessary for handling of proteins and carbohydrates within the body. Its deficiency can cause loss of taste and appetite, delayed wound healing, balness, growth retardation, heart disease, mental illness and delayed sexual maturing. It significant sources are milk, yolk, fish and meats. Zinc deficiency can caused by alcoholism, food refining, low proteins diet, cold, pregnancy and disease. Zinc deficiency reduces release of vitamin A from the liver and healing of wounds and reproductive functions are also adversely affected. Zinc is relatively non-toxic. Intestines have an efficient mechanism for disposing of the extra quantities of zinc not required by the body.

Chromium : It helps the muscles to take up sugar from the blood and also control fatty acid and cholesterol synthesis. Its deficiency leads to a condition hardly distinguishable from mid diabetes. Its sources are whole grain cereals, brewer's yeast, and liver.

Manganese : It is directly associated with the defence mechanism of the body. It activates various enzymes and helps properutilisation of vitamin B and E. Its significant sources are tea, coffee, peas, nuts and beans.

Iodine : It is necessary for proper functioning of the thyroid gland. It also acts as a catalyst to stimulate conversion of body fat to energy. Its deficiency causes goiter. Its main sources are iodized salts and seafood.

It is not considered necessary to deal here with some other traces elements like cobalt, fluorine, molybdenum, sulpher etc.

TABLE - III Mineral and trace elements content of some foods

(Amount in milligrams per 100 gms of edible portion of the food)

Food	Phosphorous	Potassium	Magnesium	Zinc	Copper	Chromium	Manganese
Cow milk	100	150	15	.4	.04	NA	.002
Dried skimmed milk	1000	1200	140	3.5	NA	NA	NA
Yogurt (curd)	150	250	[illegible]	[illegible]	NA	NA	NA
Cottage cheese	!50	55	20	2	NA	NA	NA
Processed cheese	500	85	25	4	NA	NA	NA
Whole wheat bread	250	220	150	3	.3	.01	4.2
White flour bread	100	220	25	1	.2	.008	0.7
Soya Flour	650	NA	300	NA	NA	NA	NA
Unpolished rice	300	NA	NA	NA	NA	NA	NA
Polished rice	110	NA	15	0.4	.2	NA	NA
Potatoes	NA	NA	15	0.4	.2	NA	NA
Cabbage	35	350	18	0.4	NA	.02	.1
orange	25	225	15	0.1	.1	.01	.03
Peanuts	4000	NA	180	NA	.3	NA	NA
Honey	18	55	2	NA	0.5	NA	NA
Yeast Baker's	400	620	60	1.5	1.5	NA	NA
Peas	NA	350	32	0.8	NA	NA	2.0
Wheat germ	950	820	520	NA	1.5	NA	4.0
Dried dates	NA	750	60	NA	.2	.01	NAk
Bananas	NA	360	45	NA	70	.01	.6
Apples	NA	110	NA	.1	NA	1.5	NA
Amends/cashews	NA	NA	250	NA	1.5	NA	2
Eggs	225	150	13	1.6	.1	.007	.03
Chicken	210	325	25	1	NA	.01	NA
Meat	160	280	25	4	.1	.01	NA
Fish	250	300	30	0.5	NA	.01	NA

Filter:

The indigestible residue of plants is popularly known as fiber as fiber or roughage in health related sciences. The nutritionists are becoming more and more aware of advantages of dietary fiber. The Surgeon General of USA a has recently advised Americans to double the fibre content of their diets because is linked to the prevention of the killer diseases.

The action of fibre is more mechanical and less nutritional. The fibre on entering the diagestive system absorbed liquids, mixes with other foods and swells. This mass, during its movement through the system, is kept soft by the fibre content. The nutrients are utilised by the system in a regulated mannre and the fibre rich mass with the waste materials comfortably winds its way through the intestines to elimination.

There are two types of fibres, one water soluble founds in nuts, legumes, apples, oats and barely etc. Which lower cholesterol bad blood fats and control blood sugar levels and second water insoluble fibre found in bran, whole grains and vegetables which controls costipation etc. Research has demonstrated that constopation, diarrhea, and similar conditions are greatly helped by sufficient fibre intake.

The best source of fibre are the whole wheat, unpolished rice, other whole grains and their products, and unprocessed fruits and vegetables. Refining and processing reduces the effectivenss of the fibre content and sometimes even removes the fibre altogether.

Calories

Calory requirements of a person depend upon frame, metabolic rate, age, climate and type of work he does. Calory requirements of a person doing hard manual labour could even be 50% or 100% more than that of a person with collar job doing office work only.

According to a detailed study, calories burnt per minute in various activities by a person of average metabolism of 60 kgs. (1321bs) weight would be as follows.

TABLE - IV Calories burnt in various activities.

Laying still	1.0
Sitting, standing, reading, writing eating, playing cards and handsewing	1.5
Driving jcar, tailoring	2.0
Washing Floors, sweeping and ironing	2.2
Golf	2.5
Walking 5 km. (3 miles) per hour speed	3.0
Walking 7 km. (4.4 miles) per hour speed	4.5
Walking 9 km. (5.6 miles) per hour speed	9.0
Gardening, weeding etc.	5.0
Cycling (depending upon speed)	3.5 to 8.0
Boxing, Rowing	12.0
Dancing,	5.0
Table Tennis	5.50
Tennis	6.0
Swimming 3Km (2 miles) per hour speed	9.0
Football	8.0
Other exercises	
Light	2.5
Moderate	4.0
Serve	8.0

TABLE V Daily caories requirements

Age	Calory requirement
upto 6 months	120 calories per kg. body weight.
7-12 months	100 calories per kg. body weight.
1-3 years	1200 calories per kg. body weight.
4-6 years	1500 calories per kg. body weight
7-9 years	1800 calories per kg. body weight
10-12 years	2100
13-15 years-boys	2500
13-15 years-girls	2200
16-18 years-boys	3000
16-18 years-girls	2200
Men light work	2200
Medium work	2800
Heavy work	3400
Women Light work	1900
Medium work	2200
heavy work	2800

Nutritive Values of food :

Its more or less known that a particular article of food has so many calories, proteins vitamins, minerals, enzymes and natural glucose etc. But that does not that as soon as that food article goes within you, immediately that much energy is transferred to the various parts of body. It depends upon various body system as to how much energy and other elements they can extract from that food and transfer to various systems of your body. Mind draws its power from the soul and directs all sense organs. Mind has no other power sources of its own. It is, therefore, clear that it depends upon your physical, emotional, mental and spiritual levels of that time as to how much energy etc. you can extract or draw from the food you eat.

Nutritive elements which are ordinarily present in various items are indicated in table VI given below. This table gives only the averages. The child inherits many qualities and defects of mother. In same way many deficiencies of the mother earth are found in the food produced therein. Consequently food grown in different from the averages indicated in the table given below. This table gives the various elements found in 100 gms of the edible portion of those foods.

Weight:

What should be the average weight of a healthy person? This will depend upon your age, height and body frame, then even with a heavy weight, you could be considered healthy. In the table given below, on the basis of the charts of a life insurance Corporation, for various heights and ages, two types of weights are given-one which is considered ideal for that age and height and other is the maximum weight beyond which even a person of the broadest frame should be considered unhealthy.

TABLE VII Ideal and maximum body weights for various ages and heights.

Height in cms. Ideal-Max	Age 18-22 Ideal-Max		Age 23-27 Ideal-Max		Age 28-32 Ideal-Max		Age 33-37	
150	45.5		47.0		48.3		49.4	
152	46.2	56	47.8	58	49.7	62	50.4	63
154	47.1		48.7		50.3		51.5	
156	48.0		49.7		51.4		52.6	
158	49.5	59	50.8	61	52.5	65	53.7	67
160	50.0		52.0		53.7		54.9	
162	51.2	62	53.2	65	54.9	69	56.1	70
164	52.4		54.4		56.2		57.5	
166	53.7		55.4		56.2		57.5	
168	55.1	66	57.2	69	59.9	73	60.6	75
170	56.5		58.7		60.6		62.2	
171	58.0		60.2		62.1		63.9	
		71		73		78		80
174	59.5		61.7		63.7		65.6	
176	61.0		63.3		65.3		67.3	
178	62.5	75	64.9	78	67.0	83	69.0	85
180	64.1		66.5		68.7		70.7	
182	65.7		68.1		70.4		72.4	
		80		83		88		90
184	67.3		69.7		72.1		74.1	
186	68.9		71.4		73.8		75.8	
188	70.5	85	73.1	87	75.6	94	77.8	96
190	72.1		74.8		77.4		79.6	

Height in cms. Ideal-Max	Age 38-42 Ideal-Max		Age 43-47 Ideal-Max		Age 48-52		Age	
150	49.8		50.1		50.3		50.5	
152	50.8	64	51.1	64	51.3	64	51.5	64
154	51.9		52.2		52.4		52.1	
156	53.0		53.3		53.6		53.7	
158	54.1	67	54.4	68	54.7	68	54.9	68
160	55.3		55.7		56.0		56.3	
162	56.6		57.0		57.4		57.7	
		71		72		72		72

164	58.0		58.5		58.9		59.2	
166	59.5		60.0		60.4		60.8	
168	61.1	75	61.6	76	62.0	76	62.4	76
170	62.8		63.3		63.7		64.1	
172	64.5		65.0		65.5		65.9	
		81		81		81		
174	66.2	80		66.7	67.3		67.7	
176	67.9		68.4		69.1		69.5	
178	69.6	86	70.2	87	70.9	87	71.3	87
180	71.3		72.0		72.7		73.2	
182	73.0		73.8		74.5		75.1	
		92		93		93		93
184	74.8		75.6		76.3		77.0	
186	76.6		77.4		78.1		78.9	
188	78.4	97	79.2	98	79.9	98	80.8	98
190	80.2		81.0		81.7		82.7	

The above table gives the extreme limits beyond which you should not allow your weight to go. It also gives you the ideal weight for your height and age. It is now for you decide as to hoe much reduction (or increase) in your weight is required and over what period is that reduction to be achieved. You, in your particular situation, Know the average daily calory requirement of your body and can calculate as to how many calories less you may take daily to achieve the desired reduction in weight. Then looking to the overall state of your health, and also to your own tastes, you may decide which food article in what quantity you can take every day to achieve the desired result. If some food article is good for your health but you dislike it, then with a sudden shift, your palate will not get that satisfaction and your body mechanism will not send out the required digestive juices and enzymes etc. For digestion of that food. You will thus not benefit from the change over. Let such a change be gradual and your tastes change gradually and you gradually start liking those food articles which are good for your health. Reduction in quantities can take place soonest.

Go ahead with the change required in the type of food that you eat. In taking such decisions also take into consideration the acidity/alkalinity of the foods and their cholesterol content.

ACIDIC AND ALKALINE FOOD:

With increase acidity in the stomach, many digestive problems arise. If care is not taken in this regard ulcers may even develop. It is consequently necessary that you should not eat such food which increases acidity in the stomach. Cereals, pulses and all types of meats and fish increase acidity when taken. And almost all vegetables and fruits increase alkalinity in the stomach and so decrease the acidity. Lemon, oranges, malta, grapefgruits and other fruits which have citric acid, when taken, decrease the acidity in the stomach. Unboiled milk produces alkalinity and the boiled milk and its products produce acidity.

Table below give how much acidity or alkalinity do various produce when taken. On the basis of information given in these tables and on the basis of your own health conditon, decide which of these foods you should avoid or include in your diet.

TABLE-VIII ACIDITY OF 100 GMS OF FOOD IN HC-L UNITS

Wheat, white flour and bread	75-80	Egg	110
Maize, barley and bajra	55-70	Fish	90-115
Rice	70-80	Chicken	100
Roasted gram and peas	30	other meats	100
Cheese	50-60	Chocolate	75
Cake	40	Phirni (Rice flour and milk)	90
Cauliflower	100	Freshcorn	25
Small bitter gourd	25		

TABLE IX ALKALINITY OF 100 GMS OF FOOD IN NA-OH UNITS

Unboiled milk	20	Papaya	20
Churned Yogurt	25	Coconut	75
Lemon	30	Peach	70
Lime juice	110	Apricot dried	30
Orange, grapefruit	40-50	Figs dried	1000
Malta, pineapple	30	Banana	40
Phalsa (grewisasiatica)	150	Cheeku fruit	95
Pear	20	Grapes	30
Guava	10	Brinjal	15
Jamun Black berry	40	Okra (ladies finger)	30
Lichi	70	Spinach	130
Musk Melon	130	Beet	100
Apple	25	Gourd	25
Pomegranate	40	Carrot	250
Almonds	125	Radish	25
Raisins	250	Kulfa saag	250
Coriander	150	Ice cream	5
Tomatoes	50	Soybean	50

CHOLESTEROL IN FOOD :

Cholesterol is a fat like substance which is produced mainly in the liver. It is important in the structure of body cells and hormones. Cholesterol also constitutes a building block of waxy deposits which grow inside the arteries.

Some food articles contain large amount of cholesterol. Use of such articles products cholesterol deposits in the veins and arteries. These gradually narro down resulting in high blood pressure and heart diseases. Quantity in milligrams of cholesterol in 100 gms edible portion of certain special food articles is as follows:

TABLE CHOLESTEROL CONTENT IN 100 GMS EDIBLE PORTION OF VARIOUS FOODS

Butter	280	Liver	320-420
Cheeses, Cream	110	Brain	2000
Chedder	98	Vegetables	NIL
Blue	157	Cereals	NIL
Cottage	1	Fruits	NIL
Egg Yolk	2000	Cup of whole milk	35
White of egg	460	Cup of skimmed milk	1
Sheep meat	66	cup of sharbat	6
other meats	60-100		

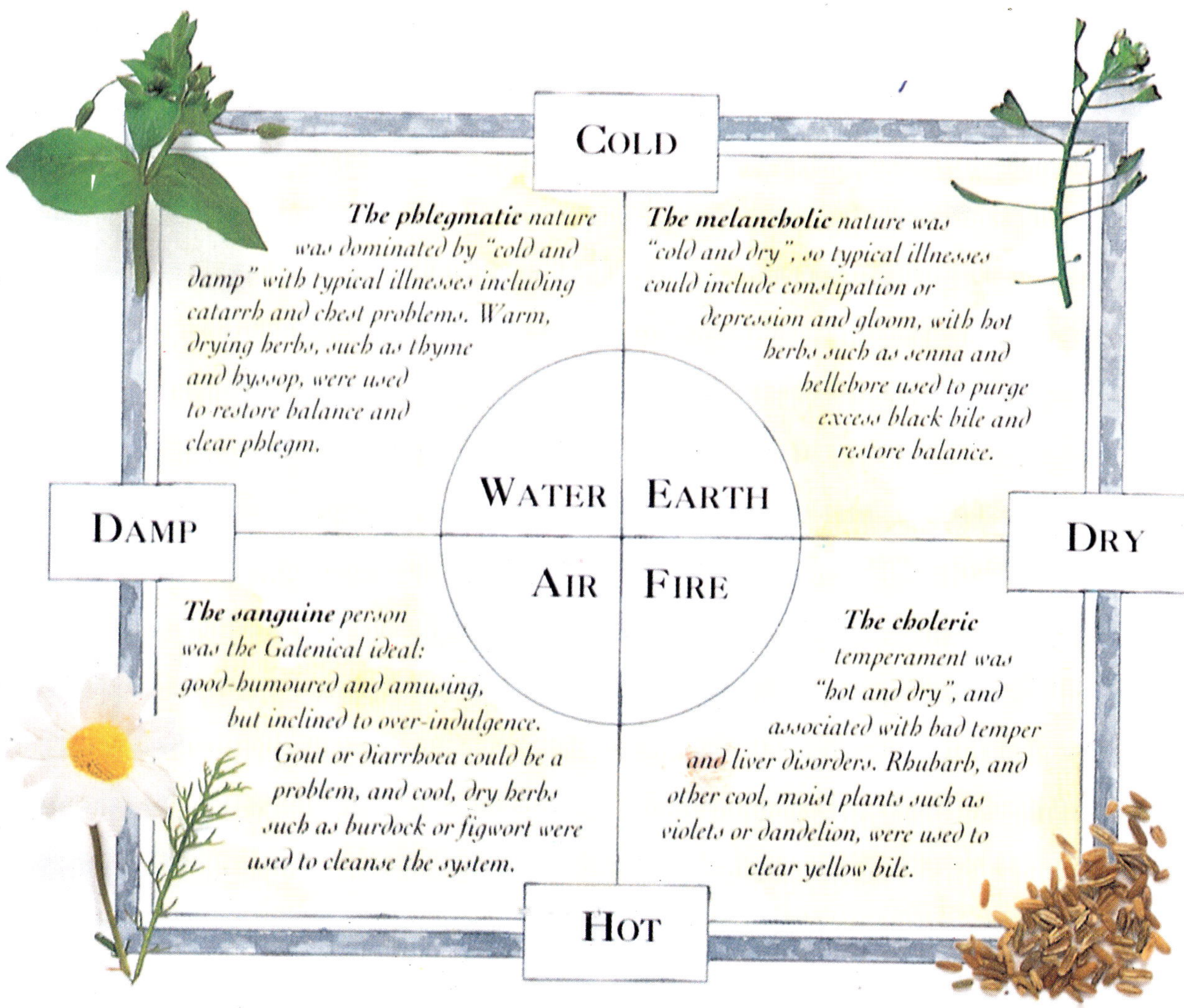

Part III

Naturopathic Treatment of Cancer

Chapter XV

The Naturopathic Perspective On Cancer

There are 107 vital points in the body. Cancers are usually located on these vital points. These vital points are junctions where the flesh, blood vessels, muscles, bones and joints meet. Our life force flows through these vital points and generates a nectar-like vital energy in each of them. Death occurs instantaneously if any of these vital centres is hit hard. Naturopathy therefore discourages biopsy, surgery or the application of rays of any sort on these vital centres.

Cancer results when there is a severe impediment of the flow of our life force or energy in any of these vital centres. These blockages are caused by chronic diseases that the body has harboured for a long period of time. Cancer is generally the end-result of a series of chronically assimilated toxic contaminations of several minor diseases, that are retained in various forms by the membranes of our body. Most of us seldom heed our minor ailments. Until our body is totally stricken and helpless, we strain it to the limit, and when it ceases to work, we abruptly leave all our so called important affairs and begin to take treatments of various kinds for its recovery. But by then, the diseases has usually crossed its primary stages and we have no choice but to deal with it in its fully grown, rampant form. The body is then entirely in its clutches with little room for manoeuvre or escape. Past negligence and ignorance is the basic cause of this state of affairs.

One of my patients had a cold and cough to begin with, which became chronic and turned into cancer. It is always our negligence toward the cure of a disease in its primary stages that lets it increase in an unabated fashion and ultimately turns it into cancer. Just as a tiny seed of a big oak tree is a microcosm of the vast tree, the smallest form of an illness contains all the potentials of a "difficult to cure" disease. The first appearance of a disease is generally a tiny one and it often seems as if no complication would result from it. But just like giving air to a little spark of fire may burn a palatial building to ashes, similarly, ignoring a tiny disease today may turn it into a hard-to-cure disease tomorrow.

When body cells are starved of their life energy, they become cancerous and begin to grow and multiply in an abnormal fashion. These cells then spread through the body in the form of primary and secondary growths. Naturopathic treatment restores the flow of our life force in all the 107 vital centres of the body, and this treatment therefore eliminates the very cause of cancer.

Cancer has three stages: (i) irritation; (ii) inflammation; (iii) induration, i.e. the process of hardening. Ulceration or the process of quick increase of a disease is really the last stage of the symptoms of cancer. A clear-cut delineation of all the above three stages is not possible, as they are all interconnected and interdependent. But ulceration can generally be called one of the manifestations of fully developed cancer.

It is thus clear that cancer originates when one gives insufficient care to one's life-style. Poor habits, irregular routine and an intemperate life-style, all sow the seeds of cancer at an early age.

A patient lying in a hospital bed often vows to take better care of his health, but these vows are generally like the promises that a student makes to study regularly next year, at the very brink of his examinations this year. Such students repent piteously before their examinations and pray to God that if He would help them to cross their ordeal this year, they would pay proper heed to their studies next year. But once they have crossed their ordeal both the student and the patient forget their promises and continue to live just as they did earlier.

Naturopaths believe that cancer is a result of the ignorance of the laws of Nature, coupled with the neglect of minor aliments. They have come to this conclusion after graphically and exhaustively examining the etiology of all the available research and scientific literature on the subject.

It is generally believed that all the research, discoveries and progress made in the field of cancer have not succeeded in reporting actual causes of cancer. This is why it is commonly believed that there is no link between living habits, diet and cancer. But according to Naturopathy, faulty living and heedless disregard of the laws of Nature result in the assimilation of toxic substances in our body, which is the first stage of cancer. When these substances are accumulated endlessly over a long period of time, the body becomes diseased and cancerous.

In the eventual analysis, the cause of cancer is in our mind and not our body, because it is the mind that forges wrong habits and initiates the disregard of Nature's laws. Just as beautiful roses have their origin not in their branches but in the soil, similarly, the origin of a disease is not in the body but in the mind.

According to naturopathy, cancer is not merely localized in the part in which it discovered. For example, the hardening of the breast or tumour in the penis or the vagina which are surgically removed are merely overt forms of its manifestation. It probably also exists in a latent from elsewhere in the body.

I once treated an elderly lady who had a cancerous tumour in her intestines. Her husband was a renowned doctor. The tumour had been subjected to several doses of radiotherapy, at the end of which the lady still complained, "The tumour has been destroyed by radium but I have irritation in my whole body. Please check what is wrong." She was right: the cancer had indeed spread to the rest of her body. I advised her to discontinue her treatment and instead, eat only natural, purified meals. These detoxified her body and she had a complete recovery after following this natural regime.

Sometimes, unabated ulceration becomes a cancer. Once, an old friend, who works in Nisargopachar Ashram, was admitted to the Sassoon Hospital in Pune for the surgical removal of a small gastric ulcer. But during surgery, it was found that his gastric ulcer was cancerous. Neither the doctor nor the patient had even suspected such a condition. The fact that he had been diagnosed to have cancer, which is supposed to be an incurable disease, caused him unbearable mental tension. He eventually died after prolonged mental torture.

How does an ulcer become a cancer? What is the mystery of this process? Replies to this question are primarily focused on our life-style. Even after a patient knows he has cancer, he continues to lead a faulty life-style because of his ignorance about its connection with cancer. This results in his bodily imbalances becoming even more chronic and makes the disease take deeper root instead of being eradicated. This is an unconscious process which is beyond the limits of normal human awareness.

Then again, one may ask how a cancerous ulcer came into being. The fact is that the ulcer did not appear all of a sudden. Hyperacidity in the body caused an outbreak of irritation which altered the cell chemistry, which in turn led to the conversion of normal cells into cancerous ones. The unchecked proliferation of these cells was speeded up by a lack of intake of certain nutrients and was aggravated by mental tension. As a result, a hard tumour of these cells began to form. It released some of its cells into the blood stream, which transported them elsewhere in the body, and thus laid the foundation for another tumour.

The renounced naturopath Dr. Tandon says:

> Cancer in its primary stages is just an inflammation of our membranes, and nothing more than this. We come often across instances when ulcers on the lip, tongue, large intestines or uterus have become cancerous. Patients who are in the clutches of this disease, all have a sufficient quantity of assimilated contaminants which irritate the local membranes on which they accumulate. The prevention of this disease will only become possible when we try to understand that our stomach (mainly the large and small intestines), is the longest, dirtiest drainage system of the world which is more dangerous than the dirty drainage systems of big cities like Bombay, London, New York and Tokyo.

Another authority, Victor B. Fleming, says:

> The first and foremost cause of cancer is the excessive assimilation of contaminated acids in our body. Of the many reasons for our body cells becoming weak, the most important are old age, sores, regular irritation and the faulty activation of some of the tissues of our body. This causes increased acidity in our cells. Just as no seed can grow in stony ground, cancer cells cannot grow in a body which is free of faulty acids. Besides, sometimes, there is an interruption in the blood circulation to important parts of our body which accelerates the growth of unhealthy cells. Eventually, due to all these reasons, our life force becomes unbalanced and the body develops "hard-to-cure" diseases like cancer.

Food and Cancer

Cancerous tumours are found more frequently in non-vegetarians than among vegetarians. Just as an excessive quantity of nitrogen creates cancerous tumours in plants, similarly, a non-vegetarian diet contains a high level of nitrogen which creates a more fertile breeding ground for cancer in the body than a vegetarian diet does. Many experimental studies and research have proved that nitrogen-containing foods contaminate body tissues much faster than other foods do, and therefore, stimulate the growth of cancer cells.

Both the intake of contaminated food and gluttonous eating habits are potential trouble makers. The outbreak of any disease is, in reality, an alarm being sounded by the body warning us that our wrong habits are creating havoc within us. But if we do not pay heed to it because of our ignorance, then our body becomes helpless to do anything else, and tissue irritation slowly builds up within it. In this manner, should acidity and irritation surpass the tolerance limits of our body, toxins and other harmful chemicals are produced. These eventually alter the basic body chemistry. When this kind of situation persists over a prolonged period, malignancies are created.

Naturopaths believe that cancer develops in those tissues in which these toxic chemicals accumulate the most. Naturopaths also give primary importance to other etiological causes, the most significant of which are imbalances in the body's metabolic and hormonal systems.

Irritation as a Principal Cause of Cancer

Cancer of the cervix, the excretory canal, the lip, the tongue, the neck and the intestines have a direct correlation with their sustained irritation by toxic chemicals over a prolonged period of time.

Irritation is not the only reason for the growth of cancer, but is one of its principal causative factors. In today's environment, we find that many are addicted to smoking and the chewing of betel-nuts and tobacco, as a result of which their lungs or their tongues become chronically irritated. Several people have sores in the delicate parts of their bodies which itch and cause them continuous irritation. These conditions predispose them to cancer, but the actual emergence of this disease is often precipitated by other factors like imbalances in their body system as a whole.

X-ray, paraffin, arsenic, edible oils, tar, etc. can only lay the foundation for cancer by causing chronic sores, when the body is already in a process of continuous degeneration and is saturated with contaminated acids which have caused an anti-clockwise circulation of its protein-linked metabolic chemicals.

The body's resistance and the capacity of its cells to fight disease decreases considerably just before the outbreak of cancer, i.e., at the pre-cancerous stage. This stage sets in sooner in persons with a delicate condition and later in persons with a high level of natural body resistance.

Chapter XVI

Testimonials of Cancer Cure Through Naturopathy

Testimonial 1

I travelled to Denmark in February 1980, to visit a well-known Naturopathic Hospital at Hyamle Garden. This hospital had been founded by the renowned naturopath, Dr. Cristie Nolfi, and is internationally reputed for its high success rate in curing cancer. Dr. Nolfi herself had cancer which she had treated with naturopathic methods with great dedication, battling against a multitude of social pressures. Even though she was a qualified allopathic doctor, she did not resort to any form of allopathic therapy other than the initial investigative tests. From the very beginning, she was confident that nature alone would cure her disease--which it did. Her story is a unique example of how a person who has been trained in the scientific disciplines of modern allopathy has rejected them in favour of naturopathy.

After being cured of cancer, she turned into a naturopath herself and has functioned as a naturopath ever since. This was an uphill task and a surfeit of problems beset her at every stage. Her own friends turned against her. They filed one legal case after another against her, had her legally punished and ultimately robbed her of the right of medical practice despite her medical certificate. But instead of being demoralized, she reacted positively to these adversities and felt happy that all the negative affiliations and connections in her life had been exposed. She met all the challenges with peace and equanimity and ultimately emerged victorious. The naturopathic centre which she set up is one of the finest in Europe.

Dr. Nolfi describes her experiences in these words:

> In the winter of 1940-41, I constantly felt dull, heavy and tired, but was unable to identify my illness. I just did not know what to do about my condition. Then in spring, I noticed a small tumour in my right breast. After much introspection, I realized that my poor digestion for the last twelve years, which was due to my faulty food habits and consumption of contaminated edibles, precipitated this condition. In addition, for the last few years, I had also had some intestinal inflammation. I was sure that these conditions had led to the growth of cancer in my body. I felt extremely guilty and remorseful about my condition, especially because I, myself, was a medical practitioner and could have easily cured it if I had paid enough attention to it.
>
> This small tumour quickly grew to the size of a hen's egg and began to look exactly like a cancerous tumour. I then consulted one of my friends, Dr. Hindhead, who was a well-known cancer specialist. He was against doing a biopsy right away, because his experience had shown that ripping open the veins during a biopsy actually increases the spread of the disease. After consulting him, I immediately abandoned the idea of biopsy. Thereafter I decided to treat myself through my diet, and started eating only fresh uncooked foods and abstained from everything that had been processed or cooked.
>
> I then began to look for a place where I could be in constant contact with mother nature. I shifted to a small island called Kattegat. Readers should remember that there are many islands near Denmark both big and small. On this secluded island, I lay in the sun for four to five hours a day, bathed several times every day and ate natural and unprocessed foods.
>
> For about two years, there was no change in my depression and lassitude, or in the size of my tumour. But I drew solace from the fact that none of them appeared to get any worse. Then slowly, but gradually, there was a perceptible change in my health. The tumour began to decrease and as its size reduced, I began to feel more energetic and refreshed.

Soon, I began to feel much healthier than I had felt for a long time.

I lived on raw foods for another year more, and continued to feel increasingly healthy and energetic. My tumour virtually disappeared. At this point I knew that the cycle of recovery was firmly established in my body, and would now continue by itself. So I modified my diet and resumed my intake of processed foods to the extent of 50 per cent of my diet. The result was disastrous. I began to feel a stretching pain in my breast which became worse as the weeks went by. After some time, the size of my tumour began to increase once again.

Thereafter, I resumed my regimen of eating only uncooked foods which alleviated my symptoms once again. My tumour almost vanished after several months of this treatment. Then in the spring of 1946, I received a parcel of dry fruits from Denmark which contained currants, dates, almonds, nuts, etc. I felt that these dry fruits would help me, and ate them all up. The result was not good because various chemicals had been used to protect and preserve these dry fruits. Three or four months after eating them, I began to get a severe pain at the site of the tumour. A minute physical examination revealed that a small tumour had again grown on my right breast. But it soon vanished as I continued with my diet of fresh foods. After it had disappeared completely for a few months, I felt extremely elated, and wanted to seek confirmation that it was completely gone.

I then committed the biggest blunder in my life and underwent the biopsy operation which Dr. M. Hindhead had cautioned me against. I agreed to it this time, because some of my doctor friends advised me that it would not harm me, as in all probability, I had no cancer. This biopsy operation was conducted in Copenhagen in January 1948. A few cancer cells were found at the site of the tumour in my right breast but were diagnosed as being in the primary stage of cancer. My cancer thus had dwindled to a very primary stage, which is normally always undetected as it is painless. However instead of making me happy, the results of the biopsy made me extremely frightened because I remembered Dr. Hindhead's warning that a biopsy operation increases the spread or cancer. Soon afterwards, in just a few months, tumours appeared in each of my breasts. After this, I took no chances again. I returned to my diet of raw foods for six months, and did not commit any negligence whatsoever this time. Soon everything became all right and my general health also improved.

My daily routine consisted of rising before sunrise and working in my small garden for several hours. This routine made it impossible for me to continue with my medical practice, so I gave it up in January 1949, and spent all time gardening. I grew my own foods using natural, compost manure. I did not even use dung, which was another natural manure, and far easier to obtain. I felt physically and mentally more active and alive than I had ever felt in my life.

My cancer was completely cured in this manner. The irony was that nobody believed me. Several experts of the modern medical system minutely checked me out, and could not find any trace of my disease. But rather than sharing my happiness, they were upset that a system which was so radically different from theirs had succeeded in curing a disease like cancer, which everybody believed was virtually incurable. They attacked me professionally and launched criminal proceedings against me for the natural death of two of my patients years ago. I was totally isolated, and did not stand a chance against so many of them. In the end, I was left with no alternative but to succumb to their wishes and give up my medical practice for ever. Thus, the chapter of my medical practice closed abruptly, and I dedicated myself to the field of naturopathy. Its results have been very successful and encouraging. The eating of uncooked foods and a few other treatments like hydrotherapy and radiation form the basis of my treatment.

Testimonial 2

"How I could get Rid of Cancer"--The story of Mariam Nesham Barzaam of Tehran (born 25 July 1931)

In April 1974, I felt some unusual sensations in my right breast. When they began to trouble me, I went to my doctor who checked me out thoroughly, and X-rayed my chest. As these investigations did not reveal anything, I ignored these sensations. Then, after about two months I developed acute pain in my breast so I ran to my doctor who diagnosed my condition as cancer and began to treat me for this disease.

I was informed on 16 September 1974 that I should undergo a diagnostic biopsy which would last for about fifteen minutes. But the doctors warned me that if, after opening me up, they felt that the cancer was widespread, they would do a mastectomy. When I gained consciousness I found that I had lost my right breast and also the functioning of my right hand.

After my breast surgery I underwent forty sessions of cobalt-based radiotherapy. X-rays of my lung were also taken after every three months.

Until March 1975 I found that there was no further change in my condition. But soon afterwards, my right thigh began to pain. This time when the doctors X-rayed me, they found that I had bone cancer. After a thorough check-up, they once again asked me to go in for surgery, in order to protect my body from a further spread of the disease. They removed my uterus and ovaries as well. But even after taking away all my reproductive organs, the pain in my right thigh persisted and began to increase. At this stage I preferred to go abroad for treatment. Since Israeli doctors made me undergo a thorough a burden they should have broken with the strain. (By then, I had begun to walk with the help of a stick.) I was again given cobalt treatment but this time on my feet. After fifteen sessions, I came back to my home in Tehran with a suitcase full of X-ray plates and prescriptions.

I was advised to undertake chemotherapy for one week every month, for six months. My weight began to increase after the first treatment and my hair began to fall from my head, and grow on my face instead.

One day, when I was peacefully taking my medicine, I chanced upon a paper which fell out of the medicine packet. It said that the medicine which I was taking, could result in twelve types of reactions, including death.

This was the turning point in my life. I firmly resolved, there and then, to stop all my medicines and leave my fate in the hands of God.

After about ten months, something momentous happened to me once again. One of my friends told me that a diet of raw foods can cure cancer. I decided to follow this advice immediately. The very next day, I went to a vegetarian shop and obtained all the information that I could lay my hands on about the nutritional elements in vegetarian food. But initially, for the first few days I ate a mixed diet of both cooked and uncooked foods. Also because I had been eating cooked non--vegetarian meals for the last forty-five years, it was difficult for me to stop them altogether.

But gradually, eating natural foods everyday infused me with fresh encouragement, and soon I began to eat only raw foods. These included fresh fruits, green vegetables, roots, honey and dry fruits.

After about two months, I felt as though there was magic in my body. There was an all-round improvement in my health. I found a new life and freshness in my body. After a few months, I went to the hospital for a body scan and X-ray. After comparing the old and new X-ray plates, the Doctor said, ''Your bones are even stronger than mine''. This occurred in April 1977. I felt elated because the cancer had disappeared in most of my body. I have preserved all my old and new X-ray plates which are an eloquent witness of the story of my troubles and my struggle with life.

The whole structure of my body has been resurrected by new diet which I consumed for nineteen months. I now have a new life in me. The insensibility in my right hand which had appeared after the first surgical operation of my right breast also vanished. All the sensations in my right hand have returned completely. This is the largest testimonial of my recovery.

This is my second year of eating only uncooked foods. I had passed through the acute pain and discomfort of cancer, radiotherapy and chemotherapy for two years. I cannot forget those days, as the trauma was really intense. I have an intense gratitude for the author of the book *Raw Diet* which gave me a new life and saved me from death.

During the last thirteen months I lost twenty kilograms of extra weight which the chemotherapy had made me gain. I am now working for a full eight hours every day in Iran Insurance Company. I can now fulfil my desire to live a happy life and remain in good health for ever.

Testimonial 3

Testimonial of Dr. Vansala, MD, Bombay, 28 June 1977.

Patient: Sushilabahn Agarwal; age 54 years; born 6 April 1923; height 4'10"; weight 86 lb.

Treatment: Papillary Adeno Carcinoma. [This is an extraordinary nasopharyngeal carcinoma, which could originate in even a minor salivary gland.]

Symptoms

1. Obstruction in the left nasal canal for the last four years.
2. Bleeding from the left nasal canal for the last seven years. (The disease started in 1965 when blood sometimes came out of the nose, mixed with mucus. She also had a temperature of 100 F and a cold. She recovered from her cold, but her fever remained for almost one year).
3. A mucous mass mixed with blood was detected in the lower part of the inside of the nose.
4. Examination of lower inner part of the nose revealed the presence of a bluish mass on the left lateral wall.

   On 16 June 1977 it was found that the mass had rapidly increased in the upper and lower part of nasal cavity. A biopsy was taken immediately which resulted in a loss of nasal canal. A pack was installed to stop bleeding, which took a full 24 hours to cease.

Tata Memorial Hospital (Cancer Department) Report

Sender: Dr. J.N. Surraiya, MS, FACT, FICS.

I endorse the view that there is a tumour of cancer in the inner nasal wall as has been diagnosed by ENT Specialist and Surgeon Dr. Chaturvedi of the Mahatma Gandhi Medical Centre and that the tumour is increasing despite the present natural treatment. The biopsy slides that I have seen definitely prove the emergence of cancer.

Keeping in view the place of the tumour, I recommend that the patient must undergo radiotherapy with tele-cobalt at the earliest.

History

The patient has been thin and frail ever since her childhood, and had frequent occurrences of constipation and headache. Her first opportunity to read naturopathic literature came at the age of 16 after which she changed her food habits and began to put soil dressings on the lower part of her body. These cured her constipation.

During the Bhudan revolution, her irregular and mismanaged dieting resulted in chronic diarrhoea Also, her participation in the physical labour associated with this movement caused intestinal troubles.

After a while, she managed to rest and control her diet once again, and thus managed to alleviate these troubles. She had typhoid in 1954 which was successfully treated by chloromycetin pills.

Her menstruation ceased between 1957 and 1959, but thereafter it become regular. She was bitten by a dog in 1962, and was given a long course of anti-rabies injections.

Her symptoms of cold accompanied by nasal bleeding started in 1965, and began to recur after every four to five months. These symptoms usually lasted for about two weeks every time.

In 1968, even the phlegm of her cough began to contain blood and droplets of blood began to flow out of her nose periodically. This was the time that she had a cough and cold and a chronic fever of 100 F for a year.

However her sputum examination report remained normal for about a year. Thereafter, her fever was cured by naturopathic treatment but her symptoms of recurring cold and nose bleeds continued to appear at regular intervals of three to four months. Besides these, her breathing through the left nasal canal became obstructed. Sometimes blood particles were seen with her cough.

In 1970 her menstruation became irregular once again, and was accompanied by heavy bleeding which lasted for several days.

In 1971 she was found to have a fibrous tumour in her uterus, for which she was given non-invasive treatment. But as the fibroid did not reduce, she was advised to have it surgically removed.

In 1973 Dr. Koticha operated upon the fibroid, which now weighed approximately 2 kg.

In 1974 a little pressing of her left breast began to result in a blood-stained discharge from the nipple. Dr. Koticha operated upon her breast and discovered two small tumours in it, which he surgically removed and sent for biopsy. Fortunately, they were found to be beginning.

By December 1975 her colds and nasal bleeding had become a very frequent occurrence.

Then in December 1976, her grandfather who was a naturopath, stopped her consumption of oil and ghee and started feeding her with a mixture of coconut, *awalah* and leafy vegetables in small quantities along with bread. However, her nasal discharges of blood and mucus continued from the nasal canal. In addition, she once again experienced an obstruction while inhaling from her left nostril.

The renowned ENT specialist and surgeon Dr. Chaturvedi in Mahatma Gandhi Hospital, Sevagram, examined her and found that the tumour inside her nose was increasing rapidly.

In January 1977, she consulted Dr. Maooskar. His treatment resulted in a stoppage of bleeding from the left nasal canal, but this remission was short-lived, as it began to recur shortly afterwards. A few months later, it soon intensified and became almost continuous. Dr. Maooskar carried on his treatment for five months. On 16 June 1977, he suggested that she undertake cancer treatment.

Dr. Sharan Prasad, a naturopath, began to treat her from 1 July 1977. At the outset, he forbade the consumption of cooked foods and milk and prescribed the following diet for her--

- 6 am 20 to 30 gm of millet juice.
- 7 am Sucking of four sweet lemons or sweet *musambi* or water of green coconut or ripe mangoes in their season (preferably very juicy mangoes) or papayas.
- 11 am 20-30 gm of germinated moong dal, green coconut (15-20 gm), and soaked dates or 10 soaked munakkas, and plenty of green vegetables (spinach, *methi*, *dhaniya*, *pudina*, *kakari*, tomato, radish, leaf cabbage, *chichira*, and plenty of *parval*, *lauki*, etc.).
- 3 pm 20-30 gm of millet juice.
- 4 pm Juicy fruits (preferably orange or sweet lime) and 20 soaked munakkas and lemon honey water.

After consuming the above diet for six months, the following results were seen in December 1977--

(a) maintenance of body weight;

(b) energy and freshness;

(c) total stoppage of bleeding from the left nasal canal;

(d) excretion of mucus in large quantities.

Unfortunately thereafter, her diet was modified a little and she was put on a "fruits only" diet. Germinated grains and coconut were not given to her any more. Her weight began to decrease with this type of diet. Shortly afterwards she developed a strong diarrhoea. There was no relief even after large intakes of fluids. Her weight began decreasing rapidly and she became very frail.

At this juncture, her naturopathic doctors were compelled to prescribe a small quantity of very thin whey mixed with water and raw goat milk. The quantity of whey was increased up to that of one kg. of milk, three times a day. She was put on this diet for three months. Thereafter the goat milk and whey were totally stopped and the patient was put on her earlier diet once again. Her naturopathic doctors were highly impressed by her steadfastness and wrote--

"The patient has an undoubted faith in naturopathy. Her mind was at peace even at the most critical of times, even though her family and friends feared for her life. This lady is an ideal patient. Such a living faith in naturopathy is very rare."

Allopathic Examination of the Patient

Shortly afterwards, she was regularly taken to Dr. Bhivapurkar, a renowned cancer specialist in Nagpur, every two to three months to find out whether her condition was improving. He reported that the size of the tumour slightly increased during the first year of the treatment, but then stopped growing and by the end of the second year it appeared to be fully under control. In the third year he stated that a layer of skin had grown over the tumour, which made it appear to be fully under control. In the third year he stated it was difficult to observe it accurately, but admitted that there was an all-round improvement in the patient every time he saw her, and felt that there was now no need to examine her again in future. Even her weight which was 63 pounds at the beginning of the treatment, had risen to 83 pounds.

At this juncture, her naturopathic doctors decided to alter her diet regime as follows--

5 am A spoonful of honey in a glass of fresh lemon water.

9 am Germinated moong dal (50-60 gm), soaked dates (20-30 gm), fresh green coconut (50-60 gm), fresh vegetables, fresh fruits (mango, chickoo, guava, papaya, banana, etc.; only one or two of these fruits at a time).

4 pm The same diet given at 9 am but with different fruits.

The large difference of time between her morning and evening meals increased her appetite, and made her eat each meal with relish. As a result of this diet, her motions became completely clear and normal, and the mucus in them kept dwindling until it disappeared completely. Her naturopaths then declared that she had been cured and wrote that "The patient appears to be very healthy. Now it is not proper to call her a patient any more. She abounds with freshness and energy and takes part in all activities of the Ashram. She works in the fields all day, cultivating vegetables which are grown with natural manure."

Herbs in Modern Medicine

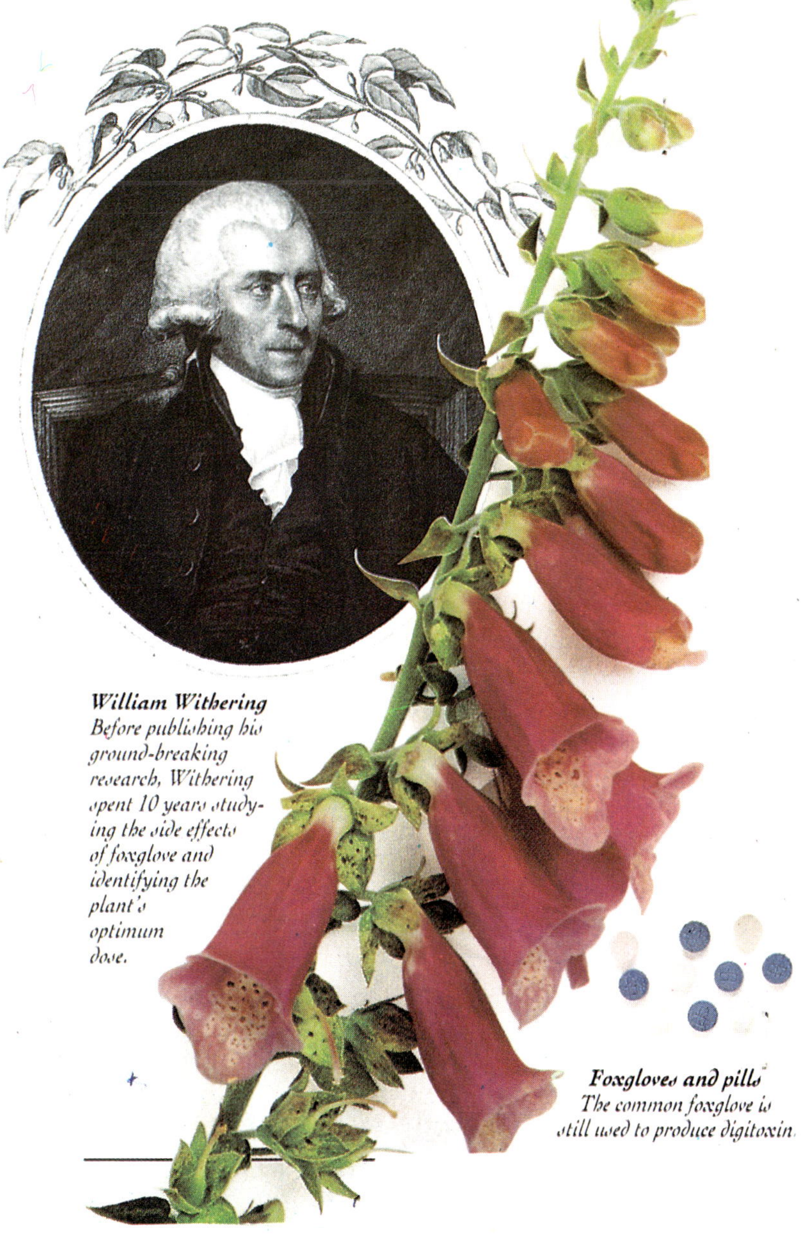

William Withering
Before publishing his ground-breaking research, Withering spent 10 years studying the side effects of foxglove and identifying the plant's optimum dose.

Foxgloves and pills
The common foxglove is still used to produce digitoxin.

JN 1775, Dr. Withering Strabs Experiments on Herbs. In 1785 he published his Medical use

Chapter XVII

Astrology And Cancer Disease

There was a time when diseases like influenza, tuberculosis and plague turned into pandemics. Now they are under control due to medical advancement. Cancer, heart troubles, high blood pressure and diabetes, however, still remain incurable.

Based upon my study of the divine science of Astrology for more than two decades, I have tried to present all viewpoints regarding cancer, based upon Indian and Western thoughts. The subject has been dealt with under the following heads:--

(i) Guidelines in classical texts

(ii) Different Rasi/Star indications.

(ii) Planets and mere planetary combinations.

(iv) Planets with Rasis.

(v) Planets with Bhavas.

(vi) Planets with Rasis and Bhavas both.

(vii) Planetary states and cancer.

(viii) Parts of body affected by cancer.

(ix) Time of appearance of the disease:

(x) Opinions of Western Astrologers and some comments of Indian astrologers on them.

(xi) Results of some statistical studies done by Indian astrologers.

(xii) Important viewpoints of some other Indian astrologers.

(xiii) My own opinion.

Considering the large number of combinations presented in the details below, readers are cautioned not to get scared to see an isolated combination in their charts indicating cancer. For eruption of a serious disease like cancer of a certain organ, really serious afflictions in the chart involving that limb must be necessary, coupled with also appropriate malefic Dasas and/or simultaneous bad transits like Sadesathi, operating at suitable times. For want of such periods in the life span of the native be can even be lucky to escape the severe effects of certain combinations. Availability of a certain isolated combination in a chart can mean, therefore, some sort of proneness only to the serious disease cancer and nothing more.

Cancer is a general name applied to all malignant tumours. It is liable to damage vital organs or tissues in the body. Both physical and psychosomatic factors could cause cancer. It appears to be largely a disease of inheritance and in some cases, acquired and in any event, Karmic. It falls under the category of Kritaantotpatti diseases, that is disease arising as a result of heredity or out of ones own doings in the previous births. Karmavipaaka has a telling reason why one falls prey to this disease. The man who suffers from cancer must have perpetrated the heinous crime of having illicit sex relations with a widowed woman in his former birth. Some ancient astrological writers are of the view that the Lagna and the 8th house, and not the 6th house, should be afflicted to suffer from Karma Vyaadhis. The 6th house according to these sages has not much to do with malignant diseases. It is not, however, possible to confirm or to contradict this opinion. It is not an easy task to discover correctly from the chart ones susceptibility to cancer, because no systematic study of the various cancers and the combinations causing the same have been so far made, yet whether one is predisposed towards suffering from a serious disease like cancer can be indicated with a fair amount of accuracy by a study of the chart as a whole. Astrology if the combinations causing the affliction of a benefic namely Jupiter or Venus, or if the Moon is strongly placed in the chart without afflictions, then by adopting suitable remedial measures, the onset of cancer can be prevented. Moderation in life and practice of Yoga can also enable one to overcome the disease.

GUIDELINES IN CLASSICAL TEXTS

In olden days, as man was closer to nature and moderate in his habits, suffering from disease was in general less than today. Many diseases in fact have their origin in the present civilization. Classical texts do not make mention of cancer. Dr. Raman has treated it as near Vrana and has given a combination applicable to cancer, which is available in Brihat Parasara Hora and Jataka Parijata as follows:

(i) If the 6th lord is a malefic planet and is situated in Lagna, 6th or 8th house, it will create Vrana on the body of the native.-- B.P.H. Bhava effects st. 104.

(ii) If the 6th lord with malefics occupies Lagna, 8th or 10th house and is devoid of benefic aspects, the native suffers from Vrana in his body.--J.P. 6.70.

One other astrologer has opined that our ancients called cancer as Arbuda or Raktarbuda, the word meaning a swelling or tumour and that Ayurveda considers it as arising from Pittadosha and naturally therefore Indian astrological texts hold the planet Mars to be mainly responsible for its eruption.

In my view, there are combinations in texts indicating Gulma or Gulmaroga, which means diseases of the spleen or abscess or tumour in the stomach. These combinations can be made applicable especially to cancer in the abdominal region.

Readers will notice that a good number of combinations quoted below from my collection have their origin in some classical texts which are only oblique combinations for cancer. For example, the Moon and Saturn in 6th house together are said to create leukaemia or blood cancer in the 55th year of one's life. Actually the combination has been given to indicate Raktakushtha or red-leprosy as per Brihat Parasar Hora.

DIFFERENT RASI/STAR INDICATIONS

(i) People born in ascendants Cancer, Virgo and Scorpio (in descending order of merit) are more prone to cancer. Other less important signs on the ascendant are Aries, Gemini, Sagittarius, Capricorn and Aquarius as opined by certain astrologers. A statistical study by Mr. Kharegat, an astrologer, indicates that people born in ascendants Taurus, Aquarius and Pisces are the least prone to cancer. Aquarius as ascendant is thus disputed regarding proneness to cancer. In my statistical analysis of 88 charts ?? as ascendant is next in importance only to cancer sign, which is of maximum recurrence.

(ii) Asterism Jyeshta has something to do with tumours. Of special import for investigation are the last quarters of Aslesha, Jyeshta and Revathi.

(iii) A person born in the first part of nadi-amsa Karikara dies of cancer in the 68th year (Karikara amsa is 6036 to 6048 in movable signs, etc.).

Planets and Mere Planetary Combinations

(i) The Sun is a karaka of any unhealthy and unrestrained growth and should be considered in cancer cases.

(ii) Affliction of the Sun along with Kalasarpa Yoga in the chart may cause cancer.

(iii) The Sun, Mercury and Venus in 4th house from Saturn during eclipse indicate uterine cancer.

(iv) If the Moon combines with a malefic, the native suffers from throat disease. With severe afflictions, throat cancer can result.

(v) Afflictions of the Moon and Venus create stomach ailments and tumours.

(vi) Combination of the Moon, Mars and Jupiter or Saturn brings about cancer in Mars Dasa, also when Mars aspects Jupiter. Generally the spleen is involved.

(vii) The Moon, Mars, Saturn, Rahu and Ketu, involved in any way with each other indicate possibility of cancer.

(viii) Out of several dicta regarding the cause of cancer, the one most dependable is that if the Moon gets afflicted heavily in any house of a natal chart by three or more malefics in any manner, there is every likelihood of the native acquiring cancer.

(ix) Saturn is invariably associated with tumours. Saturn causes tumours of the site represented by the planet associated with it in any particular case. Thus, when the Moon is involved by association or aspect with a combination of Mars and Saturn, cancer of the breasts or uterine cervix is developed.

(x) In most cases of cancer, a peculiar aspect has been observed between the Moon and Saturn. Saturn has been seen in the following positions from the Moon conjunction--4th, 5th, 7th, 9th, 10th and 11th.

(xi) A study of several charts has shown a link between the Moon and Saturn in cancer cases, the link being in Navamasa chart. In Navamasa chart, Saturn conjoined with or aspecting Moon by usual 3-7/10th aspect seems a fairly common feature in cancer cases.

(xii) The Moon in conjunction with Rahu or Ketu located in the 3rd house either from Mars or Saturn indicates possibility of cancer.

(xiii) Rahu and Ketu mainly and all other planets complementarily play a joint role in cancer disease. Chiefly the planets Moon, Mars ruling sores, ulcers and blood, Rahu and Ketu the significators of unnatural growths like an ant-hill, the abode of serpents, and Saturn who signifies the end of a man are the quick messengers of this disease. Any good aspect like that of a strong Jupiter may be able to save the patient from death by early diagnosis and treatment.

(xiv) Weak Mars if afflicted by Rahu creates leukaemia.

(xv) Mars appears to be the villain in patients having the cancer of the gall-bladder.

(xvi) Most cancer cases need surgical therapy and so Mars should be involved in cancer cases.

(xvii) Mars is connected with blood and so he must be there in blood cancer. When Mercury and Venus combine with aspect or association of Mars-Saturn combination, cancer of blood is likely.

(xviii) Mars-Mercury indicate venereal disease which can lead to cancer. Mars is karaka for all diseases in female organs. When it is afflicted by Mercury it forms ulcer which tends to cancer.

(xix) Mars-Venus in disharmony--blood cells are damaged leading to diseases like cancer.

(xx) Mars and Saturn either in conjunction or aspecting each other or in mutual 3/11 positions indicate possibility of cancer.

(xxi) Rahu or Ketu found in 3/6/8/12th house from Saturn or *vice versa*--possibility of cancer.

(xxii) Mars-Rahu in adverse positions--boils and abscesses etc. with possible malignancy. Mars Rahu are the agents which possess the power to destroy cells, especially if they are afflicted by Saturn, Rahu creates cancerous tumours.

(xxiii) Mercury-Rahu disharmony--venereal diseases which may lead to cancer.

(xxiv) Uncontrolled growth of cells in any bodily part is known as cancer. Expansion is the function of Jupiter which is an expansive planet. Jupiter is thus the planet responsible for multiplication of cells and their growth. Whenever Jupiter is afflicted cancer is caused due to malfunctioning of the process of cell division.

(xxv) Jupiter-Rahu in adverse conditions--wound or poisonous gas which attacks skin and can later on lead to skin cancer.

(xxvi) Venus becomes involved with the seat of disease in almost all patients who have cancer within the oral cavity.

(xxvii) If malignancy is any clue to the definition of cancer, it can be said that Saturn and/or Rahu must have an intimate role to play in causing this disease. Rahu is responsible for all types of malignant growths. Combination of Saturn-Rahu with aspect of other malefics may excite the cause of cancer by causing cell damage.

(xxviii) Rahu-Ketu afflictions create boils and skin eruptions which precede cancerous growth.

(xxix) For growth to be eccentric Uranus should be involved.

PLANETS WITH RASIS

(i) Sun in Taurus aspected by Saturn creates tumour-forming tendency.

(ii) Sun in Pisces aspected by malefics indicates possibility of uterine cancer.

(iii) If Mars and Saturn both are in cruel Shashtyamsas and are placed in mutual kendras in inimical signs or in conjunction with the Sun and the Moon respectively, cancer and like troubles are possible.

(iv) If the Moon is conjoined with Saturn in Rasi and occupies Navamsa of Cancer, Scorpio or Aquarius, the native will suffer from tumours.

(v) If the lord of the Drekkana occupied by Saturn is the Moon, there is a possibility of tumour; and if it is Jupiter, the ailment is in the stomach and it is hidden.

(vi) When Mars and Saturn either alone or conjoined respectively by Rahu and Ketu are placed in mutual opposition positions in signs one of which is owned by Mars or Saturn, cancer and like troubles are possible.

(vii) Cancer of spine involves 260 of Cancer and Capricorn, first degree of common signs and the planet Saturn.

(viii) For detecting cancer, the chart as a whole is to be studied to assess whether a native is susceptible to any kind of infection. All kinds of infections could be judged from the extra-Saturnine planets and from Cancer, Scorpio and Pisces signs. The last quarters of asterisms Aslesha, Jyeshta and Revati in these signs are most significant.

PLANETS WITH BHAVAS

(i) The Sun in Lagna aspected by Mars may create cancer of the spleen.

(ii) Afflictions to the Sun, Saturn and 4th house indicate lung cancer.

(iii) Saturn in 4th with Mercury and Venus when the Sun is also afflicted will either cause cancer of the oesophagus or cancer of blood (leukaemia).

(iv) Malefics in 5th house and the Sun occupying 6/8/12 houses or afflicted will cause cancer in the abdomen.

(v) The Sun in 6th house with malefic connections brings about ulcers, wounds and similar ailments. Rahu's association in these cases will definitely point to cancer.

(vi) If Mars and Saturn are in 6th house and aspected by the Sun and Rahu, a long-lasting or chronic disease develops.

(vii) Sun, Moon, Mars and 6th lord in conjunction anywhere create blood cancer.

(viii) Stomach cancer--The Sun is mostly afflicted, Rahu-Ketu axis is usually in 1-7 houses. The lord of the 6th house will be tenanted by a malefic and the lord of 6th himself would be a malefic stationed in 8th or 12th house.

(ix) The Moon, Saturn and houses Lagna, 6th, 8th, 12th seem to figure prominently in the charts of cancer patients. The maiming or disfigurement of the body due to surgery to remove corrupt tissues to save life is related to the ascendant or its lord and to the 6/8/12 houses or their lords. Saturn, characteristic of all that hardens, hinders, depletes, coagulates and suppresses, would seem to be the best fitted planet to be associated with cancer. He would also explain very well the mental anguish and depression that follow the biopsy confirming malignancy of the lump or growth. The Moon ruling the mind and also the secretions of the body system would also fit well.

(x) Lagna lord and the Moon along with 6th occupying 6/8/12 house cause bad tumours.

(xi) If evil planets are combined with the Moon, and lord of Lagna is in 6/8/12 houses with Rahu/Ketu, the native suffers from an incurable disease.

(xii) Cases of cancer can be diagnosed from the Moon, Mars, Saturn and Rahu. Any relation between the lords of 6th and 8th makes for a high intensity of the ailment. Extra-saturnine planets do not have significant influence on individual lives and so also on cancer.

(xiii) When Mars/Rahu occupies the 5th house and Saturn aspects the same from 3rd, and when Venus is in the 10th from the Moon, a hidden malady is indicated in the stomach region.

(xiv) The Moon and Saturn in 6th house create leukaemia in 55th year of life (This combination has been actually given for red-leprosy as per Brihat Parashara Hora).

(xv) Leukaemia is cancer of the blood-forming organs, principally bone marrow. The Moon and Mars, 4th, 8th and 12th houses and their lords need to be closely studied for this disease.

(xvi) The Moon and Venus in 12th, Mars occupying 6th house indicate uterine cancer.

(xvii) The Moon governs breasts and Mars controls glands. The 4th and 10th houses govern right and left breasts respectively. Therefore if 4th and 10th houses, their lords, the Moon and Mars are afflicted especially by Rahu and Ketu, there is a likelihood of breast cancer.

(xviii) If the 6th lord Moon occupies Lagna, and 4th and 10th houses are afflicted--cancer of breasts.

(xix) If the Moon, 4th lord and 10th lord are occupying 6/8/12 houses and are spoiled by malefic aspects--cancer of the breast.

(xx) There is an opinion also that afflictions of the Moon and 3rd house need consideration for cancer of the breast.

(xxi) Mars in Lagna or in 6th devoid of strength--spleen involved in cancer or like diseases.

(xxii) Lagna lord occupying Lagna, 3rd or 6th house and aspected by Mars and Rahu indicates a serious disease causing heavy expenditure.

(xxiii) Mars joining lord of 6th in Lagna, 6th, 7th or 10th house may cause cancer.

(xxiv) We can surmise the presence of cancer from the chart, should there be a relation between the three planets Mars, Saturn and Rahu, signifying cancer and between the 6th and 8th houses and their lords. In case of cancer it must also be established by investigation of 6th and 8th houses that a chronic and deep-seated disease is very much expected in the chart.

(a) Mars and Saturn combination in 6/7/8/12 houses.

(b) Mars in 6th and Saturn in 12th or *vice versa*.

(c) Mars or Saturn occupies 6th house and aspects cruelly the other planet mutually--cancer is possible.

(d) Whenever the 4th house is heavily afflicted and Mars is also associated with the same, lung cancer is expected which spreads fast.

(e) When the lord of the Ascendant and the 4th are placed in the 6th house in combustion or retrogression and are aspected by Mars and Saturn, cancer is possible.

(xxv) Mercury creates skin cancer when afflicted in Lagna or 12th or by 6/8/12th lords or by the malefic planets posited therein.

(xxvi) Jupiter, 5th house and 5th lord when afflicted badly lead to stomach cancer, cancer of liver, etc.

(xxvii) Venus rules over the ovaries and when afflicted by 6/8/12 house lords, it tends to create trouble of ovaries which can result in cancer of the same with serious afflictions.

(xxviii) Saturn with Ketu in 7th house--tumour and like troubles.

(xxix) Saturn with Rahu in 8th house--possible involvement of uterus in cancer.

(xxx) Saturn in 2nd house can indicate destruction of cells beginning with heart disease. Saturn in 4th or in 5th is an indication for stomach trouble and imbalance in stomach region starting with a heart problem and can lead to cancer with serious afflictions.

(xxxi) Especially Rahu and the lords of 6/8/12 houses are responsible for malignant growth. All other cruel planets also require attention.

(xxxii) Rahu in Lagna is a warning that hidden disease can surface.

(xxxiii) When the lord of 6th house is in conjunction or aspect of Rahu, the individual can suffer from cancer and the part affected by this disease will be known by the house aspected by it or the lord of that house.

(xxxiv) Lord of 6th house falling in Lagna, 8th or 10th house with association or aspect of malefics, especially Rahu, gives rise to vrana roga or mamsarbuda roga that is cancer (some opine that lord of 6th house should be a malefic in this combination which is however not justified in actual experience). The part indicated by the house or the house lord will suffer from cancer.

(xxxv) Rahu/Ketu should be in the 6/8/12 houses from either Lagna or Lagna lord in Rasi chart and simultaneously in Navamsa chart Rahu/Ketu should be in kendra or trikona from either Navamsa Lagna or from the position of lagna lord in Navamsa chart--possibility of cancer.

(xxxvi) The 3rd house and its lord are involved in throat cancer and 3rd and 4th houses and their lords are involved in breast cancer.

(xxxvii) Cancerous or malignant growth can be inferred from the 4th house.

(xxxviii) The 6th lord in 12th, 12th lord being in 6th--troubles of spleen and cancer of the same with further afflictions.

(xxxix) Lord of 11th house in 6th house--a complicated disease may appear.

PLANETS WITH RASIS AND BHAVAS BOTH

(i) The Sun, Ketu, Cancer sign, 5th and 6th houses figure prominently in case of stomach cancer.

(ii) If the ascendant is afflicted and if the Sun, Mercury, Virgo sign and 6th house are afflicted by malefics, there is a possibility of cancer of gall-bladder.

(iii) The planets Sun, Mars and Ketu, Virgo and Scorpio signs, 6th and 8th houses would feature in the cancer of the colon and rectum.

(iv) The Sun, Mars, Mercury, Virgo sign, 6th house and its lord need to be examined for cancer of bladder. Blood in the urine is a warning of this cancer. Usually the Sun and Mercury together with the lord of 6th house are severely afflicted by Mars, Saturn and Rahu-Ketu axis.

(v) The planets Sun, Moon, Mars, watery signs, 4/8/12 houses and their lords if afflicted by Rahu create leukaemia or blood cancer.

(vi) Cancer disease is mostly detected when the Moon is afflicted with Saturn, Rahu or adverse planetary position is present in Lagna or in cancer sign.

(vii) Mars in 5th and Saturn in 8th house subject to disturbing vibrations especially when the Moon is heavily afflicted in Uttara, Hasta, Chitta, Swati, Punarvasu, Mrigasira and Aswini stars, the virulence of the ailment decreasing from the 1st star to 7th one indicate disease like cancer.

(viii) The planets Moon, Mars, Venus and Rahu, Taurus and Aquarius signs and 2nd, 11th houses are involved in throat cancer.

(ix) The Moon, Jupiter 3/4/6/9 signs, 4th and 6th houses are closely involved in lung cancer. It is seen that in cases of lung cancer common signs are in the 6th and/or watery signs in 8th house.

(x) Weak Moon and Rahu related to 5th and 7th houses and sign Scorpio is involved in the cancer of the uterus. There is another opinion also that Virgo sign and 6th house are concerned with the uterus and Mars **and** Venus are the chief planets to be considered for this purpose.

(xi) There is a danger of cancer of the uterus or breast if Saturn and Uranus occupy 6th or 8th house in watery signs and if the combination is joined with or in bad aspect of the Moon, Mars, Venus or Neptune.

(xii) The planets Moon, Venus, Watery signs and 8th house and 8th lord are involved in cancer of the kidneys, bladder or prostate.

(xiii) If the lord of the sign occupied by the Moon is weak and if conjoined with Lagna lord occupies 6/8/12 houses, then an emaciating disease develops, cancer being an emaciating disease.

(xiv) Mars rules over blood and wounds, and wounds and the like (vranas in general) come under 6th house and Virgo sign.

(xv) In case of cancer of the skin, Mars and Rahu have dominant positions afflicting the lagna or 6th house in Cancer sign.

(xvi) Studies have revealed that the cancer patients have Aslesha asterism related to their lagna or the 6th house and afflicted by Mars. This asterism falls in Cancer sign, second half part.

Variations

(i) Cancer sign in 6th and occupied by Mars and Saturn (or one of them in 6th and other in 12th house) indicates cancer and like troubles.

(ii) The 6th house, Cancer sign, Mars and Saturn in them or afflicting them is a signal for cancer disease. Aslesha asterism is known as a Sarpa asterism indicating snakes.

(iii) Mars and Saturn conjunction in 6th house in Aridra or Swati stars (falling in Gemini and Libra signs respectively) indicates possibility of cancer. It will be seen that these stars are controlled by Rahu in Vimshottari scheme. Similar investigation can be made with Satabhisha star also falling in Aquarius, which is also controlled by Rahu.

(iv) Mars in Scorpio Lagna without aspect of Jupiter or Venus creates tumour and the like. Leo Lagna, with Mars in Scorpio sign or Scorpio navamsa, creates the same result.

(v) Afflictions by Mars, Rahu in watery signs and connected with 6th house, such as lords of Lagna and 6th in one house conjoined with Mars, creates glandular tumours.

(vi) Saturn in Lagna in Virgo sign aspected by Mars will cause during the Period and subperiod of the lords of 6th and 8th (Saturn and Mars themselves) an abdominal swelling and kidney disease etc. This combination has been found to exist in some cases of abdominal cancer.

(vii) Lords of the ascendant and the 6th house in the 10th house aspected by Mars and Saturn predispose one to cancer of the breasts. With Aquarius as Lagna, the chances are more.

(viii) Mercury in Aries or in Scorpio as Lagna can promote diseases of the rectum. Mercury afflicted in Scorpio, along with mars and Rahu, can trigger off cancer of colon and rectum.

(ix) Cancer of the genitals comes under the 8th house, Scorpio sign and Mercury. The last degrees of Aries and first of Taurus, Mars and Saturn are also to be considered.

(x) Gadaavali says that mercury in Scorpio causes cancer of genitals if Scorpio happens to be 4th, 6th or 11th house and if lagna lord is debilitated, combust or in the company of Rahu in a saturnine sign.

(xi) Cancer of the rectum and of the prostate seems to be connected with Scorpio and the 8th house. A node in the 8th may signify piles; if it is in the star of Mars, fistula may result; but if Saturn and Ketu are together in 8th one may be disposed towards suffering from cancer of the rectum or of prostate. When the Lagna or the Moon-sign is Scorpio with Saturn therein, and lord of the 6th is in the 10th, the native is exposed to cancer of the rectum. Scorpio is the natural signifier of the rectum and the situation of Saturn therein can cause irritation to the organs of elimination resulting in their cancer.

(xii) If Jupiter occupies the 6th house in conjunction with or aspected by malefics or combines with a malefic navamsa or is in debility in Capricorn, the native will suffer from cancer.

(xiii) Breast cancer refers to Venus, the 6th house and the signs Aries, Gemini, Cancer and Libra.

(xiv) A native with Sagittarius as Lagna with 6th lord Venus occupying the 10th house has been seen to suffer from tongue cancer and the cancer was traced to syphilis of the tongue, lord of 2nd also being in Lagna.

(xv) Saturn's affliction in the 6th house in Rahu's star indicates possibility of cancer.

(xvi) Saturn in 12th creates sores and eruptions slow to heal. In Aslesha (Cancer sign 2nd half) in 12th it causes tumours, blood poisoning and destruction of cells.

(xvii) Devakeraleeyam says that if a native is born in Nadiamsa Viswambhara in Scorpio Lagna and if Saturn is in his sign of debility along with 8th lord (that is Saturn and Mercury occupy 6th in Aries), the native suffers from bodily weakness and other complications of cancer. (Viswambhara Amsa in Scorpio is from 8036 to 8048).

(xviii) Rahu or Ketu in Lagna, malefics in 6th house--cancer of the stomach. (Ascendant should be here of 3/5/8/12 signs; in these signs Scorpio should be exempted as 6th lord is Lagna lord also.)

(xix) The 6th lord in Lagna in the sign of his enemy, joined with or aspected by the lords of the 8th and 12th houses, causes malignant growth.

(xx) Cancer of gall-bladder points to 8th house and Scorpio sign. (This can apply to urinary bladder also).

(xxi) Cancer of hips involves 6th and 9th houses, Virgo and Sagittarius signs.

PLANETARY STATES AND CANCER

In one textbook importance has been given to the states of planets in determining the exact part and nature of afflictions. It says that all planets in sleeping state (*sayana*) cause serious illnesses like cancer, tumour, leprosy and other *prarabha vyadhis*. The Sun in sleeping state causes tumour of the brain and eyes or even paralytic attacks as a result of cancer except when the Lagna is Aries or Leo and the Sun is in an angle therefrom. The Moon in sleeping state causes brain tumour and lung cancer and also internal bleeding due to bursts when the Moon occupies the 6th house except for Sagittarius Lagna. Mars in sleeping state sharing 6/8/11 houses with Saturn causes cancer as a consequence of eczema or syphilis except for Aquarius, Pisces or Leo Lagnas. In eating state (*bhojana*) in such a situation he causes amputation due to cancer or decay of parts. In certain cases Mars placed in such a position causes suicide resulting from unbearable cancer pains. Mercury in sleeping or eating state in 6/7/8 houses with Saturn, causes cancer of the urinary or genital organs. Jupiter in eating state in 6th or 8th owned by the Moon or Venus causes various types of ulcers, acne, gangrene and bleeding which can lead to cancer. Venus causes cancer of the throat, gums and tongue, etc., if he is the 2nd lord in the 6th or in 12th in sleeping state. In sleeping state Venus causes ear cancer if he is placed in the Sun-Rasi which happens to be the 3rd or 6th house or when Venus occupies the 10th whose lord is in debility. Saturn often causes intestinal and bone cancer. Rahu and Ketu cause cancer of many types in different states. Saturn and Rahu in 4th house normally cause breast cancer in women born in Leo or Capricorn Lagnas provided Saturn is in *sayana* state and Rahu in *nidra* or *aagamana* state. Venus and Rahu in Lagna, 5th or in 7th house cause ovarian tumour and cancer in females if they are in *sayana* and *nidra* states respectively. The Sun, Moon and Mars in 6th house cause ophthalmic tumour or cancer when the Moon and Mars are combust and in *bhojana* or *sayana* states.

PARTS AFFECTED BY CANCER

Cancer being degeneration of cell, its localization should be scanned from the part attributed to the afflicting sign or planet. Parts of the body affected can be known also from the Lagna lord, Karaka planets, etc. Different planets control different parts. When these planets become *marakas* or get afflicted otherwise, the part shown by them based upon the distribution given by Varahamihira depending on rising lagna--*drekkana* will be also useful to determine the part of the body. To identify the part affected, a guideline is also to check the zodiacal sign occupied by Rahu when it is conjunct with Saturn or aspected by him. The part indicated by the sign will be affected. Twenty-seven asterisms also hold a more meaningful clue here. Each asterism is associated with a vital part or organ. If any asterism occupied by Lagna, the Moon or the Sun is occupied or aspected by Rahu and Saturn, the corresponding part could be affected. There is an opinion that more importance needs to be given to the aspect of Saturn than conjunction to pick up the clue. To establish malignancy in cancer charts, the houses where the three planets Mars, Jupiter and Uranus are placed should be noted. The weakest among these houses indicates usually the site of malignancy. This will be further substantiated by the lord of the 6th or 8th by its presence or aspect on that house. During the transit of Rahu, malignancy has been observed over the part, established as above. This can be confirmed further based upon the

age of the native at that time and the part of the body involved. For example, considering the cancer of prostate, transit of Rahu over that part of the native somewhere after 60 years of age would be only the right time. The different planets when they are responsible or *karakas* for cancer create the disease in the following organs:

The Sun. Head, stomach and intestines.

The Moon. Face, chest, breasts, spleen and blood.

Mars. Head, neck, throat, reproductive organs, rectum, blood and bone marrow.

Mercury. Face, mouth, nose, lips, navel, lower stomach and skin.

Jupiter. Tongue, nose, ears, liver and thighs.

Venus. Throat, eyes, reproductive organs, testicles and ovaries.

Saturn. Teeth, gums, palate, arms, legs and bones.

Rahu/Ketu. Abdomen and spleen.

TIME OF APPEARANCE OF THE DISEASE

Cancer may appear in Rahu Dasa, Sun Bhukti provided Rahu and the Sun are in mutual association or aspect in the 6th or 8th house. Symptoms of cancer develop in either Dasa or Bhukti of Rahu or Ketu which are the chief significators of this disease. Rahu Dasa, if Rahu occupies a sign of Saturn, that is Capricorn or Aquarius, is likely to cause cancer. Saturn Dasa is also qualified if Saturn is weak or sufficiently afflicted. The 6th lord or the occupant of the 6th house, from agna or from the Moon, can bring about this trouble in his Dasa, so also any planet badly afflicted in Rasi and aspected by the 6th lord or by the occupant of the 6th house.

OPINIONS OF WESTERN ASTROLOGERS

Kharegat, a well-known astrologer of India, statistically studied 344 cases of cancer. He states that much attention has been paid to the astrological signification of cancer disease by Western astrologers using the tropical, that is Sayana, positions of planets, as stated below. Kharegat's comments on each of these significations have been give based upon his study of 344 charts.

Carter

C.E.O. Carter while commenting on cancer in his book, *An Encyclopaedia of Psychological Astrology*, states:

> Cancer is not, as is often assumed, a disease especially connected with the Moon or with the sign of the same name, although, of course, it frequently attacks the stomach. The typical indications are that the Sun is nearly always related both to Jupiter and to Saturn, either by aspect or by sign. Thus it may be in aspect with both, or in aspect with one either or from a sign of Jupiter. The aspect with both, or in aspect with one either in or from a sign ruled by the other. For example, it may be in Sagittarius in aspect with Saturn, or Saturn may aspect it from a sign of Jupiter. The aspect need not be evil, but if it is not, then the Sun is usually in bad aspect to Mars, Uranus or Neptune as well. Neptune seems sometimes to take the place of Jupiter and this planet is frequently in aspect, no always evil, to Mars or Saturn or both. In cancer cases about 25th degree of Virgo-Pisces is a common area of affliction (Sidereal equivalent 30 of Virgo-Pisces).

Kharegat's comment: Carter's observations are fully borne out in the majority of cases studied.

Wemyss

The indications in the horoscope are the degree of growth 160-170 Taurus-Scorpio blended in affliction with 270 Cancer-Capricorn and their rulers.

Kharegat's comment: This indication is not supported by the majority of cases studied. When it is applicable, however, Mars, Saturn, the Sun or Neptune enters into the configuration.

Ebertin

He bases his indications only on the intrinsic nature of the planets and some mid-points in their mutual hard angle aspects. According to him, the sickness axes, the two mid-points Sun/Neptune and Sun/Saturn are aspected by malefics and by the personal points like Rahu, Sun, Moon, Ascendant, M.C. or their mid-points. He further quotes an astrologer Konig who proposed a formula for detecting cancer cases, namely, Neptune=Mars/M.C. Or =Saturn/M.C.

Kharegat's comment: Out of Ebertin's two sickness axes, the more frequently affected by malefics appears to be Sun/Neptune which is contacted not only by malefics but by personal points as well. As regards Konig's formula, it appears only in a few cases studied. Nevertheless, if the aspects of these mid-points considered not only to Neptune,

but to 250 of Pisces and to Jupiter and malefic Mars, Saturn, Uranus, the formula becomes valid in 84 per cent of the cases.

Write

The founder of Uranian system of Astrology gives the formula, Saturn divided by Hades minus Neptune as a point that is contacted by the personal planets by hard angle aspects.

Kharegat's comment: As the ephemeris of Hades, a hypothetical planet is readily available, the formula is of limited value.

Emylee L. Hughes

In an article entitled "The Astrological Predisposition and Occurrence of Cancer" Hughes gives a formula similar to the Arabic points: the part of Cancer=Ascendant divided by Neptune minus Jupiter. This point according to the author is activated by aspect in eevery case.

Kharegat's comment: All the hard and soft angle aspects are considered and the orbs used are rather wide. Restricting the orb to 50 and not using doubtful aspects like quintile and biquintile, it is certainly true that in 90 per cent of cases studied, it is aspected by malefics or personal points.

Robson, another Western astrologer says that the Moon is found heavily afflicted in cancer cases.

Comment of Dr. B. Raman

In the view of Raman, another well-known Indian astrologer, Western astrologers lay emphasis on afflictions in Cancer sign which should be in Lagna for suffering from cancer. He comments:

> Cancer occurs with great frequency in females because of the great suspceptibility of the breasts and uterus to this disease. This is perhaps one of the reasons for the sign Cancer being associated with the disease cancer in Western Astrology. While in our humble opinion, there is not much evidence to support this theory there is no doubt that Moon's affliction in Cancer sign can lead to a lot of stomach and intestinal disorders.

Comment of Dr. P.S. Sastri

Commenting on Carter's finding, Dr. Sastri says;

> Since cancerous growth destroys the vital cells, Carter was led to believe that in all such cases, afflictions of the Sun from Jupiter and Saturn are found. But the cells come under Saturn and Mars and their maintenance depends on the Moon and to some extent on the Sun and Jupiter. We therefore find affliction to and from Saturn and Mars and any kind of malignant growth involves Rahu. Blood being corrupted in such cases, we need to examine the luminaries and Mars as well as 6th house. Merely because Mars or Saturn or both are in 6th or 8th house does not imply cancer. In fact, Saturn in these houses can be a great asset warding off many ailments has to be considered along with the house of longevity. Since cancer can attack any part, one has to examine the planets and houses governing these parts. We also emphasize the importance of Rahu because of the poisonous nature of this ailment.

Comment of Kothari on Carter

It is felt that there may be much correlation with signs ruled by Saturn and Jupiter, and the Suns placement as opined by Carter. However, it is observed that Rahu-Ketu axis plays a sinister role in the horoscopes of potential victims of cancer disease. There is a considerable scope to narrow down the field of study and finally trace out the exact degrees of zodiac which might have been activating cancerous growth in certain parts of the body. Mr. Carter is of the opinion that 25th degree of Virgo-Pisces (Sayana) is a common area of afflictions as that degree seems to be connected with swollen conditions, generally tumours and growths. The star Labrum is situated at 25035 Virgo corresponding to Nirayana 205. This is the star of 4th grade and partakes qualities of Venus and Mercury, the planets which are commonly afflicted in cancer disease. There is another star near the above degree, the name of the star being Zavijava and its location being 2602 Virgo (Nirayana 2032). The faint yellowish star is predominantly of mars-mercury character and is said to be involved in case of diabetes, especially if planets are afflicted around this degree and they are 6th from the Moon. There are some other degrees around the one indicated by Mr. Carter, which are positively sensitive and might be indicators of cancerous growth when under severe affliction. Such degrees together with names of stars which tenant those degrees. Their qualities and possible effect on human parts are given below. Similar sensitive degrees could also be traced in other zodiacal signs involved in this disease.

Star Copula, Sayana 23058 Virgo, Nirayana 0028 Virgo: A cluster of stars with character of Venus and the Moon when under severe affliction, it indicates long drawn illness and danger to eyes.

Star Markeb, Sayana 27048 Virgo, Nirayana 4018 Virgo: A star having qualities of Saturn and Jupiter. When under severe affliction, particularly with the Moon and Neptune around the degree, shows intestinal troubles.

Star Zaniah, Sayana 3043 Libra, nirayana 10013 Virgo: A star with qualities of Venus and Mercury. When under severe affliction with the Moon around the degree, indicates illness arising out of impurities of blood.

Star Vindemiatrix, Sayana 8050 Libra, Nirayana 15020 Virgo: A star with qualities of Saturn and Mercury. When under severe afflictions may indicate troubles with intestines and kidneys.

Star Algorab, Sayana 12020 Libra, Nirayana 18050 Virgo: A star with qualities of Mars and Saturn. When under severe affliction with Mars, Saturn, Neptune involved around the degree may indicate disorders of spleen, kidney and liver. Mercury, Venus and the Sun around the degree under severe affliction from Rahu-Ketu axis and also Neptune may cause troubles in the leg.

STATISTICAL STUDIES BY INDIAN ASTROLOGERS

Kharegat's Study

Kharegat studied statistically 344 cases of malignant cancer out of which in 293 cases the ascendant was known, and in 51 cases only the date of birth. Based upon his study he arrived at the following conclusions.

With aspects as considered by Indian Astrology--

(i) At least two of the signs, Cancer, Scorpio, Pisces or Libra, are afflicted by the aspect or conjunction of lords of malefic houses or of malefics.

(ii) Mars is in the first half of the zodiac that is from Aries to Virgo.

(iii) Following Jaimini, if we locate the sign (or house) of Arudha of 6th house, it is found afflicted by at least two malefics if not more.

(iv) The Sun is afflicted by any of the rulers of the 6th, 8th, or 12th from the Sun-sign, and the rulers of the 6th and 8th or the 6th and 12th are usually in aspect.

(v) Saturn aspects Mars or vice versa especially in the Navamsa chart.

(vi) In Navamsa chart, the Sun is in the 1st, 5th, 7th, 9th, or 11th from Jupiter.

(vii) Cancer Saham is almost always afflicted. (Cancer Saham = 2 x Ascendant x Moon. This is a very sensitive point and aspected by malefics or other personal points like M.C. the Sun, the Moon, sickness, mid-point Saturn/Neptune or Ascendant/M, in 99 per cent cases. The Saham point is most often in the 8th from the Sun).

With aspect as per Western astrology--

(i) About 25 per cent Sayana Pisces (that is 30 Nirayana Pisces) is almost always aspected by malefics or by the death axis mid-point Saturn/Mars.

(ii) Part of Cancer sign is aspected by malefics or by personal points (that is MC, the Sun, the Moon.

(iii) The points Mars/MC or Saturn/MC are aspected by malefics or personal points.

Of course, all the above indications cannot be expected to be present before predicting the disease. Cancer usually attacks in later middle age or old age, hence it is necessary to find out the longevity of the subject before pronouncing that this disease is present as some of these combinations may also cause accidents, etc.

Tables I and II give the sign positions of planets in different houses from lagna for the cancer cases studied. An inspection of Table I will show that the Sun is most often in Sagittarius and Taurus, the Moon in Leo and Sagittarius, Mercury in Virgo, Venus in Scorpio, Mars in Cancer and Leo. Saturn in Gemini and Libra. Uranus in Virgo, Libra, Scorpio and Capricorn, Rahu in Capricorn, Aquarius and Pisces. As for the Ascendant, people born in Cancer are most likely to succumb to this disease, whereas people born in the signs Taurus, Aquarius and Pisces are the least likely to suffer from it. Considering house positions of planets in Table II the significant positions are: The Moon in Lagna or 2nd

but rarely in 8th house; Mars in the 7th and 8th; Jupiter in 2nd and 5th; Saturn in 5th; Rahu in Lagna; Neptune in 9th and 10th and Pluto in 7th, 9th and 11th. Jupiter, whatever be his position in the chart or ownership of signs, always acts as a malefic in cancer cases. In fact Mars, Jupiter and Saturn aspect each other by houses or by being in the sign of the other. This is understandable, as Jupiter is the planet of growth and Mars and Saturn are destructive forces. Sometimes Neptune takes the place of Jupiter as 3rd factor.

Study by Surendra Pai

Pai studied 173 cases (males 90, females 83). Assuming aspects of Mars as 4,7,8; Jupiter 5,7,9; and uranus 5.7.9 the following has been seen in cancer cases:--

(i) All these three planets interlinked by their aspect on each other; or

(ii) All these three planets cast their aspect at a particular house; or

(iii) Two of these three planets in conjunction and aspected by the 3rd; or

(iv) Two of these three planets in conjunction and aspecting the 3rd planet.

Out of 173 cases, Cancer aspects were observed in 162 cases and not observed in 11 cases. The four types of aspects mentioned above were observed in 112 of the 173 cases and in 50 cases the aspect was observed in only two planets (Uranus and Jupiter in 6 cases; Uranus and Mars in 29 cases; Jupiter and Mars in 15 cases). However in all such cases, another aspect either square, 1500 or 2100, 600 to 720 was observed with the 3rd planet. Conclusions from the above are:

(i) In the birth charts of people who suffer from cancer, there exists a definite aspect among the planets Jupiter, Mars and Uranus. This is termed as cancer aspect.

(ii) Also the Moon is aspected by Saturn thereby indicating that the individual will have to face evil.

Besides the existence of cancer aspect among the three planets, the following other factors also need to be present for actual suffering:

(i) At birth the Moon should conjoin either Rahu or Ketu.

(ii) The individual should be going through the period of Rahu during his life span.

(iii) In case of leukaemia, it was further observed that the Moon also participated in cancer aspect along with other three planets.

Subsequent to the first study, a thought was given to the group where only two planets were aspecting each other whereas the third one out of these three was not participating. One thing common in such charts was noticed that the third planet which is not involved in the aspect is usually placed in the zodiacal sign whose lord is seen participating in this aspect along with the other two already involved.

Further study was conducted on 840 cases of cancer given by the Project Director of Cancer Research of the American Federation of Astrologers. It was found that in more than 86 per cent of the cancer cases, the cancer aspect among all the three planets was observed.

Study by Kathore

Study of a large number of charts of cancer victims (exact number not mentioned) reveals the following general pattern of planetary positions and signs as per Nirayana system:

(i) Mutable signs 3/6/9 and cardinal signs 4/10 are found mainly rising as Ascendants.

(ii) Lord of Lagna is invariably afflicted by Saturn and/or Rahu. Lord of Lagna is usually placed in 6/8/12th house and so afflicted.

(iii) Majority of charts with cancer disease have Kalasarpa Yoga. At times Saturn would be seen just outside the Kalasarpa Yoga.

(iv) The Sun, the Moon, Mercury and Venus are either in conjunction with or in square with Rahu-Ketu axis. Besides, the above planets are either seen by Mars and Saturn or are in square or opposition to these planets.

(v) The Sun is always in conjunction, square or trine aspect with Rahu-Ketu axis.

(vi) The Sun is always seen in group with Mercury and Saturn, Mars and Venus, or Mars and Saturn. The Sun is the planet for all unrestrained growths and as such should have prime consideration in cancer cases.

IMPORTANT VIEWS OF SOME OTHER INDIAN ASTROLOGERS

Bepin Behari

Pisces is said to be related to Portugal which was the lowest incidence of cancer, both for males and females. If the individual has strong Pisces sign, the susceptibility of cancer is certainly greatly reduced. Scotland having the highest cancer incidence comes under the sign Cancer ruled by the Moon as well as under Libra ruled by Venus. These two planets should be carefully watched for perversity; and afflictions of the Sun, the different kind of disease which also involves decomposition of certain organs, the germ for which, however, has been isolated. Cancer is still, however, a mysterious affliction.

I.R. Shankar

The 6th house reveals possible illness and the 8th house is investigated for deep seated disease. The 12th house is also important as it throws light on hospitalization and convalescence. Since cancer is described as growth of cells, we will have to correlate growth idea with the planetary significance. Jupiter is the planet which signifies growth. However, Jupiter is very much a symbol of tradition and convention and any growth associated with Jupiter should be healthy. As a significatory therefore Jupiter is ruled out when it comes to cancerous kind of growth. The shadow planet Rahu is astrologically associated with morbid and erratic growth and swelling causing pain and discomfort which is despised. Rahu is therefore the key symbol to signify cancer disease. Equally important is Saturn who symbolizes decay and death. Saturn is also a karaka for chronic diseases. The role of Mars also cannot be overlooked as cancer could also be of ulcer type and blood cancer. Ulcer, wounds and blood are all signified by Mars.

J. N. Bhasin

He is of the following opinion leaving aside all the statistical studies:

A part of the body suffers when the following four factors representing it are afflicted in a chart: (1) The house representing the part; (2) the lord of this house; (3) the sign bearing the same number as the house and (4) the lord of this sign.

In case of cancer also this is applicable. The affliction should be caused by the malignant and disease-causing planets Saturn and Rahu and/or their dispositions. Where a simple explanation is possible why should we bring in any complex reasoning? The disease of cancer, whatever its type, can be explained on the basis of the sudden and malignant influence of Rahu and of Saturn on the limb involved. Why go to kalasarpayoga or to the location of Mars in the first half of the zodiac, etc.? It is also unreasonable to hold that the signs 4/7/8/12th only are afflicted in case of cancer. It is not so. Only the signs relevant to the type of cancer involved are found afflicted. Also the houses connected with the part involved are important. For example--5th house for stomach cancer, 7th house for uterus, 3rd house for cancer of rectum, 2nd house for face, 11th house for blood cancer etc.

Dr. P.S. Sastri

Cancer is an infection of the blood and blood comes under the Moon and Mars, and also under the Sun. The maintenance of the cells is regulated by the Sun, the Moon and Jupiter. Any affliction to these comes from Mars and Saturn. Rahu governs any form of malignant growth. The disease to which one is subjected to is to be read from Lagna, Lagna lord 6/8/12th houses. While Mercury indicates ulcers, Mars suggests tumours. Cancer which is primarily indicated by Rahu finds its place because of other planets involved. A badly afflicted Moon suggests the possibility of cancer. Cancer proper appears to fall in the opening degrees of Virgo and Pisces signs.

Dr. Sastri in another article says--

Cancer appears to have connection with Aries and Libra 230 and 240, Cancer and Capricorn 40, Virgo and Pisces 150. [It is not clear if these degrees quoted by Dr. Sastri are Sayana or Nirayana. In case of Virgo and Pisces at least it is not near 250 Sayana of Virgo-Pisces given by western astrologer Carter]. Other indicators are afflicted Jupiter and Saturn, and the signs Aries, Taurus, Cancer, Libra and Capricorn. From analysis we find that the planets involved in cancer cases are the Moon, Mars, Saturn and Rahu, particularly the last three. The importance of the lords of 6th and 8th, Lagna and Badhaka planets also cannot be underrated. The planets and the houses governing the different parts are all involved in the diagnosis of cancer. It is observed that we cannot generalize and lay down any specific rules leading to cancer. Each case has to be examined separately on its own merits. [Some specific degrees given by Dr. Sastri are kidney refers to 20 of fixed signs and generally to 100 of Taurus and Scorpio, spine refers to 260 of Cancer and Capricorn and 10 of common signs, lungs refer to 40 of Aries and Libra in addition to 3rd house and Gemini sign.]

MY VIEW

Cancer is a disease like any other disease and diagnosed accordingly, using well-established principles of medical Astrology. There is no need to treat cancer as a disease different from others for astrological predictions and to seek some specialized planetary combinations. Cancer is an abnormal and unchecked growth of cells connected with any part, the growth being not innocent but poisonous and malignant. Thus, blood cancer (leukaemia) is the abnormal growth of white blood cells.

In my view no foolproof and generalized combinations indicating cancer can be laid down by any amount of statistical studies. Statistical studies have value in their own place but are of limited importance, and each chart will have to be examined on its own merits for predictions. I agree therefore with the approach of the late astrologer Bhasin, who followed four factors as given below.

A part of the body suffers, whether due to cancer or any other disease, when the following four factors representing the part are afflicted in a chart:

(i) the house representing the part;

(ii) the lord of this house;

(iii) the sign bearing the same number as the house; and

(iv) the lord of this sign.

In case of cancer also this is applicable. The afflictions should be caused in 6/8/12th house, by 6/8/12th lords, by malefic planets Mars, Saturn or Rahu and/or by their dispositions. Extra-saturnine planet Uranus, which is known as a planet of eccentricity, can be considered in addition to others, to cause afflictions. Only the signs, houses and planets relevant to the type of cancer and the limb involved in the same will be found afflicted. Mild afflictions will cause mild suffering involving the limb whereas severe afflictions, coupled with suitable malefic Dasa periods and bad transits like Sadesathi, can cause serious incurable disease like cancer involving the said part. General strength of Lagna, its lord, the Moon and the Sun also should be considered before venturing predictions.

Jupiter is a planet of growth but in my opinion it is a giant benefic and therefore a planet of healthy growth by nature and cannot lead to malignant growth unless he becomes a functional malefic, is weak and severely afflicted. On the other hand very weak and afflicted Moon and the Sun can create unhealthy growths.

Kalasarpa Yoga is put forward as a yoga available in charts of patients suffering from cancer. I never advocate a partial yoga as yoga and therefore even if six planets are on one side of Rahu-Ketu axis and seventh planet is out on other side I will not call the chart as having a kalasarpa Yoga is not common, but in case a full Kalasarpa Yoga exists in a chart, it is a sort of unbalance in general and therefore for health also and coupled with afflictions may result in cancer.

Specific degrees of certain signs are advocated as indicating cancer, if afflicted. This method may be useful for research in Sayana system, but in Nirayana system, it will not useful due to different values of Ayanamsa used in preparing charts. Also considering predictions based on these degrees, decision regarding orbs of influence on both sides of these degrees will be a problem.

Chapter XVIII

Naturopathic Treatment of Cancer

The courses of treatment given below work in the first stage of cancer. Treatment must be followed for six weeks.

CHILDHOOD LEUKEMIA

Time	Diet	Treatment
6 am	lemon 1	strolling
1-2 pm	hot water	250 gm
8 am	orange 2; green water 250	cold-hot hip-bath
9 am	curd	200 gm with 10 basil leaves
10 am	soup; grape juice 250 gm	massage sun-bath, enema as required
12 noon	coconut water 200 gm	cold bath 3 to 5 min.
1 pm	khichri (dal + rice mixture);	orange 2-3
4 pm	soup of fresh almonds	
7 pm	2 oranges (sucked)	hot mud pack on belly for 20 min.
9 pm	250 gm boiled vegetables with 100 gm	light night walk steamed bio-basmati rice

Yogasanas

- Shavasana (the corpse pose); before sleeping
- Nadi Shuddhi Pranayama
- Deep breathing practice.

LEUKEMIA IN ADULTS

Time	Diet	Treatment
6 am	lemon 1; lukewarm water 250 gm	stroll 1 km
8 am	soup 25 gm; milk 100 gm; raw brown sugar; green water 25 ml	sun bath
10 am	soup (50+50) gm; (any porridge) with milk	enema (as required); oil massage except belly
12 pm	coconut water 200 gm	cold bath for 3-5 min.
1 pm	khichri 100 gm	
4 pm	millet soup (5+5)	
6 pm	soup 100 gm; milk 100 gm; raw brown sugar; orange (2-3) on feeling hunger	
7 pm	curd 200 gm with 10 basil leaves	
8 pm	250 gm green vegetable soup with mushroom	
9 pm	boiled rice 300 gm	light night walk

Exercises

Shavasana before going to sleep.
Deep breathing practice.

LYMPHOMA

Time	Diet	Treatment
6 am	lemon 1, water 250 gm	stroll 1-2 km
8 am	cabbage soup 100 gm; avoid milk; raw brown sugar 10 gm	sponge 5 days a week
9 am	soup 100 gm; no milk; curd 200 gm with 10 basil leaves; raw brown sugar 10 gm	sun bath
12 pm	coconut water 200 gm	cold bath 5 min.
1 pm	khichri 300 gm	
4 pm	green water 200 gm	
6 pm	soup 100 gm; no milk raw brown sugar 10 gm	rest treatment; on fever cold water bandage on head and stomach
7 pm	lemon soup 250 gm	deep breathing practice
8 pm	on hunger, weakness or insomnia 2-3 oranges or papaya 250 gm	enema 3 days in a week; strolling
9 pm	curd with basil leaves	

Exercises

Shavasana before sleeping.

CANCER OF THE BRAIN

Time	Diet	Treatment
6 am	half lemon with lukewarm water, 250 gm	stroll 1-2 km
8 am	honey 25 gm; hot water 250 gm; basil leaves 10	cold mud pack on head and stomach

Time	Diet	Treatment
9 am	soup 200 gm; curd 200 gm with 10 basil leaves; raw brown sugar 10 gm	oil massage except belly
11 am	coconut water 200 gm;	sponge with lukwarm water
12 noon	orange 2; khichri 250 gm or as per hunger	hot and cold hip bath with green leaf
1 pm	curd with basil leaves	
4 pm	buttermilk	
5 pm	buttermilk	
6 pm	curd	
8 pm	boiled vegetables 300 gm	light walk

Exercise

Shavasana before sleeping.

CANCER OF THE MUSCLES (RHABDOMYOSARCOMA)

Time	Diet	Treatment
6 am	lemon, honey, with lukewarm water 250 gm	
10 am		sun-bath
9 am	soup 250 gm; raw brown sugar 25 gm	enema 3 days a week
11 am	coconut water 300 gm	
12 noon	round gourd dish 25 gm; orange 2; khichri 300 gm	lukewarm water bath
3 pm	buttermilk with basil leaf	
5 pm	green water 200 gm	
7 pm	papaya 250 gm; orange 2; turnip, cabbage salad	
8 pm	coconut water 200 gm	hot mud pack
9 pm	boiled vegetables 300 gm (such as parval, plenty of strolling round gourd, ladyfinger, coriander, mint, cabbage)	

Exercise

Shavasana before sleeping.

MALIGNANT MELANOMA (CANCER OF THE SKIN)

Time	Diet	Treatment
6 am	lemon 1 with lukewarm water 250 gm	stroll 1 km
8 am	honey 25 gm; milk 250 gm; fresh fruit juice 250 gm	
9 am	curd 200 gm with 10 basil leaves; porridge 200 gm	sun bath
11 am	vegetable dish 100 gm; boiled carrot 50 gm	
12 pm	grape juice; curd 200 gm with 10 basil leaves; 10 soaked raisins	light cold bath

Time	Diet	Treatment
1 pm	green water khichri 250 gm	
3 pm	onion-tomato soup 250 gm	
6 pm	papaya 100 gm; coconut water; round gourd dish 50 gm; draksh 50 gm	
7 pm	fresh almond soup	deep breathing practice
8 pm	barley soup 250 gm	
9 pm	boiled vegetables 350 gm	light night walk

Exercises

Shavasana before sleeping.

NEUROBLASTOMA (CANCER OF THE SKIN)

Time	Diet	Treatment
6 am	lemon; honey 25 gm; luke warm water 250 gm	stroll 1-2 km
8 am	fresh vegetable soup 250 gm;	sun bath
12 noon	light ?strach 20 gm; whey 100 gm; vegetable dish 100 gm; boiled carrot 50 gm	oil massage; cold bath
2 pm	khichri 250 gm; fresh almond soup 100 gm	
3 pm	soup 100 gm; milk 50 gm; orange 2	
4 pm	green water 200 gm	
6 pm	round gourd dish 50 gm; whey 100 gm; papaya 250 gm; draksh 50 gm; coconut water 200 gm	enema (twice a week)
7 pm	papaya 250 gm; vegetable soup 250 gm	deep breathing practice
9 pm	unpolished ricewith boiled vegetables; curd 200 gm with basil leaves	stroll 1-2 km

Exercise

Shavasana before sleeping.

CANCER OF THE BREAST

Time	Diet	Treatment
6 am	lemon 1; honey 20 gm; water 250 gm	strolling 1-2 km
8 am	fruit shake 250 gm	sun bath
10 am	coconut water	massage and hip bath
12 noon	khichri 300 gm; light starch 40 gm; whey 150 gm vegetable dish 150 gm; butter 5 gm; boiled carrot 5 gm; milk 25 gm; orange 2	
2 pm	fresh almond soup 250 gm	
4 pm	green water 250 gm	Pranayama
6 pm	papaya 200 gm; simple vegetable dish 50 gm; draksh 100 gm whey 150 gm	

Time	Diet	Treatment
7 pm	buttermilk	steam bath
9 pm	fresh bio basmati unpolished rice with green vegetables	light walk

Exercises

Shavasana before sleeping.

CANCER OF THE LUNG

Time	Diet	Treatment
6 am	lemon 1; honey 20 gm; water 200 gm	morning walk 1-2 km for a week
8 am	curd 200 gm with 10 basil leaves	sun bath
11 am	green water 200 gm	simple bath
12 noon	bread 1 slice; khichri 20 gm; butter 10 gm; whey 150 gm; vegetable dish 250 gm; boiled carrot 50 gm; sauce 10 gm; cucurbit gourd 20 gm	cold mud pack on head; cold hip-bath for 2 min.
1 pm	khichri liquid 300 gm	
3 pm	basil-chaulai decoction 100 gm; milk 25 gm; orange 2	
5 pm	buttermilk	
6 pm	coconut water	evening walk
7 pm	papaya 200 gm; grape 10 gm; whey 200 gm	
8 pm	fresh almond soup	light night walk
9 pm	boiled vegetable with bio basmati rice (brown)	'Yoga nidra' for 30 minutes

Exercises

Shavasana before sleeping.

SECONDARY TUMOURS OF THE LUNG

Time	Diet	Treatment
6 am	lemon 1; honey 20 gm; lukewarm water 200 gm	stroll; enema on constipation
8 am	basil-chaulai decoction 100 gm; milk 50-100 gm	sun bath; massage cold mud pack on belly for 20-30 min.
10 am	soup tomato 100 gm with onion 2	simple bath
11 am	water 200 gm +whey 250 gm; tomato 200 gm; millet 10-20 gm	cold mud pack on head
4 pm	soup millet+tomato	cold mud pack for 20 min.
6 pm	papaya 200 gm; grape 250 gm basil-chaulai decoction 200 gm milk 100 gm	
8 pm	curd 200 gm with basil leaves; boiled vegetables 300 gm	light night walk; bath before bed

Exercises

Shavasana before sleeping.

CANCERS OF GASTRO-INTESTINAL TRACT

Time	Diet	Treatment
6 am	lemon 1; honey 200 gm; lukewarm water 200 gm	stroll 1-2 km
8 am	grape juice 250 gm	enema twice a week
9 am	cashew nut soup 250 gm	sun bath
11 am	apricots spouts 250 gm	oil message
12 noon	green water	
1 pm	khichri 300 gm	
3 pm	fresh wheat grass juice (do not take anything for half an hour thereafter)	
6 pm	butter milk 250 gm	Pranayama
7 pm	green vegetable salad 300 gm	light walk
9 pm	boiled rice with green vegetables 300 gm	

Exercises

Shavasana before sleeping.

ORAL CANCER

Time	Diet	Treatment
6 am	lemon 2; honey 20 gm; water 200 gm	stroll; sunbath; massage; enema on constipation
8 am	basil-chaulai decoction 100 gm; milk 50-100 gm	cold mud pack on belly for 20-30 min.
9 am	green water	simple bath
10 am	soup, tomato 100 gm with onion 2	
11 am	water 200 gm +whey 250 gm; tomato 200 gm; millet 10-20 gm	cold mud pack on head
4 pm	soup millet+tomato 300 gm	
6 pm	papaya 200 gm; grape 250 gm basil-chaulai decoction 200 gm	
8 pm	curd 200 gm with basil leaves boiled vegetables 300 gm	cold mud pack for 20 min.
9 pm	whey 100 gm	light walk

Exercises

Shavasana before sleeping.

CANCER OF THE CHEEK

Time	Diet	Treatment
6 am	lemon 1; honey 200 gm; lukewarm water 200 gm	stroll 1-2 km
8 am	grape juice 250 gm	enema twice a week
9 am	cashew nut soup 250 gm	sunbath
11 am	apricots sprouts 250 gm	oil massage
12 pm	green water	
1 pm	khichri 300 gm with fresh spinach soup 250 gm	
3 pm	fresh wheat grass juice (do not take anything for half an hour thereafter)	
6 pm	buttermilk	Pranayama
7 pm	green vegetable salad	light walk
9 pm	boiled rice with green vegetables (plenty of parval, carrot, cabbage, mint, chulai, buck wheat)	

Exercises

Shavasana before sleeping.
Other asanas as prescribed by doctor.

CANCER OF THE TONGUE

Time	Diet	Treatment
6 am	lemon 1; honey 20 gm; luke warm water 200 gm	stroll 1-2 km
8 am	basil-chulai decoction 100 gm; milk 100 gm	
9 am	green water 250 gm	sunbath
11 am	coconut water 250 gm	body massage
12 noon	porridge 20 gm; dish 150 gm; butter 10 gm; millet 20 gm; sauce 10 gm; whey 10 gm	hip bath
2 pm	fresh fruit juice 280 gm	
3 pm	orange 2;	enema (twice a week)
4 pm	green water 200 gm	
6 pm	papaya 20 gm; maize basil-chulai decoction 100 gm; milk 100 gm	
9 pm	khichri liquid curd 200 gm with basil	light night walk leaves

Exercises

Shavasana before sleeping.

CANCER OF OESOPHAGUS

Time	Diet	Treatment
1.	Juices for 10 days; 200 gm to 1000 gm throughout the course	stroll up to 4-5 km 4 times first day
2.	Curd and fruits: mango, papaya, fig., currant, date, etc., for one month; curd up to 1-2 kg	
3.	Normal diet: for 15 days 12 porridges; vegetable dishes; butter 10-20 gm; coconut 10 gm; curd 200 gm	
3 pm	orange 2-3; coconut water 200 gm	enema (if required)
6 pm	milk 500 gm; fruits 400 gm	
7 pm	curd with basil leaves	
8 pm	grape juice 500 gm	
9 pm	fresh almond soup light food; boiled green vegetables 300 gm (cabbage, cauliflower, carrots, beans, etc.)	light night walk

Exercises

Shavasana before sleeping.

CANCER OF THE STOMACH

Time	Diet	Treatment
6 am	lemon; water 200 gm; a spoonful of honey in one glass of fresh lemon water	stroll
8 am	whey-curd 200 gm with 10 basil leaves	enema (once a week)
9 am	germinated moong dal 50 gm; soaked dates 10; fresh green coconut 50-60 gm; fresh vegetables (carrot, cabbage, spinach, beans); fresh fruits (mango, chickoo, guava, papaya, banana; only one or two fruits at one time)	sunbath
10 am	butter milk 250 gm	sun bath and oil massage
11 am	green water 250 gm	simple bath
12 noon	coconut water 250 gm	
2 pm	oranges 2	
4 pm	fruits	hip bath
7 pm	fresh almond soup 250 gm	cold mud pack
9 pm	milk 200 gm	light night walk

Exercises

Shavasana before sleeping.

CANCER OF THE COLON AND RECTUM

Time	Diet	Treatment
6 am	lemon 1; hot water 200 gm	strolling; sunbath; massage except belly
8 am	orange 2; sweet lemon juice 250 gm	hot-cold hip bath
9 am	green water	

Time	Diet	Treatment
10 am	fresh vegetable soup 200 gm	
12 noon	whey 250 gm; vegetable dish 200 gm; tomato 100 gm	simple bath
4 pm	soup (10+10)	stroll
6 pm	milk 250 gm; currant 20 gm; papaya 200 gm; orange 2-3	hot mud pack on belly continue with wet mud pack
7 pm	green vegetable salad	
9 pm	boiled rice with boiled green leafy vegetables, bottle gourd, cauliflower, carrot	light night walk

Exercises

Shavasana before going to sleep.

PRIMARY CANCER OF THE LIVER

Time	Diet	Treatment
6 am	lemon 1; hot water 200 gm	stroll; sunbath; massage except belly
8 am	orange 2; grape juice 250 gm	hot-cold hip bath
10 am	millet soup 150 gm	
11 am	coconut water 250 gm	
12 noon	whey 250 gm; dish 200 gm--tomato 100 gm; onion 1	simple bath
4 pm	barley soup 200 gm;	stroll
6 pm	milk 250 gm; currant 20 gm; papaya 200 gm; orange 2-3	hot mud pack on belly and continue with wet mud pack
7 pm	green vegetable salad	
9 pm	boiled rice with boiled green leafy vegetables; bottle gourd, cauliflower, carrot	light night walk

Exercises

Shavasana before going to sleep.

SECONDARY CANCER IN LIVER

Time	Diet	Treatment
6 am	lemon 1; honey 20 gm; water 200 gm	stroll; sunbath; massage; enema on constipation
8 am	basil-chulai decoction 100 gm; milk 50-100 gm	cold mud pack on belly for 20-30 min.
10 am	soup: tomato 100 gm with onion 2	simple bath
11 am	water 200 gm +whey 250 gm; tomato 200 gm; millet 10-20 gm	cold mud pack on head
12 noon	green water 200 gm	
1 pm	khichri 250 gm	
4 pm	soup millet+tomato	
8 pm	cold mud pack for 20 minutes	
5 pm	coconut water 300 gm	
6 pm	papaya 200 gm; grape 250 gm; basil-chulai decoction 200 gm; milk 100 gm	cold mud pack on before bed bath
8 pm	curd 200 gm with basil leaves; boiled vegetables 300 gm	light night walk.

Exercises

Shavasana before sleeping.

CANCER OF THE GALL-BLADDER

Time	Diet	Treatment
6 am	lemon 2; honey 20 gm; water 200 gm	stroll; sunbath; massage; enema on constipation
8 am	basil-chulai decoction 100 gm; milk 50-100 gm	cold mud pack on belly for 20-30 min.
10 am	soup: tomato 100 gm with onion 2	simple bath
11 am	water 200 gm + whey 250 gm; tomato 200 gm; millet 10-20 gm	cold mud pack on head
4 pm	soup millet+tomato	
8 pm		cold mud pack for 20 min.
6 pm	papaya 200 gm; grape 250 gm basil-chulai decoction 200 gm milk 100 gm	
8 pm	curd 200 gm with basil leaves; boiled vegetables 300 gm	before bed bath light night walk
9 pm	buttermilk 250 gm	

Exercises

Shavasana before sleeping.

CANCER OF THE PANCREAS

Time	Diet	Treatment
6 am	lemon 1; honey 20 gm; water 200 gm	stroll; sunbath; massage; enema on constipation
8 am	basil-chulai decoction 100 gm; milk 50-100 gm	cold mud pack on belly for 20-30 min.
10 am	soup: tomato 100 gm, onion 2	simple bath
11 am	water 200 gm +whey 250 gm; tomato 200 gm; millet 10-20 gm	cold mud pack on head
12 noon	green water 230 gm	
1 pm	fresh vegetable soup with steamed rice	

Time	Diet	Treatment
4 pm	soup millet+tomato	
8 pm		cold mud pack for 20 min.
5 pm	coconut water 240 gm	
6 pm	papaya 200 gm; grape 250 gm basil-chulai decoction 200 gm milk 100 gm	
7 pm	green vegetable soup 200 gm	light night walk
8 pm	curd 200 gm with basil leaves before bedbath boiled vegetables 300 gm	
9 pm	spinach, cabbage, cauliflower and chulai dish 300 gm	

Exercises

Shavasana before sleeping.

CANCER OF THE BONE

Time	Diet	Treatment
6 am	lemon 1 with lukewarm water 200 gm	
7 am	orange 3; grape juice 100 gm	stroll 1-2 km
10 am	vegetable soup 300 gm	sunbath
11 am	coconut water 200 gm	
12 noon	boiled vegetables 300 gm; tomato	massage except belly; hot-cold hip bath
2 pm	orange 3; soaked raisins 10	simple bath
5 pm	millet soup 300 gm	cold hip bath
7 pm	papaya 300 gm boiled carrot 300 gm	stroll; hot mud pack
8 pm	buttermilk	
9 pm	khichri with green vegetables 300 gm ; coconut water 200 gm	light night walk

Exercises

Shavasana before sleeping.

EWING'S SARCOMA

Time	Diet	Treatment
6 am	lemon 1; honey 20 gm; water 300 gm	stroll; sunbath; massage
8 am	sweet lemon juice 170 gm	
9 am	whey 250 gm	hip bath
12 noon	whey 250 gm; germinated salad moong 30 gm; 100 gm; vegetable dish 250 gm	hot-cold hipbath
2 pm	green water	
3 pm	orange 3; grape 250 gm	
6 pm	fruits 300 gm; salad 100 gm	massage of head and feet
7 pm	lemon water 190 gm	
8 pm	pulse extracts	
9 pm	curd 200 gm with 10 basil leaves	

MULTIPLE MYELOMA

Time	Diet	Treatment
6 am	lemon 1; honey 20 gm; luke warm water 300 gm	stroll; enema twice a week
9 am	basil-chulai decoction 100 gm; milk 50 gm; raw brown sugar 20 gm; fresh carrot juice 100 gm	sunbath; massage steam-bath
10 am	lemon water 200 gm	
12 noon	boiled vegetable dish 250 gm; salad 100 gm; ripe juicy mango, grapes, papaya, figs; fresh cheese	
4 pm	orange 3	simple bath
7 pm	soup 250 gm; papaya 250 gm; salad 100 gm	stroll
9 pm	boiled vegetables 300 gm steamed rice; curd 350 gm	

CANCER OF THE UTERINE CERVIX

Time	Diet	Treatment
6 am	lemon 1; hot water 200 gm	stroll; sunbath; massage except belly
8 am	orange 2	hot-cold hip bath
10 am	millet soup (10+10)	
12 noon	whey 250 gm; vegetable dish 200 gm; tomato 100 gm	simple bath
4 pm	barley soup (10+10)	stroll
6 pm	milk 250 gm; currant 20 gm; papaya 200 gm; orange 2-3	hot mud pack on belly and continue with wet mud pack
7 pm	green vegetable salad (parval, cabbage, carrot, cucumber, pumpkin	
9 pm	boiled rice with boiled leafy green vegetables, bottle gourd, cauliflower, carrot	light night walk

Exercises

Shavasana before going to sleep.

CANCER OF THE UTERUS

Time	Diet	Treatment
6 am	lemon & orange; sip hot soup	stroll
8 am	curd 200 gm with 10 basil leaves	
9 am	fresh apricots; coconut water	
12 noon	cashew nut soup; 300 gm water	sunbath
2 pm	rice soup	

Time	Diet	Treatment
4' pm	butter milk;	hot-cold hip bath
7 pm	corn soup with brown steamed rice	light walk
8 pm	green water 200 gm	
9 pm	steamed rice with vegetable soup 400 gm	

CHORICARCINOMA OR CANCER OF THE PLACENTA

Time	Diet	Treatment
6 am	lemon 2; honey 20 gm; water 200 gm	stroll; sunbath; massage; enema on constipation
8 am	basil-chulai decoction 100 gm; milk 50-100 gm	cold mud pack on belly for 20-30 min.
9 am	green water 200 gm	
10 am	soup: tomato 100 gm, onion 2	simple bath
11 am	water 200 gm + whey 250 gm; tomato 200 gm; millet 10-20 gm; green leafy vegetable salad	cold mud pack on head
12 noon	coconut water 300 gm	
4 pm	soup millet+tomato	
8 pm		cold mud pack for 20 min.
6 pm	papaya 200 gm; grape 250 gm basil-chulai decoction 200 gm milk 100 gm	
8 pm	curd 200 gm with basil leaves; boiled vegetables 300 gm	before bedbath light night walk
9 pm	mushroom soup	

Exercises

Shavasana before sleeping.

CANCER OF THE TESTES

Time	Diet	Treatment
6 am	lemon 1; honey 20 gm; lukewarm water 200 gm	stroll 1-2 km
8 am	basil-chulai decoction 100 gm; milk 100 gm	subath
12 noon	porridge 20 gm; vegetable dish 150 gm; butter 10 gm; millet 20 gm; sauce 10 gm; whey10 gm	hip bath
2 pm	porridges 280 gm; fresh cheese 20 gm	
3 pm	orange 2; green water	enema (twice a week)
6 pm	papaya 20 gm; maize basil-chulai decoction 100 gm; milk 100 gm	

Time	Diet	Treatment
9 pm	khichri liquid; curd 200 gm with leaves	light night walk basil

Exercises

Shavasana before sleeping.

Nadi Shudhi Pranayama.

CANCER OF THE PROSTATE

Time	Diet	Treatment
6 am	lemon 1; honey 20 gm; water 200 gm;	stroll; sunbath; massage; enema on constipation
8 am	basil-chulai decoction 100 gm; milk 50-100 gm	cold mud pack on belly for 20-30 min.
10 am	soup: tomato 100 gm, onion 2	simple bath
11 am	water 200 gm + whey 250 gm; tomato 200 gm; millet 10-20 gm	cold mud pack on head
2 pm	coconut water 200 gm	
4 pm	soup: millet+tomato	
8 pm		cold mud pack for 20 min.
6 pm	papaya 200 gm; grape 250 gm; basil-chulai decoction 200 gm; milk 100 gm	
7 pm	coconut water 250 gm	
8 pm	curd 200 gm with basil leaves boiled vegetables 300 gm (parval, cabbage, cucurbit, round gourd, pumpkin, cucumber etc.)	before bedbath light night walk
9 pm	steamed rice 300 gm; curd + basil leaves 5	

Exercises

Shavasana before sleeping.

CANCER OF THE PENIS

Time	Diet	Treatment
7 am	lemon juice with water	stroll
9 am	fresh wheat grass juice mushrooms; carrot soup	
11 am	fresh vegetable juice; cabbage; radish 500 gm	sun bath
12 noon	khichri with papaya soup	
1 pm	coconut water; brussels sprouts, broccoli, sprouted moong	
3 pm	orange 3; soaked mnakkas 10; sweet lime juice	
5 pm	buttermilk 200 gm	
6 pm	curd with basil leaves	

Time	Diet	Treatment
7 pm	cashew soup 300 gm water	light walk
8 pm	green water	
9 pm	germinated lentils 30 gm; cabbage 40 gm; beans 30 gm; or tomato soup 200 gm	

Exercises

Shavasana before sleeping.

CANCER OF THE URINARY BLADDER

Time	Diet	Treatment
7 am	lemon juice with water	stroll
9 am	fresh wheat grass juice; mushrooms; carrot soup	
11 am	fresh vegetable juice; cabbage; radish 500 gm	sun bath
12 noon	khichri with papaya soup	
1 pm	coconut water; brussels sprouts, broccoli, moong sprout	
3 pm	orange 3; soaked raisins 20; sweet lime juice	
5 pm	buttermilk 200 gm	
6 pm	curd with basil leaves	
7 pm	cashew soup; water 300 gm	light walk
8 pm	green water. 200 gm	mud pack (cold)
9 pm	germinated lentils 30 gm; cabbage 40 gm; beans 30 gm; or tomato soup 200 gm	

Exercises

Shavasana before sleeping.

CANCER OF THE KIDNEY

Time	Diet	Treatment
6 am	1 spoon honey in lukewarm water 250 gm	stroll
8 am	brussels sprouts with cabbage-cauliflower soup 200 gm	
11 am	buttermilk 300 gm; germinated pulses 30 gm; green coconut 30 gm; papaya 240 gm	sun bath
2 pm	coconut water 250 gm; grape juice 100 gm	
5 pm	curd; orange 3 with basil leaves	
7 pm	cucumber; garlic onion with green cabbage 300 gm	
8 pm	sweet carrot or orange juice 300 gm	mud pack (cold)
9 pm	boiled steamed basmati brown rice with sweet corn soup 200 gm; green vegetable salad	light night walk

WILM'S TUMOUR

Time	Diet	Treatment
7 am	lemon hot soup	stroll 1-2 km
8 am	curd 200 gm with 10 basil leaves	
9 am	millet soup; water 200 gm; cabbage salad	sun bath
11 am	butter milk; germinated pulses 35 gm; soaked dates or soaked munakkas 10; green vegetables	
12 noon	coconut water 200 gm	cold bath for 5 min.
1 pm	brown steamed rice 300 gm	
2 pm	sweet lemons or orange juice 250 gm	
3 pm	coconut water 250 gm	
5 pm	butter milk 150 gm	
7 pm	green water 100 gm	mud pack (cold)
8 pm	mushroom garlic onion soup; water 300 gm	
9 pm	millet juice; fresh almond soup 250 gm; fresh grape juice 250 gm; parval soup	light night walk

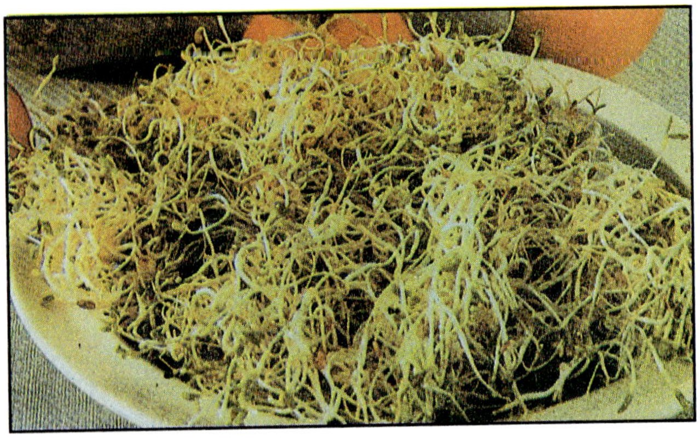

ALFALFA

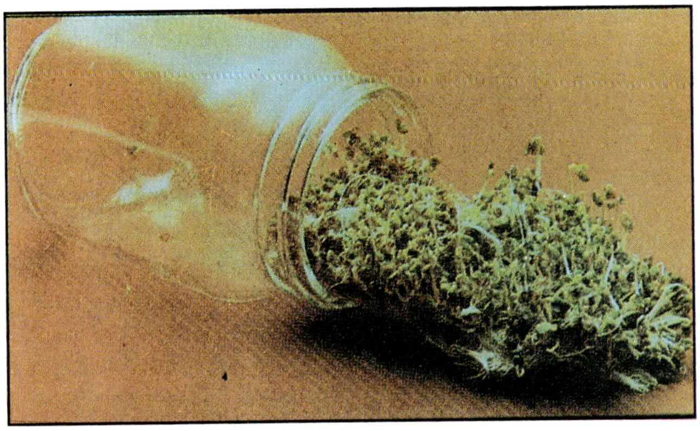

RADISH

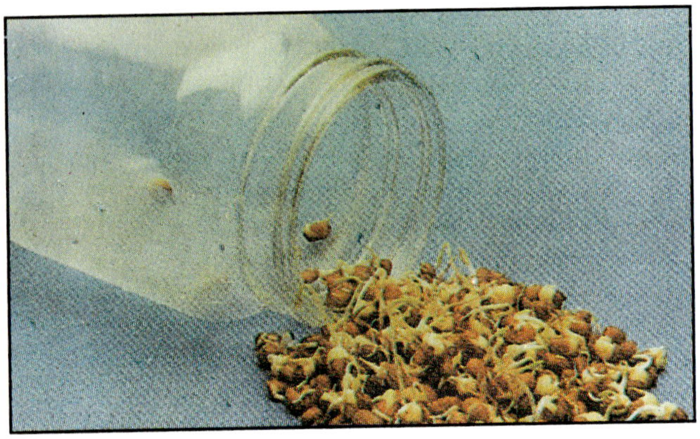

ADZUKI BEAN

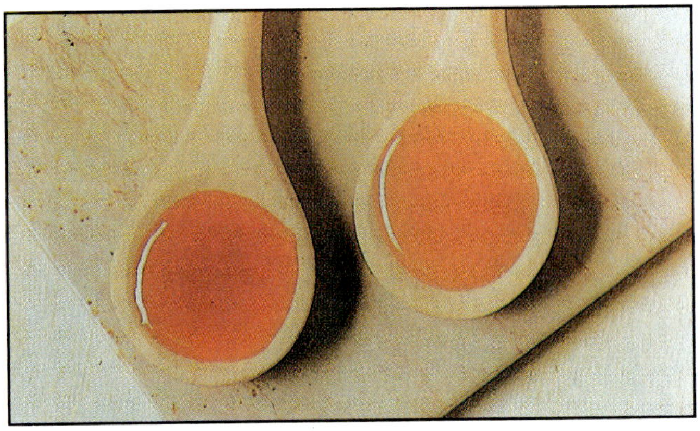

HONEY

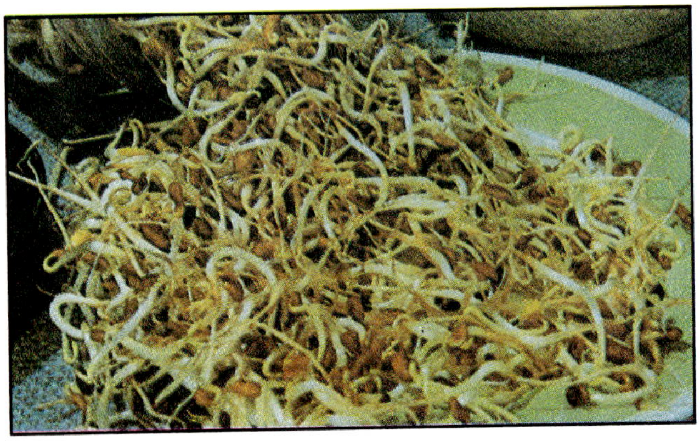

FENUGREEK

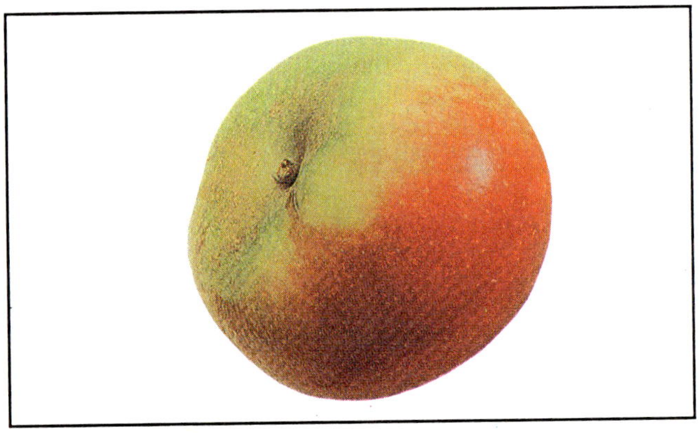

APPLE

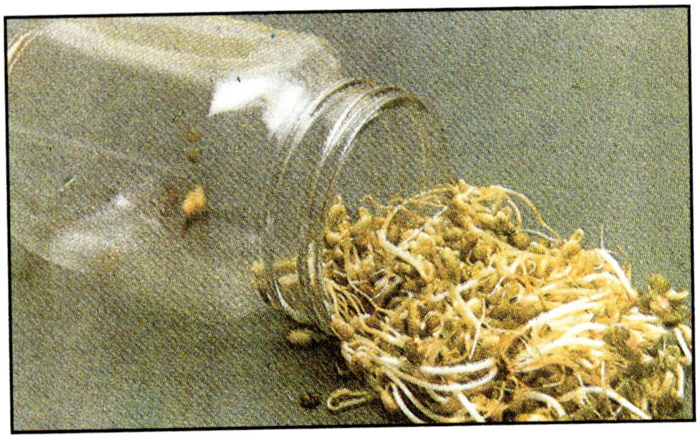

MUNG BEAN

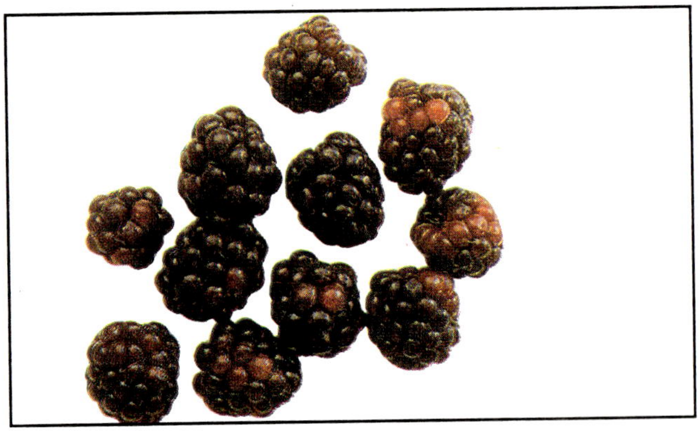

BLACKBERRIES

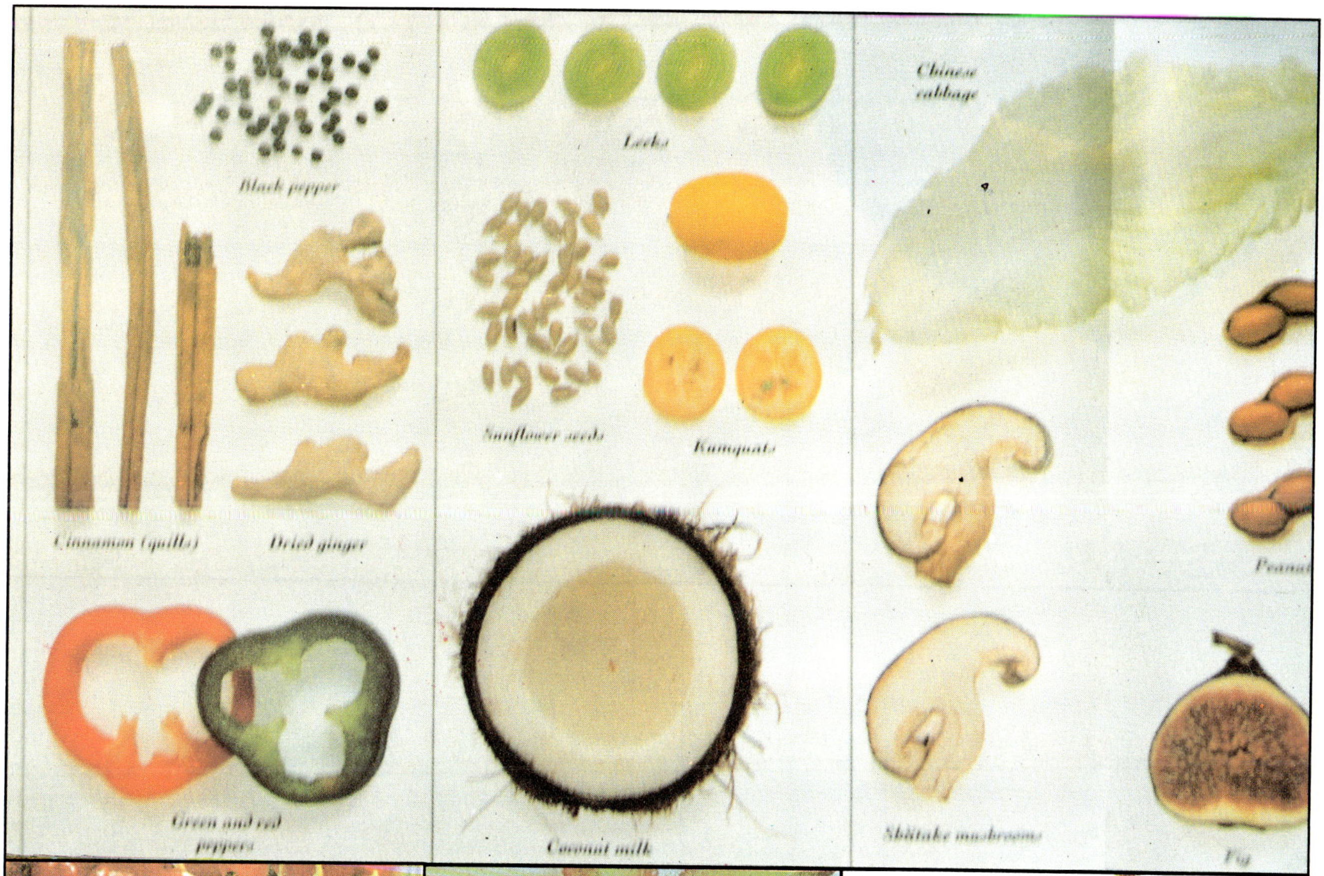

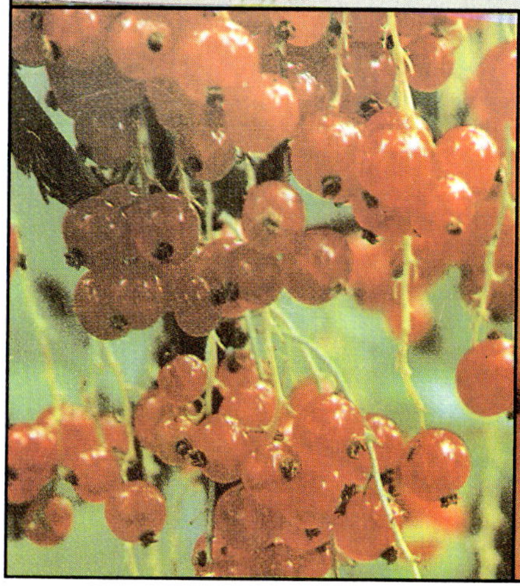

CURRANTS

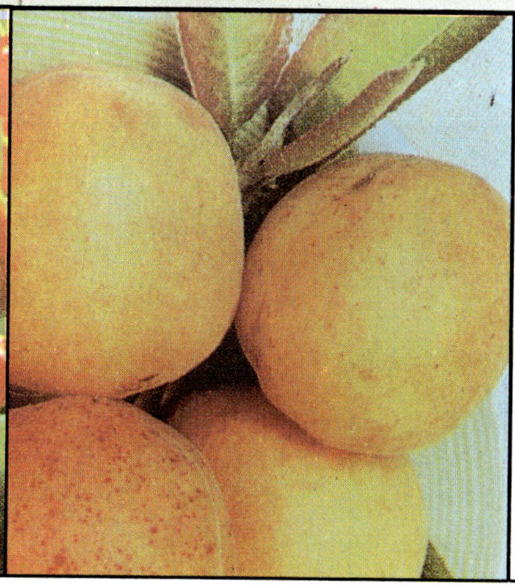

APRICOTS

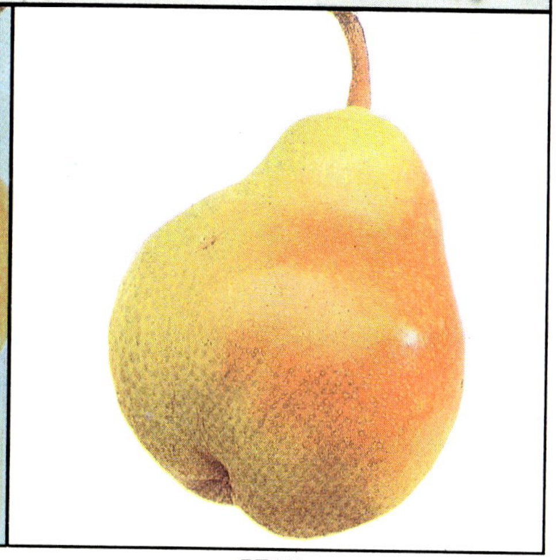

PEAR

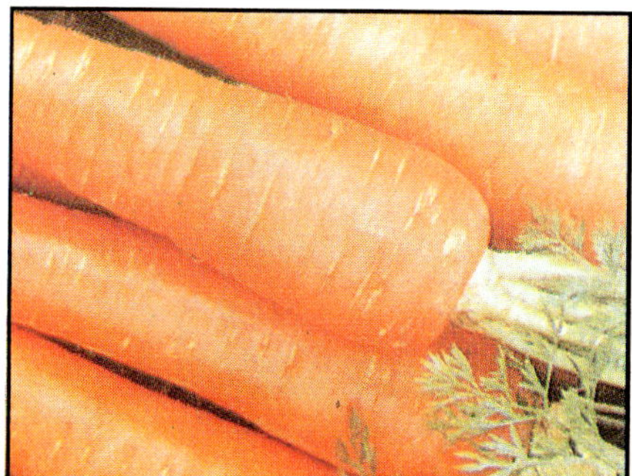

CARROTS

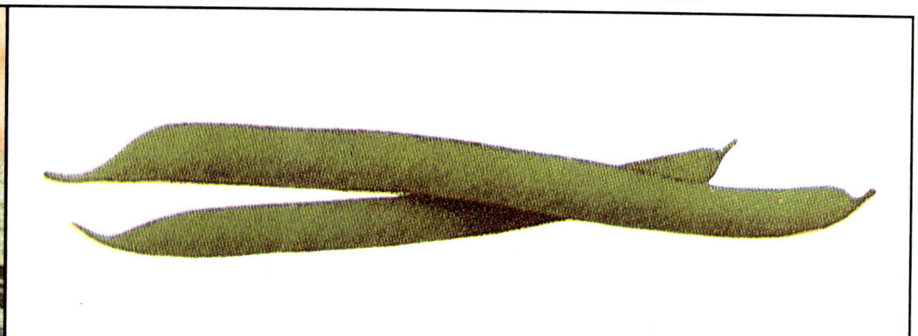

FRENCH BEAN

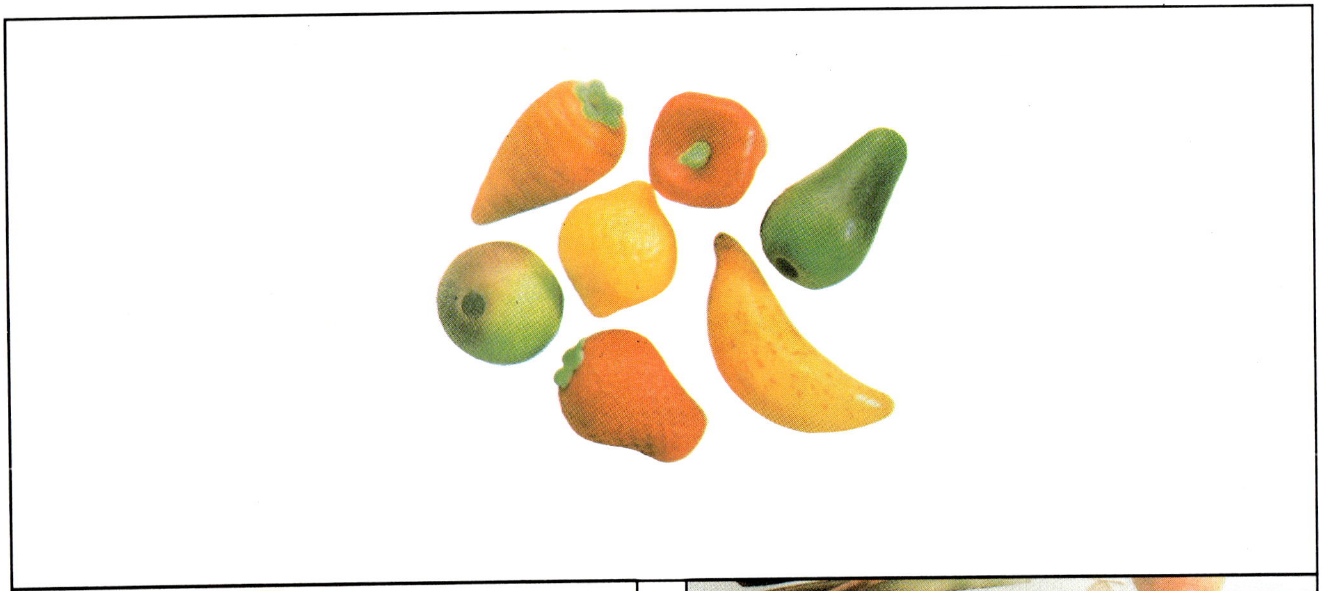

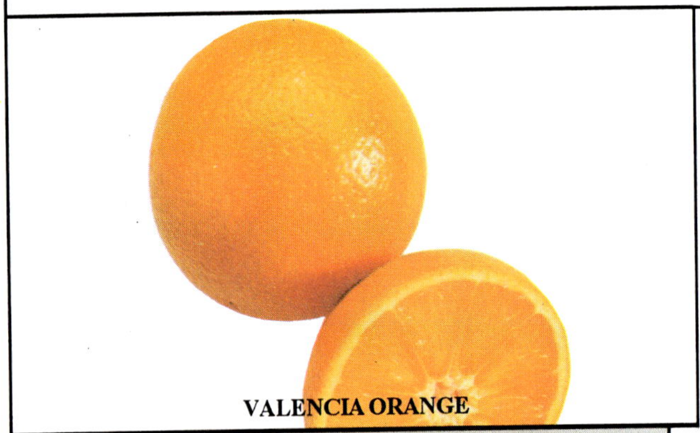

VALENCIA ORANGE

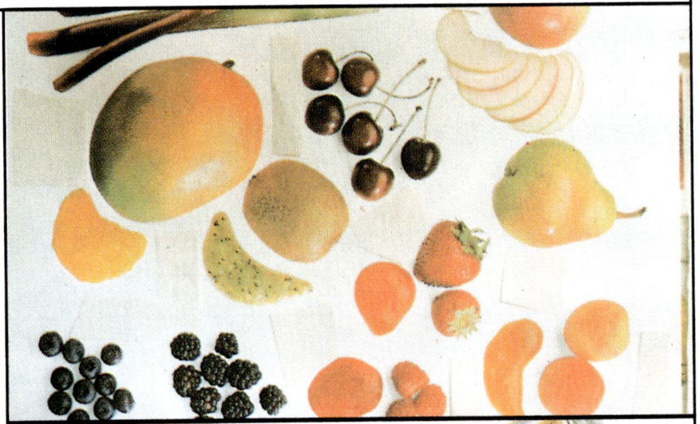

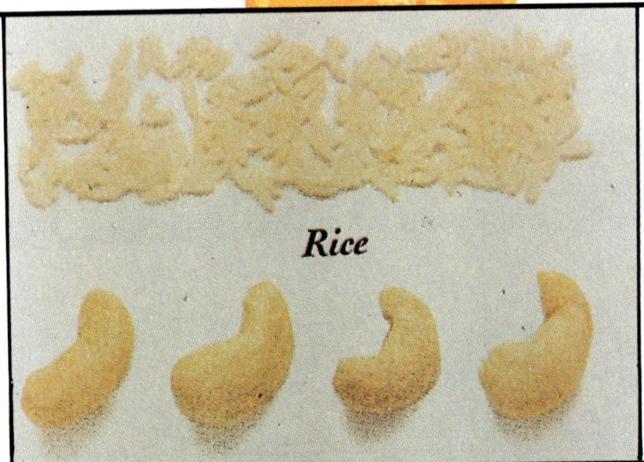

Rice

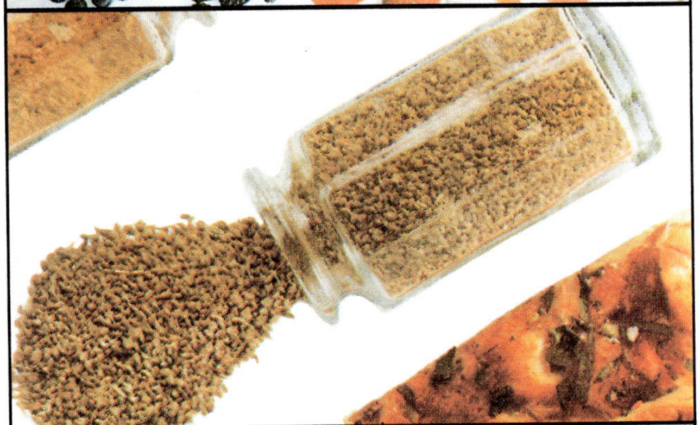

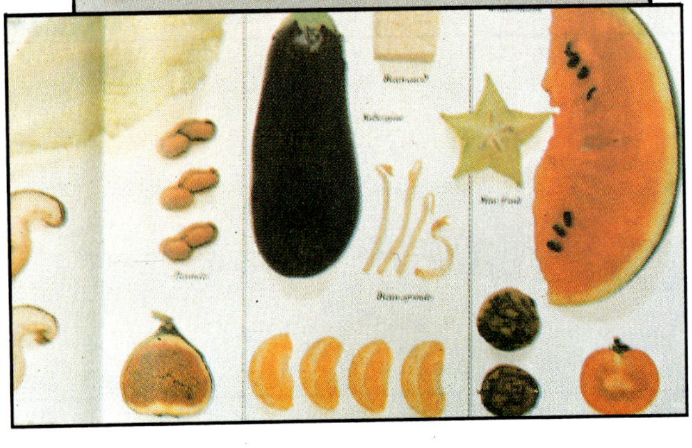

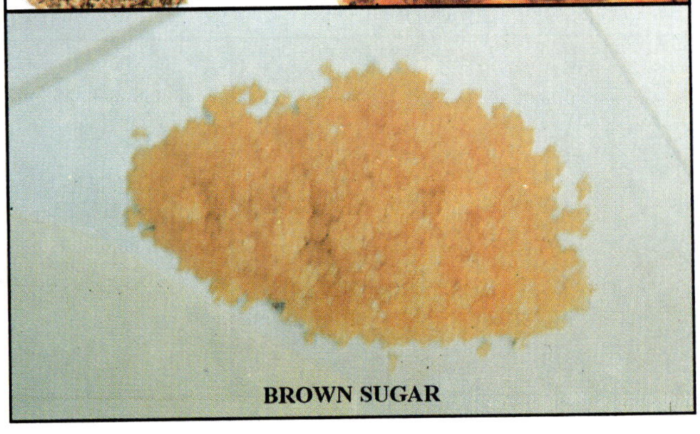

BROWN SUGAR

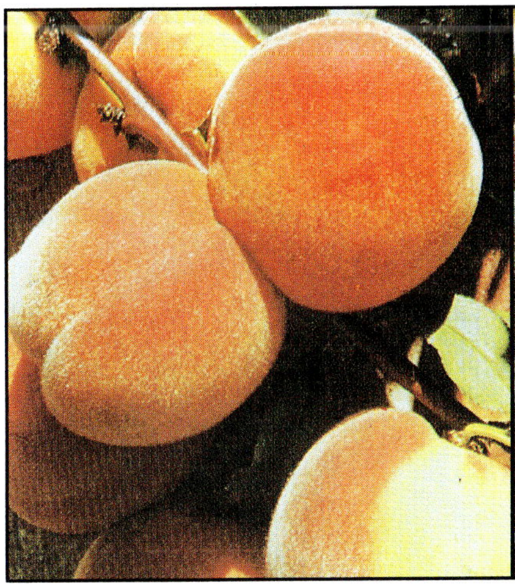

PEACHES

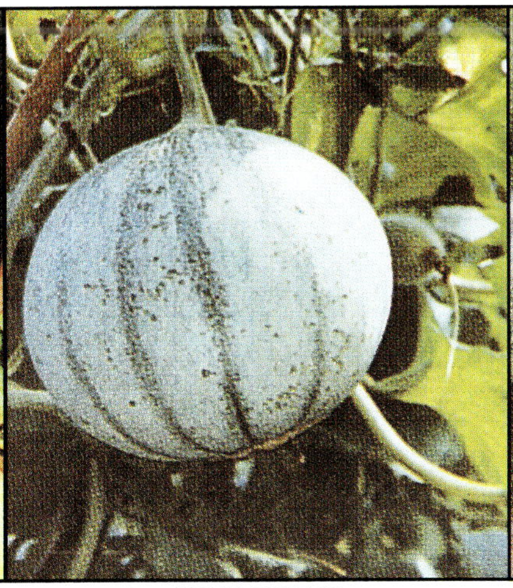

CHARANTAIS

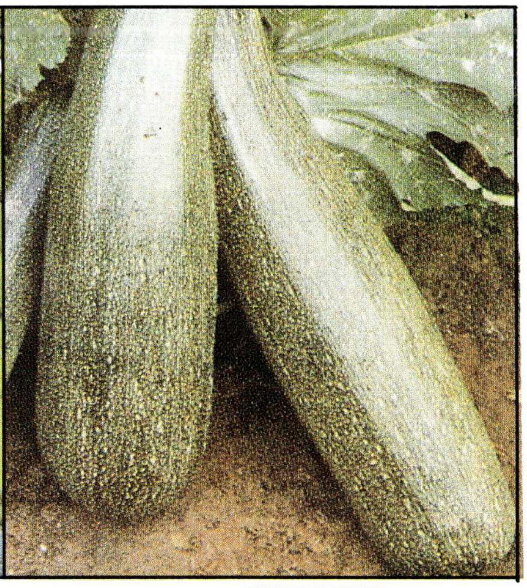

CUCUMBER

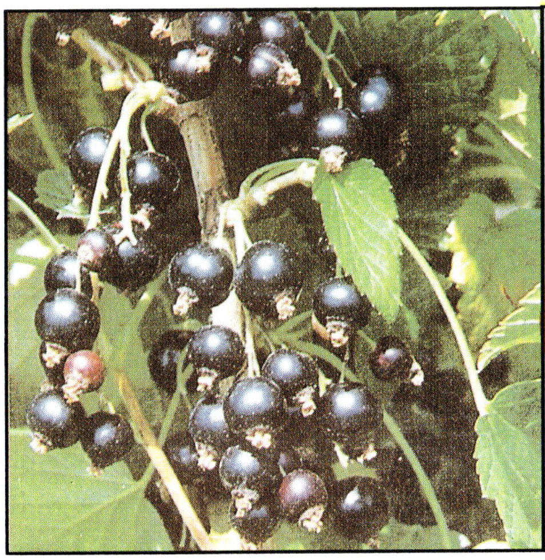

BLACKCURRANTS

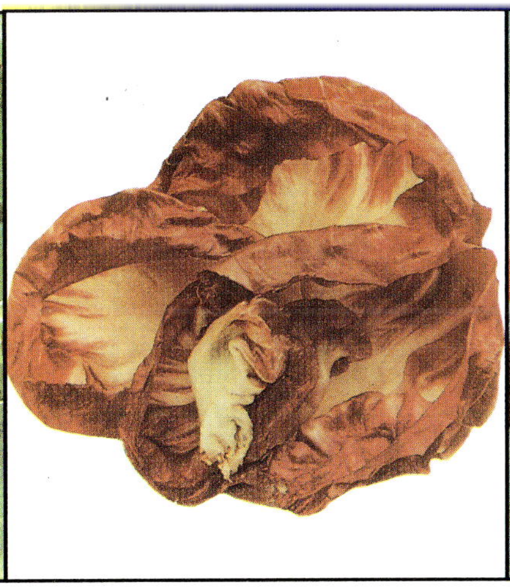

RADIOCCHIO

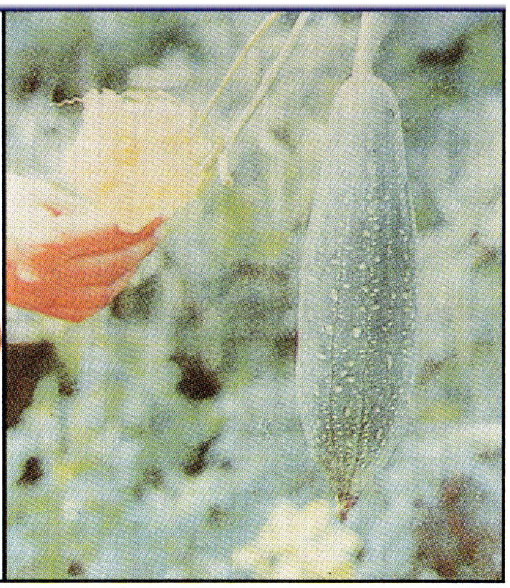

CUCURBITACHEAE

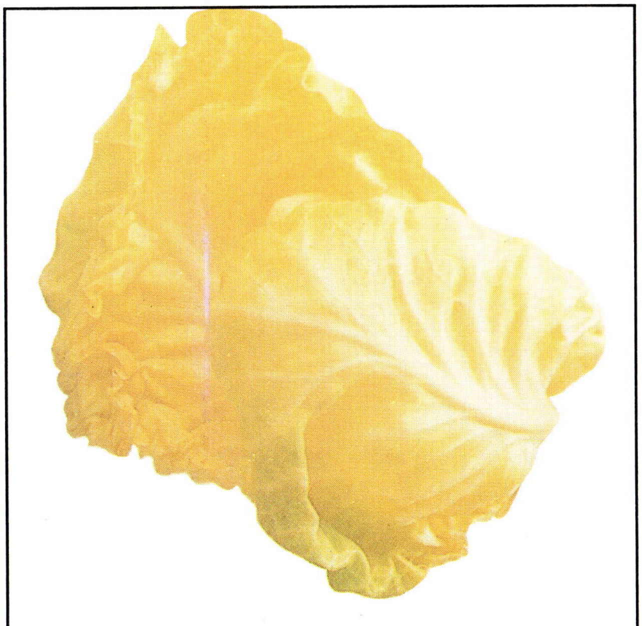

CABBAGE

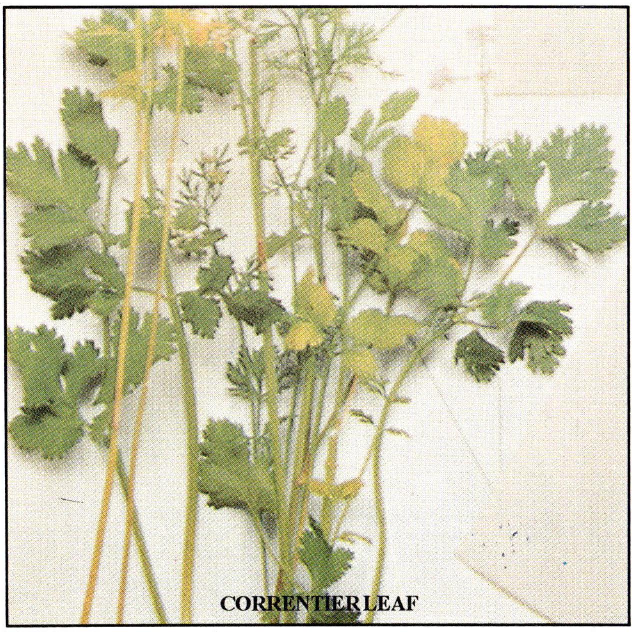

CORRENTIERLEAF

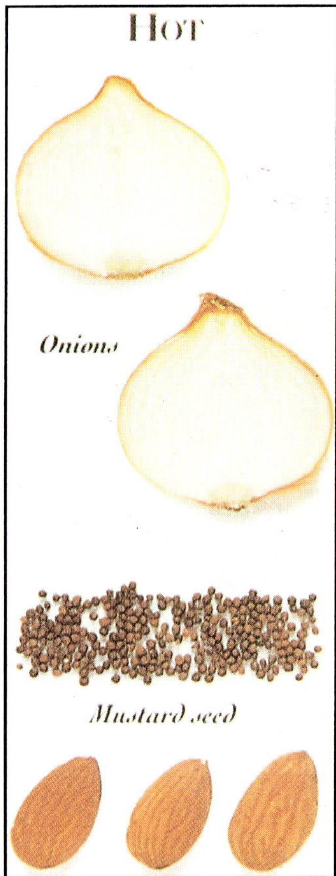

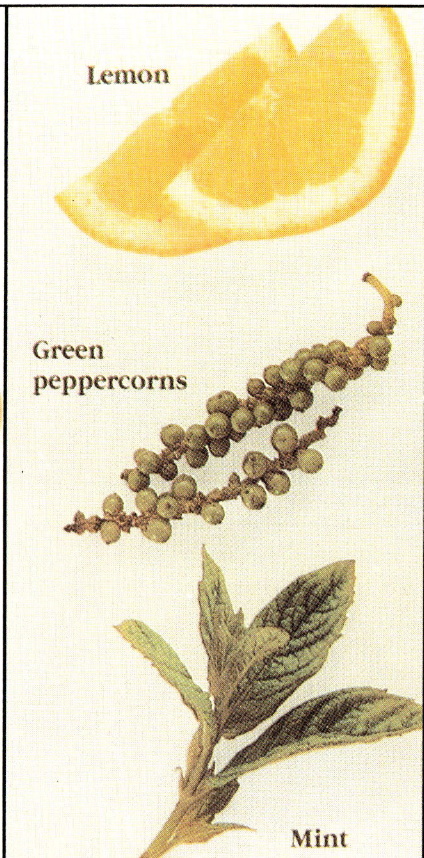

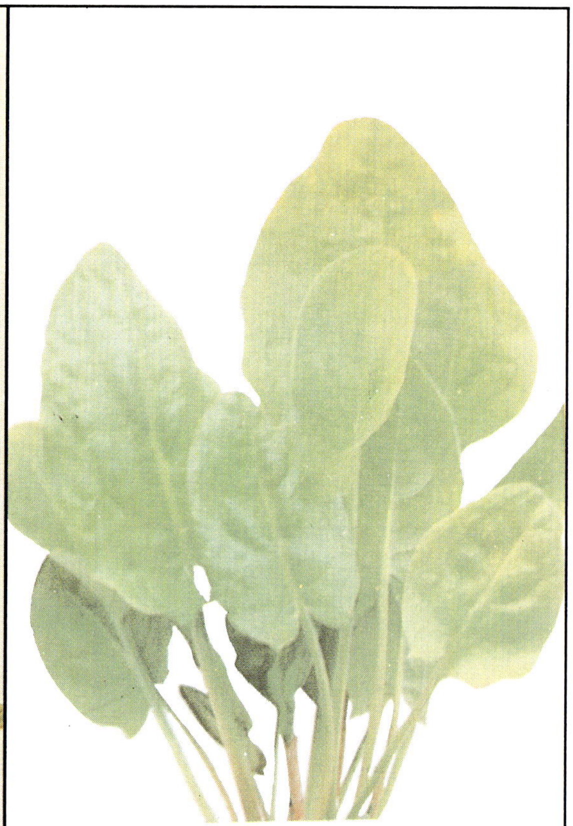

SPINCH

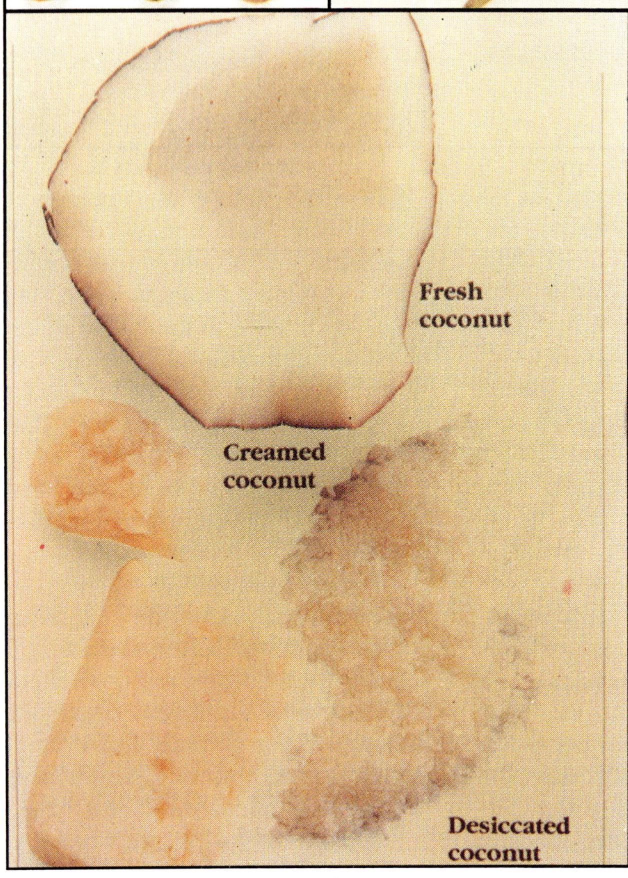

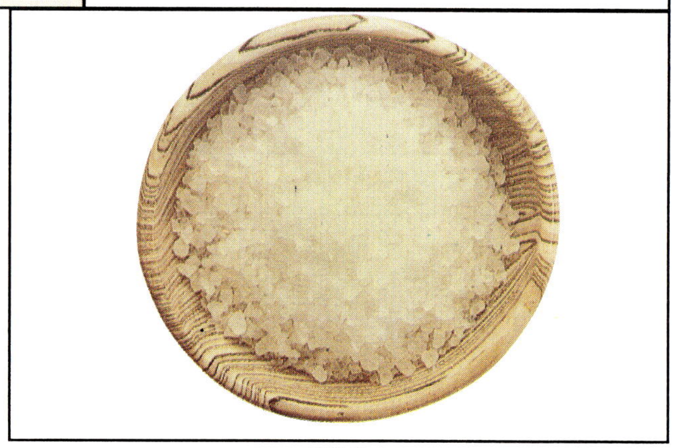

SALT

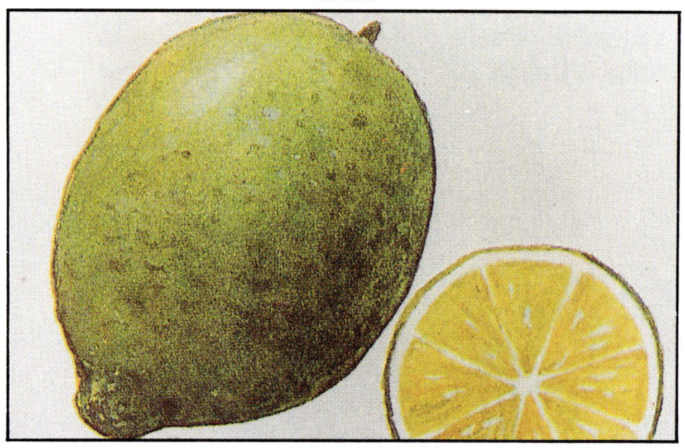

LEMON

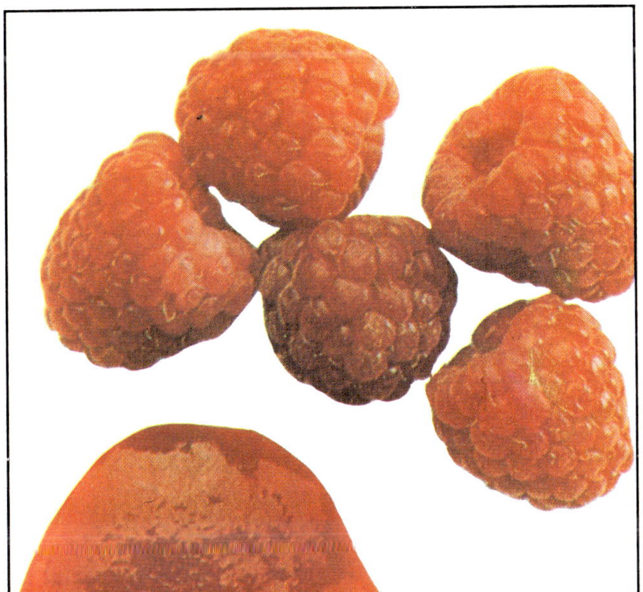

LEMON

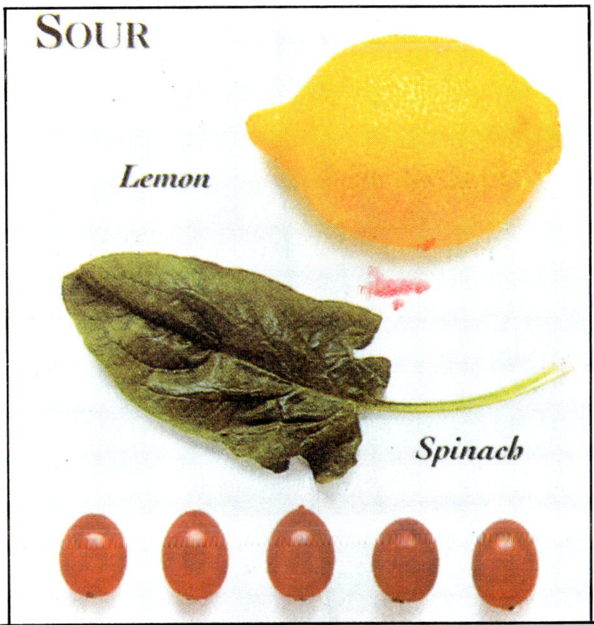

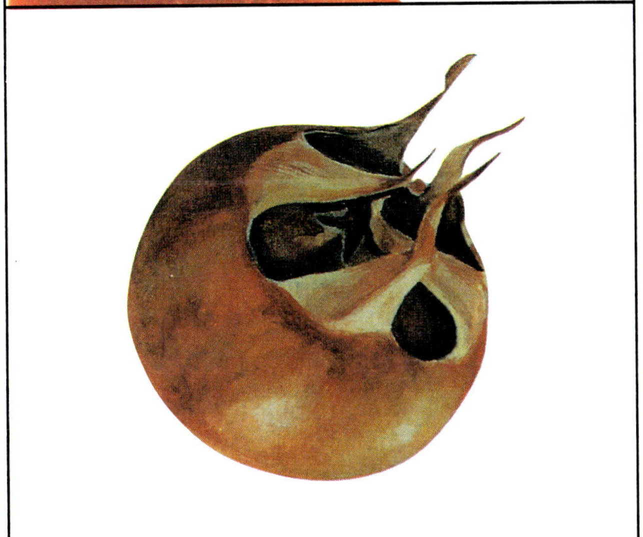

POMEGRANATE

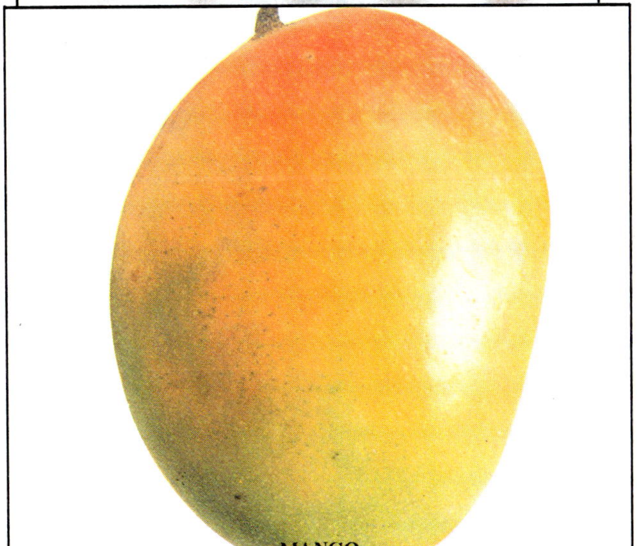

MANGO

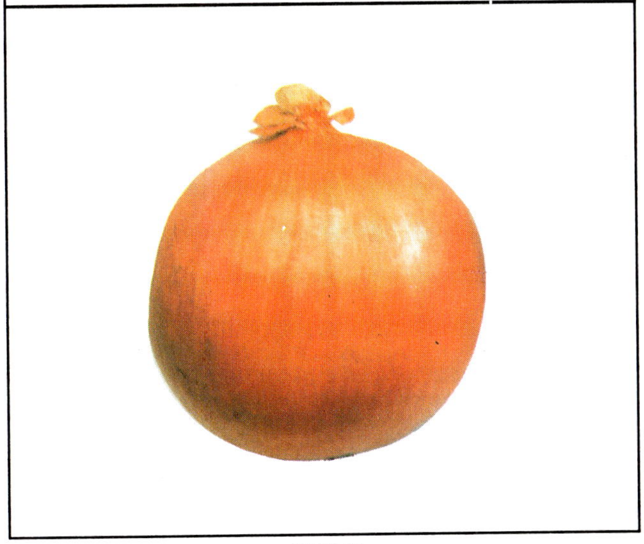

ONION

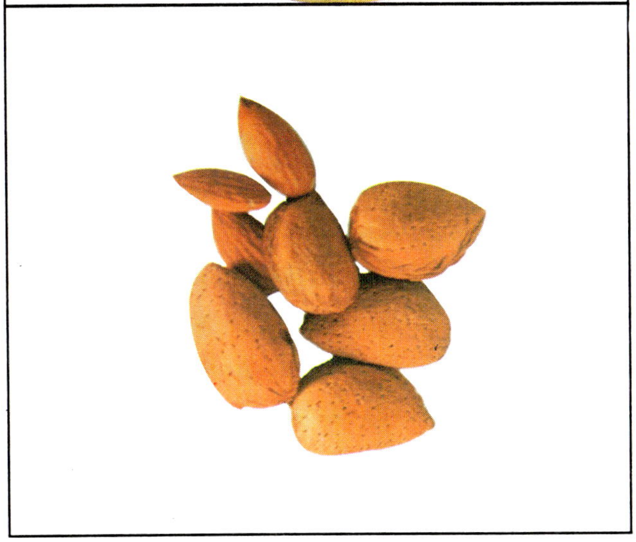

ALMONDS

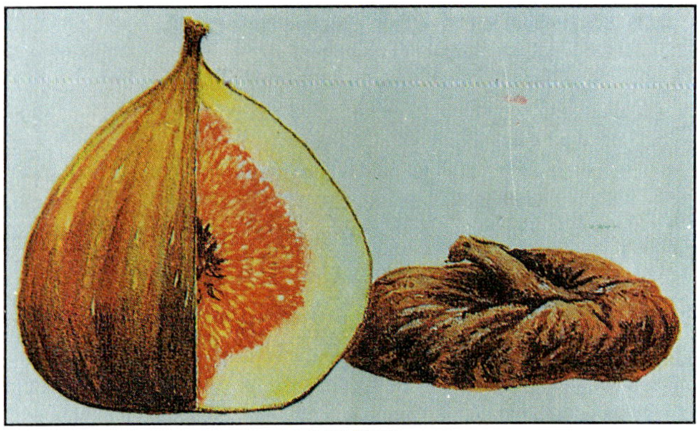

LEMON

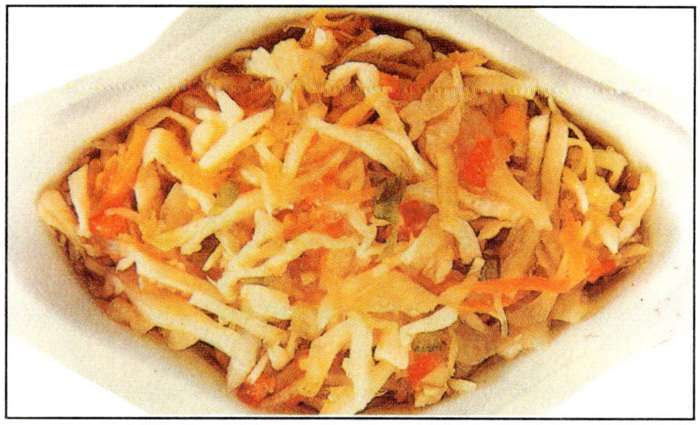

GREEN VEGETABLE

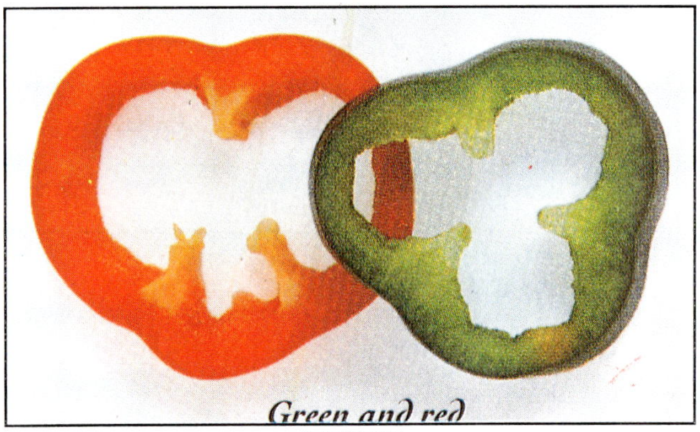

PEPPERS

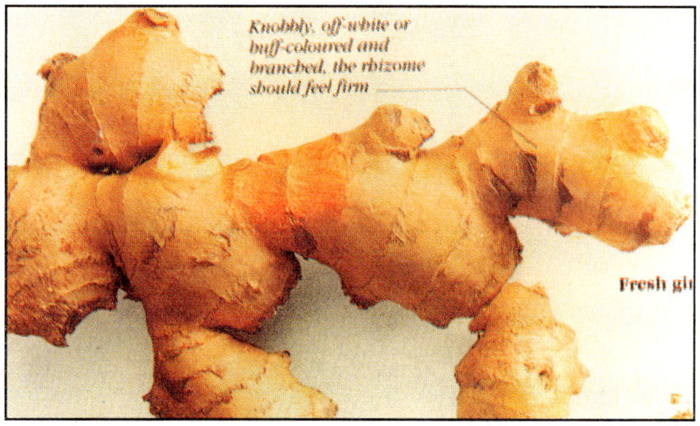

GINGER

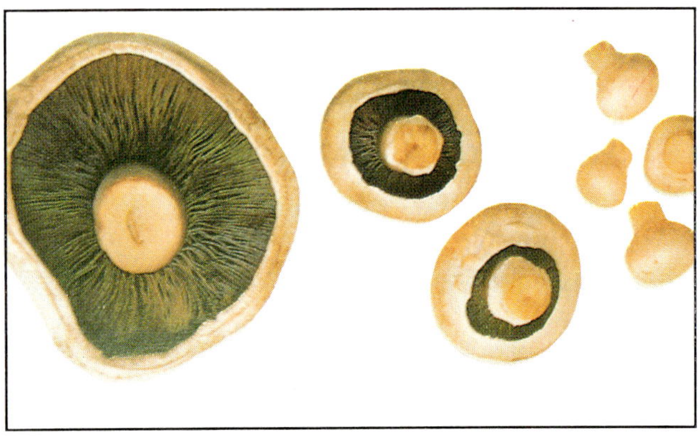

MUSHROOM

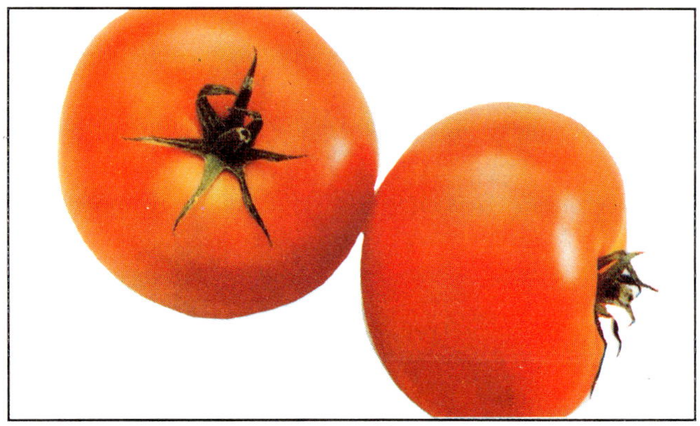

TOMATO

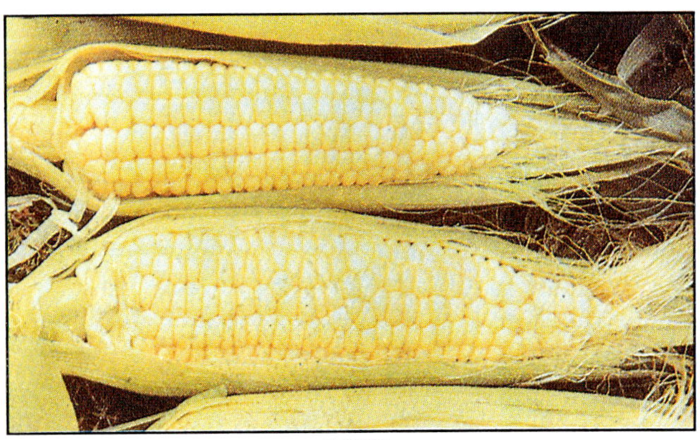

CORN

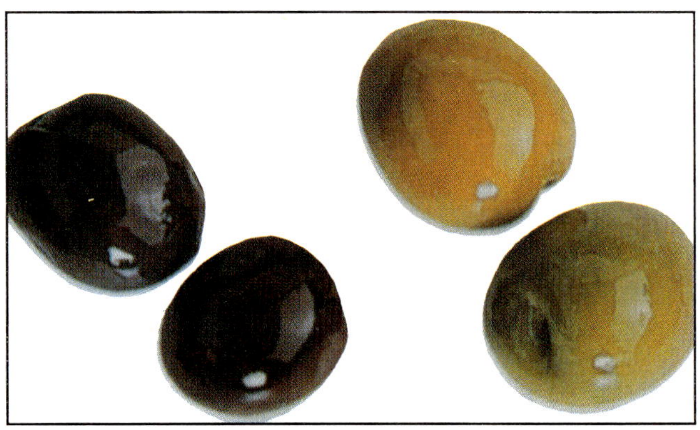

OLIVE

CHAPTER XIX

Yoga Practice For Cancer Prevention And Cure

THE PATH OF KUNDALINI YOGA

Kundalini Yoga is the path to self-knowledge. It helps one to awaken his inner consciousness and elevate it to the plane of the Ultimate Reality--the highest level of inspiration, illumination and bliss. It is the process of arousing the divine power that lies dormant within us, so that it can purify our consciousness and merge it with the eternal current of the Supreme Consciousness.

Everything in the cosmos has been created by the Ultimate Reality. His pure, divine energy exists in all forms of life in the universe. In human beings, the seat of divine consciousness and illumination, called Shiva, resides in the crown of the head. We are unaware of its existence because it is enveloped and completely concealed by gross layers of cosmic energy in the form of our karma from past lives, and the different states of our consciousness. The energy of spiritually unevolved human beings is not pure or strong enough to penetrate these sheaths and they, therefore, live in the darkness of ignorance.

Kundalini shakti is the only force that can forge a pathway through these layers of cosmic energy and make the individual consciousness unite with the Supreme Consciousness. This is symbolically described as the union of Shiva with Shakti. Kundalini shakti in the primary cosmic power of the Almighty with which He creates, maintains and dissolves the universe. It is the source of all the energy and matter in the cosmos and is capable of assuming any form or state. It exists in all forms of life and non-life.

The kundalini is the *prana shakti* or the life force in human beings. All the functional activities of the body and mind are correlated to and sustained by kundalini shakti: all our thinking, desiring, speaking, eating, working, hearing, breathing, hormonal secretions, transformation of food into flesh, urine, bones, semen, etc. receive their energy from kundalini. Human vitality increases or decreases in proportion to the energy emitted by the kundalini.

The kundalini is usually described as a coiled serpent sleeping at the bottom of the spine. The serpent symbolizes the all-powerful energy of creation, while the bottom of the spine is regarded as the seat of primary ignorance. It is the location of the grossest sheath of cosmic energy that envelops the Ultimate Reality. The consciousness of the average human being operates at this level. Its grossness governs his behaviour, making him restless, moody and emotional. His focus of attention is the turbulent external world, and all his thoughts and actions are based on its violent tremors. Only when he begins to probe inwards, and takes his awareness from the gross to the subtle layers of consciousness, is he able to perceive the serenity, tranquillity and bliss that lie within himself. The closer he gets to his inner core, the more enlightened he becomes. But this inward journey will be successful only if the kundalini shakti is awakened, because it will not be possible to penetrate the centres of cosmic energy that surround the divine consciousness without its primal power.

The kundalini can be awakened if its cosmic energy is heated by deep, focused meditation over a prolonged period of time. When the great shakti of kundalini is awakened, internal heat, light and sound are generated as the cosmic energies of the inner layers of our consciousness are released. The kundalini snake figuratively begins to uncoil and travel upwards to the seat of divine consciousness in the crown of the head. The process of kundalini awakening happens through *chakras* (wheels of energy) flowing through *nadis* (pathways)

Chakras

In meditation, the chakras are visualized and experienced as circular movements of energy vibrating at different frequencies. There are several centres of cosmic energy in our body. Of these, seven principal ones span the full spectrum of our consciousness from the gross to subtle. They are the *mooladhara*, *swadhishtahan*, *manipura*, *anahata*, *vishuddhi*, *ajna* and the *sahasra* chakras. It is through these chakras that the shakti of the awakened kundalini flows. Each chakra is a storehouse of a different form of cosmic energy, and together, they represent the totality of the cosmic energy of the universe. The chakras contain all the different types of knowledge that exist in the cosmos. All the energy embedded in our unconscious and the accumulated karma and experiences of our previous lives, both good and bad, positive and negative, painful and pleasant are also stored in the chakras.

The Seven Cakras

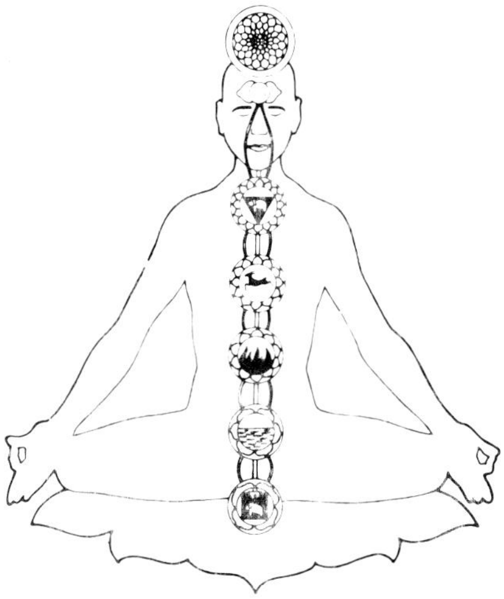

Levels of Consciousness

VIEW FROM THE FRONT

All our mental, psychic and karmic energy keep flowing into the chakras, thereby blocking them either partially or totally. They need to be fully opened before the kundalini can be awakened. This opening brings to the surface an explosion of these unconscious experiences and not everybody is adequately prepared to handle them. Only those who have well developed reasoning and understanding are able to cope. Therefore, before one embarks on the process of awakening and manifesting the great force of the kundalini, it is extremely important to purify and strengthen the mind. Each chakra has a trigger point or *chakra-kshetram* in the front of the physical body and a *bija mantra* (seed mantra) associated with it. Concentration on the trigger point and meditation on the bija mantra leads to the awakening of each chakra.

Mooladhara Chakra

Mooladhara is the lowest chakra in man's spiritual evolution, and its influences are at the root of our whole existence. The kundalini's great potential lies dormant in this chakra, and until it is awakened, man is unaware of the divine consciousness within himself. His behaviour is solely guided by his instinctive responses to the external world, his emotions and desires.

Mooladhara chakra is visualized as a lotus flower with four deep crimson petals. Its trigger point in the male body is the perineum (the area between the anus and the scrotum) and in the female body on the posterior side of the cervix. The sense of smell is associated with mooladhara, and it is here that psychic smells are manifested. Its sensory organ is the nose and its organ of activity is the anus. All the passions, complexes, guilt and agonies of human beings as well as the lower associations of past lives are stored in the mooladhara. Sexual consciousness also emanates from here. Mooladhara is the base from which the *ida*, *pingala* and sushma nadis emanate.

Mooladhara awakening is often accompanied by itchy sensations around the anus, and sense of smell becomes so acute that offensive odours are difficult to bear. When the kundalini awakens in mooladhara, there is a simultaneous awakening of the unconscious field of human existence which a person may have been completely oblivious of. The first experiences are levitation of the astral body, i.e. the sensation of floating upwards in space, leaving the physical body behind, clairvoyance, control of the body, breath and mind, the ability to produce any smell for oneself or others, freedom from disease and cheerfulness. This is also a crucial period of development, since all repressed emotions, especially those of a more primal nature, surface. Passions mount and one becomes irritable and unstable, and exhibits violent behaviour swings. During this period of intense psychic and emotional upheaval, the guidance of a qualified and understanding guru is essential.

Swadhisthana Chakra

Mooladhara contains strong physical emotions and associations, while the swadhisthana is the storehouse of mental emotions like desires, impressions, perceptions, experiences and associations from the present and past lives. Both chakras are associated with the unconscious mind.

The swadhisthana chakra can be experienced as being black in colour, as it is the seat of primary ignorance. It is traditionally depicted as a six-petalled vermilion or orange red lotus. The element of this chakra is water, symbolized by a white crescent moon within the pericarp of the lotus. The sense connected with this chakra is taste and its sense organ is the tongue. The organs of activity associated with it are the reproductive organs, kidneys and the urinary system.

Manipura Chakra

Manipura (lit. city of jewels), is the centre of dynamism, energy, will and achievement. It is the main reservoir of prana and regulates the digestion and heat of the body. It radiates and distributes pranic energy throughout the human framework. Its element is fire and its colour is bright yellow. It has ten petals and its trigger point is the navel. The sense of of sight is connected with this chakra; its organs of knowledge are the eyes and the organs of action the feet. These two organs are closely interlinked because vision and wilful action are interdependent. When this chakra is blocked, one is in poor health, depressed, and suffers from lack of motivation and commitment in life. The opening of manipura is important for anyone who wishes to enjoy life more fully.

As long as it does not reach manipura chakra, the kundalini can slip back into the mooladhara and go back to sleep, awakening and reawakening many times. But having once reached manipura chakra, it cannot descend down to the lower chakras.

Meditation on manipura chakra leads to the unfoldment of knowledge of the entire physical system. When this centre is purified and awakened, the body becomes disease-free and the fear of fire disappears. The meditator also acquires great material wealth. Only when the meditator reaches manipura chakra is he able to visualize the infinite state of divine consciousness. It stretches before him endlessly, full of beauty, truth and auspiciousness. As long as the evolution of the kundalini is in the planes of the mooladhara and the swadhisthana, a person is guided, in some degree, by his mental and emotional problems. But transcending these planes, he will see the bliss, noble views, perfect ideas and greater possibilities ofhuman consciousness. Naturally, whatever he thinks or does will be influenced by this higher vision. This is why the psychic powers that come with the awakening of manipura are benevolent and compassionate, while those which manifest in the lower chakra are still tinged with emotions.

Anahata Chakra

Anahata chakra is "the space within the heart", the centre of spiritual love. It controls the mind and the emotions. The kundalini remains at this chakra for a long time after it ascends from manipura. It is a delicate centre because it is directly connected with the part of the brain responsible for creativity and fine arts like painting, singing, etc.

Its element is air and its trigger point is at the level of the heart behind the breast bone. Its colour is blue and it has ten petals. The skin is the sense connected with this chakra and its sense organs are the hands.

The anahata chakra can only be awakened if there is total surrender to the mantra and to the guru (master). Anahata chakra can also be aroused by pure, selfless devotion to the Almighty.

Before anahata chakra awakens, there may be frequent pain in the chest or irregular heartbeats. But rather than feeling ill, one feels healthy and active and requires little sleep. Noises or sounds coming from other dimensions may be heard along with buzzing or humming sounds and the music of a flute.

Fate governs the lives of people only until the kundalini reaches anahata chakra. The meditator who has reached anahata is able to shape most of his destiny because he will have exhausted most of his karma by the time he reaches this chakra. The meditator becomes clairvoyant and psycho-kinetic, and develops the ability to heal others either by touch or by generating his own spiritual energy. His speech becomes inspired and he can spontaneously compose poetry. Non-attachment to worldly matters develops. With the discovery of true freedom, all dualities in life become meaningless.

Vishuddhi Chakra

Vishuddhi is the centre of purification of bodily secretions. It is visualized as a violet-coloured lotus with sixteen petals. Its element is ether-space which is more subtle than air. Its trigger point is the base of the throat where there is a small depression.

Vishuddhi receives thought vibrations from other people's minds. It is also the legendary "fountain of youth" in which the vital life essence secreted by the *bindu* (described later) is retained and utilized, becoming the nectar of immortality. As long as vishuddhi chakra remains inactive, this fluid runs downwards, unimpeded, to be consumed in the fire of the manipura, resulting in decay, degeneration, and finally death in body tissues. When this chakra is opened, cool soothing energy can be felt and the drops of the nectar of life can be experienced. Opening of the vishuddhi brings about full knowledge of the past, present and future. The sense of hearing becomes very sharp but through induction and not the ears.

Bindu Visarga

Bindu is the origin of creation or the point where Oneness first divides itself to produce the world of multiple forms. It secretes the nectar of life and is directly connected to vishuddhi chakra. The kundalini does not pass through this chakra but awakens it through vishuddhi.

The bindu's element is ether. Its trigger point is the small depression at the back of the head where Hindu men traditionally wear a tuft of hair. The bindu has no petals but is symbolized by a tiny crescent moon on a clear, moonlit night. The cosmic sound of "aum" is heard at the time of its awakening. The meditator who awakens his bindu can arrest his ageing process and also maintain the nutrition and vitality of his body without breathing.

Ajna Chakra

Ajna chakra is the point of confluence where the three *nadis--ida, pingala* and *sushumna* merge into one stream of consciousness and flow up into the Sahasra chakra in the crown of the head. Ajna is also known as the third eye, the centre of intuition or the command chakra. Direct mind-to-mind communication between the meditator and his earthly and astral masters takes place in this chakra. This chakra is more active in females than in males.

Ajna chakra is silver blue and has two petals. Its trigger point is the eyebrow centre where Hindu women traditionally wear a vermilion dot, the mercury from which is supposed to stimulate this chakra. This chakra's element is ether.

The sense organ, the organ of sense perception and the organ of action associated with ajna chakra are all considered to be the mind. This is because the mind perceives knowledge directly without any inputs from the other senses. Similarly, the mind can actively manifest without the aid of the physical body. The mode of operation of this chakra is thus purely mental.

In kundalini yoga, ajna chakra is the focal point of *mantra japa* because the strengthening of mind alone will make the meditator strong enough to face the explosions of intense feeling, emotions and painful karma that occur when the kundalini passes through the lower chakras. Only by the strength of reason and will power can this onslaught be contained. It is, therefore, advisable to purify the mind before attempting to open the chakras. When ajna chakra is strengthened by mantra japa it channelizes the meditator's pranic energy downwards to awaken mooladhara chakra.

Ajna chakra bestows the ability to fully comprehend all cause-effect relationships, the ability to enter another's body at will and to become an all-knowing and all-seeing being. The different results accruing out of meditation on the various chakras are collectively realized by meditating on this chakra alone. The meditator acquires all the cosmic *siddhis* when his kundalini reaches this chakra. Highly evolved persons place their life-force (*prana-shakti*) in ajna chakra at the time of death. This ensures their salvation.

Sahasra

Sahasra is not a chakra but the destination of the kundalini's ascent through the chakras. It is the seat of Divine Consciousness. One's union with the Almighty takes place here. The mind gets absorbed into the Supreme Consciousness which alone remains thereafter. The meditator goes into a state of samadhi or divine awareness at the time of this union.

Nadis

The nadis are the pathways of pranic energy in our body. Breath is the external manifestation of prana and can influence its flow. There are 72,000 nadis in the body. Ten of these are more important, and three of them the most important. These are: *ida, pingala* and *sushumna*.

The blue-coloured ida (lunar nadi) controls our mental processes and the red-coloured pingala (solar nadi) our physical actions. The golden-coloured sushumna (spiritual nadi) stays asleep until it is awakened by the practices of pranayama. Kundalini shakti travels upwards to sahasra through sushumna. Ida and pingala function alternately. Ida is activated when breathing takes place through the left nostril, and pingala when breathing takes place through the right nostril. Ida activates the left hemisphere of the brain and the pingala the right. Our thoughts are thus controlled by our nadis.

The spiritually unevolved cannot exercise any control over the activation of their nadis, and transport their thoughts. They are enslaved by their thoughts and are puppets of the feelings and emotions that they generate. Mood swings like depression, anxiety, elation, etc. come and go unchecked and rule their behaviour.

The practices of pranayama enable one to regulate the flow of his prana, thereby giving him control over his thoughts and actions. They can enable him to make ida and pingala flow simultaneously, thus activating both hemispheres of the brain together, giving him access to double the brain power that he normally has, which opens up new dimensions in his thinking and living. The simultaneous activation of ida and pingala alone can awaken sushumna and the kundalini can rise up through the chakras only when sushumna opens.

Ida, pingala and sushumna begin in mooladhara chakra and terminate in sahasra chakra. Sushumna flows through the inner central canal in the spinal cord and ida and pingala flow on either side. The three nadis intertwine at each chakra, where ida the pingala switch sides.

VEDIC MEDITATION

Vedic meditation is a process of deep relaxation and absorption--both physical and mental, at a level which few of us experience, even in sleep. Meditation brings excellent health and can alleviate and cure many ailments. Bio-feedback mechanisms have proved that during the relaxation induced by Vedic meditation, delta waves are emitted by the brain, which are identical to those produced in deep, dreamless sleep. Tranquillity marks this state.

A practised meditator can reach this mental state at will, without going to sleep. This leads to a purification of the mind. Complexes, phobias and prejudices break down. A process of re-programming of the mind begins. The ego becomes superfluous. The centre of consciousness now operates from the self instead of the ego. The petty desires of the mind become meaningless; the meditator realizes that they are false because they are temporary and transient. The focus of energy and concentration becomes the soul and its eventual union with the Almighty. The meditator becomes absorbed in a state of unalloyed contentment and peace.

Vedic meditation is the catalyst of this transition to transformation. It involves the following processes:

(4) Shavasana

All of us build up stresses and tensions in the course of living. These lock up a certain portion of our vital energy in various parts of the nervous system. They inhibit all movement of energy towards the inner consciousness. They also leave us with very little extra energy to even attempt any kind of inward movement. Anyone who does not relax after a period of tension cannot release his blocked energies and will slowly burn up his nervous system. Sleep is nature's natural restorative process. But if tensions are deep seated, sleep too, does not remove them.

The process of meditation begins with relaxation, with *shavasana*. Shavasana means the death or corpse pose which is symbolic of total emancipation from all pain and agony, worry and worldly bondage, liberation and release.

The practice of Shavasana completely relaxes the body, and releases the energy locked up in the nervous system. It involves lying motionless on the ground, flat on the back, with the eyes closed. The hands rest alongside the body with the palms facing upward and the legs and feet lying slightly apart. The body should be completely still. The attention is slowly rotated from one part of the body to the other, until each part has been systematically concentrated upon, turn by turn.

This process takes the focus of attention and concentration away from the stresses and strains of the mind, and directs it to the muscles and joints. When the flow of thought moves out from one part of the body to another, it draws out with it the nervous energy. Also, when the focus of attention shifts from the mind to the body, the tensions of the mind no longer hold centre-stage, so their chatter slowly becomes fainter and finally stops, leaving the mind quiet and peaceful.

Deep relaxation occurs when the mind is completely quiet and calm, though remaining fully conscious, and the body is still and motionless. This state is seldom reached in sleep. The pathways of energy are free of all blocks, and *prana* can easily flow beyond the realms of normal awareness into the subconscious and unconscious. It gives us access to the creative and more subtle states of our minds.

Only in a state of deep relaxation can the practice of meditation channelize our *prana* to the core of our being, making us aware of the inner, eternal truth within.

(B) Pranayama

Prana is our life-source and vital energy which is a microcosmic element of the pure and eternal energy of the Almighty that pervades the universe and all forms of creation. The core of our individual prana is as pure as the universal prana. But it is surrounded by the gross sheaths of the mind and body, and the different states of our consciousness. Each of these sheaths locks up large portions of our *prana*, and consequently, the amount of *prana* available to us for our interaction with the day-to-day world is very little. The practice of pranayama enables us to penetrate these sheaths and reach the more sublime states of our consciousness. It also releases the latent *prana* stored within them, and thus makes all our activities (meditative or otherwise), infinitely more powerful and successful.

Shavasana initiates the meditative process and the journey towards the depths of our inner being; Pranayama stimulates the flow of our *prana* from one dimension of consciousness to another.

The flow of *prana* is regulated and controlled by our breath. Deep, rhythmic breathing in certain ratios of inhalation, retention and exhalation, activates the flow of *prana* and makes it move from one dimension of awareness to another. The practice of pranayama for just a few minutes can raise an individual's energy level and take him into the inner realms of his being. It shifts the focus of his consciousness from outer to the inner world--a state in which the stresses, strains and tensions of life disappear. Pranayama makes the mind introverted and more powerful. Eventually, the practice of pranayama in which the retention of breath is six times as long as the inhalation, awakens the core of our inner cosmic energy.

Pranayama must be learned from an experienced teacher. If practised incorrectly, it can awaken negative currents of *prana*.

(C) Mantra

The pranic energy in each of our states of consciousness vibrates at different frequencies. To progressively move form one stage of awareness to another, towards the deepest core of our being, we need to be able to harmonize ourselves with the vibrations of each of these states. The simplest method of achieving this is by meditating on a mantra.

A mantra is energy encased in a sound structure. Every mantra contains within its vibrations a certain power. Concentration on, and repetition of, a single mantra results in its energy being elicited to carve out a pathway to the vital pranic energy in the innermost depths of our consciousness. It is crucial to have the right mantra, preferably one tailored to each individual's level of vibrations and given to him or her by an experienced teacher.

The core of Vedic meditation is the verbal or mental repetition of a mantra. It is a method of channelizing one's consciousness from the lowest to the highest level of pure thought. At the ultimate or final level, a state of bliss prevails. One does not enjoy bliss, but becomes bliss itself.

There are many forms of yoga which show the path to self-awareness and to finally reach the state of union with the Ultimate Reality, but of all of them, Mantra meditation is the only one which does not produce any negative reaction while being practised. The two most important factors in meditation are to have a proper mantra, and to meditate upon the right mantra. This is because when you start the journey toward evolution, a lot of hurdles, both psychic and emotional, can come in your path. Sometimes, you may feel very lonely or even start crying. You may feel very tense or might experience other unexpected complications in your life. But through proper guidance from a person who has gone through these experiences, you will be able to surmount all these difficulties and eventually achieve your goal of union with the Almighty.

The universe is the creation of the Supreme Soul, the Almighty. This means that the Creator is infinitely more powerful that all that He creates. The Creator is the originator and everything in this universe emanates from Him. We are all part of his creation, the *Brahmanda*. Our ultimate objective is union with the Ultimate Reality of the universe.

The Supreme Soul, or the 'Paramatma' creates individual souls or atmas. Some of them, by virtue of their meditation, prayers and other purification processes, become 'Maha Atmas'. Only Maha Atmas can finally achieve union with the Paramatma, and thus attain the goal of *moksha* or salvation from worldly bondages.

The frequency of the sound "aum" is in harmony with the vibrations of the Paramatma. Proper breathing through the practice of pranayama and meditation on a mantra which encapsulates "aum" create strong vibrations which can forge a pathway to union with the Ultimate. This union is forged through the kundalini shakti.

Advanced Meditation and Awakening of Kundalini

Kundalini is the cosmic power present in all human beings. It is not a material force like electricity or magnetism. It is a spiritual potential, shakti, or cosmic power. It lies dormant unless awakened by meditation. Once awakened, kundalini achieves for the meditator the ultimate illumination, and is the source of all knowledge and bliss. It is pure consciousness, and is *prana shakti*--the supreme force. It is by this shakti that the world exists. As the Patanjali Yoga Sutra puts it, "Creation, preservation and dissolution are in her".

The mysterious kundalini lies at he base of the spine. In kundalini meditation, the divine power that lies dormant in every human being is aroused and pulled upward through the *chakras* or the psychic centres of the body. At the top of the head, the seat of the highest consciousness, the union of the individual and the absolute consciousness takes place. This is expressed symbolically as the union of Shakti, or kundalini, with Lord Shiva. When this occurs, the individual reaches *moksha*, the highest state of evolution and freedom from birth and death. He becomes the embodiment of all the knowledge of the universe, and is able to look into the past, the present and the future; nothing is hidden from him. It is the state of supreme enlightenment.

The kundalini can be awakened by many methods. The practices of shavasana, pranayama and mantra all awaken it and help it to begin its ascent through the chakras. It is important to maintain a delicate balance between these practices. After kundalini is awakened, union with the Ultimate Reality of the universe takes place.

The chakras can only be awakened by *bija* or seed mantras. Each *bija* mantra represents the vibration of energy associated with each chakra. These mantras are not only sounds but are also thought forms that permanently exist within the subtle depths of the *Brahmanda*. Some examples of *bija* mantras are "hrim", "tam", and "dham". They are chanted along with "aum" and other mantras. They cannot be understood intellectually, but slowly reveal themselves when the practitioner reaches the levels of awareness and consciousness at the periphery of each chakra. Every correct and proper intonation of a *bija* mantra is invested with power or energy which release tremendous amounts of *prana* in the practitioner, which then slowly surges up to open each chakra. Also, every *bija* mantra has a unique intonation tone or pitch, a musical note, a colour and an astrological significance. The *bija* mantras alone can unlock the true and full significance of the chakras.

The Role of the Guru

The word 'guru' is a combination of two Sanskrit roots, 'gu' (light) and 'ru' (darkness). The guru leads from the darkness of the transient, day-to-day superficial existence in the world, to the supreme light of the inner consciousness of the Almighty.

This light exists within each of us, but we cannot find it unless we are shown the path by a teacher who has already traversed it and knows the short-cuts and pitfalls along the route. The teacher gives the students the wick, the oil for the lamp, and the means of lighting it, but ultimately all students must light their own lamps and enlighten themselves. Lord Buddha said, "*Atma-deepo bhavo*"–"Be thine own light".

Every practice of Vedic meditation is fraught with danger and can lead to the generation of a negative force field of *prana*, that results in psychic disorders and destruction if not practised properly. This can cause irreversible damage to the body, brain and nervous system. Meditation on the wrong mantra is the most harmful process of all. Only a true guru, who has elevated himself through the rigorous disciplines of yoga, pranayama and meditation, can lead his students along the right path, progressively revealing deeper truths to them as they proceed towards self-realization and *moksha*.

At times, students may seek practical advice on how to harmonize and balance their careers, finances, health, interpersonal relationships, etc., with their spiritual progress. A true guru also gives practical wisdom and guidance on temporal matters such as these.

The guru exists for one thing alone--to help sincere students kindle the light within themselves. He is totally selfless, giving all he has and expecting nothing in return.

There are very few real spiritually evolved gurus in this world, who can shed light on all the stages of evolution to *moksha*. Many of them live in inaccessible jungles and mountains and can only be contacted telepathically. The majority of real gurus are disembodied souls who have reached their final destination but have given up their physical bodies. They guide true seekers telepathically from the astral plane. Sometimes, a seeker may receive guidance from several gurus. Sincere students will always receive the guidance of a guru till they reach their final destination of *moksha*.

YOGA NIDRA

Yoga Nidra is a method of inducing deep relaxation and preparing the mind and body for meditation. It is a state of sleepless sleep where one is on the borderline between sleep and wakefulness. It is a state of inner awareness and contact with the subconscious and higher consciousness. It is a method of introspection. It has been used by yogis since time immemorial to bring them face to face with the inner self.

A resolution or a *sankalpa* made at the beginning and end of yoga nidra goes deep into the subconscious, and is very powerful for changing behaviour, getting rid of old habits and curing certain mental illnesses.

Yoga nidra is practised lying in shavasana. The mind should retain acute attentiveness throughout. Do not slumber and do not try to understand or rationalize any of the words--they would exhaust your mind and send it to sleep.

A speaker or a narrator is needed in the initial stages of the practice. For this reason, it is a good idea to put the instructions on tape. Later on you will remember the instructions and be able to practise alone.

Technique

* Lie down comfortably and relax the whole body.
* Stop all physical movement and prepare for yoga nidra.
* Make your resolution and repeat it mentally three times.
* Relax your body again, but remain alert.
* Become aware of your relaxation. The mind, body, senses, intellect, all aspects of your personality and entire being should be in a state of relaxation as it happens at night during sleep.
* Now take your awareness out of your mind into your body. Rotate it to the parts of the body named. Become aware of each part of your body as named, and then relax it. Do not struggle. Relaxation is an automatic process which comes with awareness.
* Remember not to fall asleep.
* Take your awareness to the thumb of your right hand--your right hand thumb, your right hand thumb, and relax it.
* Go to the second finger of your right hand, third finger, fourth finger, all five fingers together, the palm of your right hand, the back of your right hand, your whole right hand. Become aware of your whole right hand and relax it completely.
* Your right wrist, forearm, right elbow, upper arm, shoulder, armpit, collar bone--Relax your whole right arm.
* Right breast, right side of the stomach, right thigh, right knee, calf muscle, right ankle, right foot, bottom of the right foot, right heel, the instep of the right foot, big toe, second toe, third toe, fourth toe, all five toes, whole foot.
* Relax the whole right side of your body--right arm, right torso, right leg and foot.
* Now become aware of the left side of your body. Left thumb, first finger, second finger, third finger, fourth finger, all five fingers, palm, back of the left hand, the whole left hand.
* Your left wrist, forearm, left elbow, upper arm, shoulder, armpit, collar bone--Relax your whole left arm.
* Left breast, left side of the stomach, left hip, left thigh, knee, calf muscle, ankle, and now your whole left foot.
* Left ankle, top of the left foot, left heel, bottom of your left foot, the instep of your left foot and then your toes. Big toe, second toe, third toe, fourth toe, fifth toe, and now all five toes.
* Become aware of the whole left side of your body and relax it completely--Left arm, left torso, left leg and foot.
* Now relax both sides of the body together--both arms, both torsos and both legs.
* Now go on to your back--first the right side of the back--right buttock, go higher to the part of your back behind the right stomach, the right waist, behind the right lung, the joint of the right arm and the back and behind the right shoulder. Now relax the whole right back.
* Now go to the left side of the back. Left buttock, behind the left side of the stomach, left waist, behind the left lung, the joint of the arm and the back and behind the left shoulder.
* Now relax the whole back.
* Now go to the spine, go to the end of the spine in the perineum. This is the *moolasthana chakra*. Become aware of it.

* Go to the tailbone, and become aware of the energy centre in it. This is the *swadishthana chakra*. Become aware of it.
* Go to the energy centre behind the navel. This is the *manipura chakra*. Become aware of it and relax it.
* Go to the energy centre at the joint of your neck and the spine. This is the *vishuddhi chakra*.
* Go to the energy centre in middle of your head, behind the centre of your eyebrows. This is the *agna chakra*.
* Now become aware of the energy centre at the top of your head.
* Go to your forehead. Right eyebrow, left eyebrow, eyebrow centre, bridge of the nose, right nostril, left nostril, upper lip, lower lip, chin.
* Right cheek, right temple, right ear, right side of the head, right side of the neck.
* Left cheek, left temple, left ear, left side of the head, left side of the neck.
* Whole neck, both shoulders, chest, stomach.
* Now become aware of the whole right side of the body and feel it relaxing. Then become aware of the whole left side of the body and feel it relaxing. And now become aware of your whole body and feel it relaxing.
* Focus on your breathing, feel your breath going in and out, in and out, in and out, in and out, in and out, in and out.
* Now become aware of your resolution once again. Become aware of the outside world. Hear the sounds of the outside world.
* Wiggle your toes and move your hands and feet.
* Open your eyes slowly. Your yoga nidra is now successfully completed.

MUDRAS AND BANDHAS

Mudras are physical and mental attitudes that facilitate bringing about controlled psychic states and occurrences. The system of mudras is very diverse, including many types of practices ranging from positions of the hands to very complex and subtle methods of concentrating the mind. *Bandhas* are a group of inner locks designed to hold *prana*, or psychic energy, within certain areas of the body so that its pressurized force can be directed and utilized. Together the systems of mudras and bandhas form the basis of many of the important meditational techniques. Without their knowledge and practice an aspirant is very limited in the extent to which he can progress.

Mudras and bandhas are very powerful tools. They should be learned very gradually and carefully to avoid any possible harm. If any difficulty is experienced while attempting to practise the mudras or bandhas, or if any minor physical imbalance is noticed after practice has been initiated, you should stop their practice and seek expert guidance.

Below are described Gyana Mudra, Chin Mudra, Nasagra mudra, Yoni Mudra, Khechari Mudra, Shambhavi Mudra, Agochari Mudra, Akashi Mudra, Vajroli Mudra, Ashwini Mudra, Moola Bandha and Jalandhara Bandha.

Gyana Mudra

* Assume a meditative asana.
* Fold the index fingers of both hands so that they touch the inside roots of their respective thumbs. (*Alternative*: Touch the tips of the thumb and index finger.)
* Spread the other three fingers of each hand so that they are lightly apart.
* Place the hands on your knees with the palms downward and your three unbent fingers and thumb of each hand pointing towards the floor in front of your knees.

Chin Mudra

Chin mudra is performed in the same way as gyana mudra except that the palms of both hands face upward while placed on the knees.

Benefits for both. Gyana mudra and chin mudra are simple but important psycho-neural finger locks which make the meditative asanas such as padmasana, siddhasana, siddha yoni asana, sukhasana, vajrasana and others, complete and more powerful by redirecting the nervous impulses from the hands upward to the body.

Nasagra Mudra

Nasagra mudra ("the attitude of the nose") is utilized during most pranayama practices. Its purpose is to enable the practitioner to close one of the nostrils so he can inhale or exhale through the opposite one, as instructed by the rules of pranayama.

* Sit in a meditative posture.
* Place your left hand on your left knee in gyana or chin mudra.
* Hold the right hand before the face.
* Locate the tips of the middle and index fingers of your right hand together and place them on your forehead at the centre of the eyebrow. Keep these fingers straight.
* The thumb should be beside the right nostril and the ring finger beside the left nostril. (These fingers are used to close off the nostrils. The little finger is not used in any way.)
* The right elbow should be nearly vertical. (Some practitioners who do a lot of pranayama use a strip of cloth tied around their neck to support the right elbow.)
* Nasagra mudra can also be practised with the hands reversed.

Yoni Mudra

Yoni mudra ("the source attitude") is also known as Shanmukhi mudra ("the attitude of nine gates"). It is helpful in the practice of kundalini yoga.

* Sit in padmasana, siddhasana or siddha yoni asana.
* Inhale slowly and deeply.
* Retain the breath inside and raise your hands to your face. Close the ears with the thumbs, the eyes with the index fingers, the nostrils with the middle fingers and place the ring and small fingers above and below the lips to seal the mouth.
* Retain the breath inside for as long as is comfortable while concentrating on bindu chakra.
* Then release your middle fingers from against the nostrils and slowly exhale and inhale.
* Reseal your nostrils and continue in this way.

Precautions. This mudra involves kumbhaka (breath retention) and so it should be taken up very gradually and carefully.

Benefits. This mudra is most useful in inducing the state of pratyahara, or sense withdrawal. It helps the mind to turn inward to see itself.

Khechari Mudra

Khechari mudra ("the attitude of flying upward") is a basic practice used in the advanced techniques of meditation, and its mastery is a prerequisite for anyone wishing to practise kundalini yoga. Khechari mudra has a raja yoga form and a hatha yoga form. The latter should never be attempted without the direct guidance of an experienced guru.

Raja Yoga Form

* Close the mouth.
* Roll the tongue backward so that the normally lower surface touches the upper palate. Try to bring the tip of the tongue as far back as possible without strain.
* One may optionally perform ujjayi pranayama in this position.
* Perform for as long as possible. Beginners may find discomfort after a short time. They should relax the tongue for a few seconds and then repeat the tongue lock.
* With practice, the tongue will automatically ascend into the sinuses to stimulate many vital nerve centres in the brain.

Hatha Yoga Form

* The tendon beneath the tongue must be slowly cut week by week by surgical methods or with a sharpened stone.
* Massage the tongue for long periods daily by milking it. Butter, oil or any other type of lubricant may be used to make this easier.
* This process should be continued for many months until it is possible to touch the eyebrow centre with the tip of the tongue.
* When the tongue has reached the required elongation, full khechari mudra can be practised.
* Turn the tongue backward towards the back of the mouth.
* Carefully slide the tongue through the back and upper cavity in the palate, as far as it will go.
* In this way, the air passages are effectively blocked, and the centre known as lalana chakra is awakened.

Breath

* Beginners can breathe normally during the practice of khechari mudra. Over a period of weeks and months they should gradually try to reduce the

respiration rate, until after about two months or more the number of breaths per minute is only five to eight.

* With further careful practice, preferably under expert guidance, the respiration rate can be further reduced.

Precautions. If khechari mudra is performed during physical exercise, a bitter secretion may be tasted. This can be harmful. The practitioner is advised to discontinue this mudra if this bitter secretion is tasted.

Benefits. This mudra was regarded as very important in ancient yogis texts. This mudra has very subtle influences on the human being. In the back cavity of the palate are various pressure points and glands which have extensive control over the activities of the body. The secretions from these are stimulated by the folding of the tongue. This gives extensive health benefits to the body. Saliva is also produced which removes the feeling of thirst and hunger.

Yogis who are buried under the ground for long periods of time perform khechari mudra for the whole duration. This allows them to retain their breath for as long as they wish, without harming themselves.

This mudra awakens the kundalini shakti and also helps to preserve the vital energy of the body. In its full form this practice can cause the astral body to detach itself from the physical body. The consciousness thereby dwells in the akasha, the space between the astral and physical planes.

Shambhavi Mudra

Shambhavi mudra (''the attitude of Lord Shiva'') is also known as bhrumadhya drishti (''eyebrow centre gaze'').

* Sit in any meditative pose, make your back erect and place the hands on the knees in chin or gyana mudra.
* Look at a fixed point before you.
* Then look upward as high as possible, without moving the head.
* Concentrate and focus the eyes on the eyebrow centre.

Benefits. It is a powerful technique for awakening ajna chakra--the seat of union between the lower and higher consciousness. Physically it strengthens the muscles of the eyes. Mentally, it brings about calmness of the mind and removes stress and anger.

Agochari Mudra

Agochari mudra (''the unknown attitude'') is also known as nasikagra drishti (''the nose tip gaze'') and is used in many techniques for meditation.

* Sit in any meditative pose.
* Hold the spine erect and the head facing forward.
* Focus the eyeballs on the tip of the nose.

Precautions. Do not strain the eyes--slowly increase the duration over a period of weeks and months.

Benefits. This mudra, like Shambhavi mudra, develops the power of concentration. It awakens mooladhara chakra. It brings about introversion and takes the practitioner into the psychic and spiritual planes of consciousness.

Akashi Mudra

Akashi mudra (''the attitude of inner space'') is a very powerful practice, and must be learned slowly and carefully.

* Sit in any meditative pose.
* Fold the tongue back against the upper palate (Khechari mudra).
* Practise Ujjayi pranayama and Shambhavi mudra.
* Simultaneously bend the head backward, but not fully: the head should not lean on the top of the shoulders behind the head.
* Breathe slowly and deeply.

Precautions. At first Ujjayi pranayama may irritate the throat in this inclined position of the head, but with practice it will become more comfortable.

Benefits. When perfected this mudra makes the mind go into a trance--not a trance as understood in the West but in the yogic sense where the practitioner achieves a state of heightened consciousness. It brings about mental calm and tranquillity.

Vajroli Mudra

In an aspirant of meditation there is a tendency for the spiritual energy to leak out through the sexual system; this is the root cause of sexual desires and urges. Through the practice of vajroli mudra (''the attitude of the thunderbolt'') the sexual energy gate in the body is controlled, allowing the aspirant to control his *prana* and to harness it for spiritual awakening. Vajorli mudra is also the name of the *nadi* at Swadhisthana chakra through which the *prana* related to sexual energy travels.

There are two forms of Vajroli mudra. The advanced form is only for male aspirants, and can be dangerous if practised incorrectly.

Simple Form

* Sit in any meditative asana.
* Place the hands on the knees, close the eyes and relax.
* Try to draw the sexual organs upward by pulling and tensing the lower abdomen and contracting the urinary system. This contraction is similar to that which is made when one has an urge to go for urination, but wishes to retain for some time.
* The testes in the male, and the vagina in the female, should move up a little.

Advanced Form

The advanced form should not be attempted without the guidance of a competent guru or permanent injury may result.

* A silver tube about twelve inches long is inserted into the urethra.
* Through this water is drawn upward.
* When this is perfected, milk is drawn through the tube.
* After this is developed, honey and then mercury are drawn up.
* After prolonged practice these liquids can be drawn into the urethra without using the tube.
* At first the tube or catheter should only be inserted for one inch. The distance should be increased gradually to 12 inches.

Benefits. Vajroli mudra is effective for establishing brahmacharya. Through it the practitioner is able to control vital energy that is normally lost with the discharge of semen. When perfected the practitioner is able to retain this vital energy when semen is discharged. This energy can then be transformed or sublimated for higher yogic practices.

Ashwini Mudra

Ashwini Mudra (''the attitude of the horse'') is an important practice which should be learned before one attempts Moola bandha.

Stage 1

* Sit in any meditative pose.
* Relax the whole body and close the eyes.
* Contract the sphincter muscles of the anus for a few seconds.
* Next relax the sphincter muscles for a few seconds.
* Repeat the process as many times as possible.

Stage 2

* Sit as in stage 1.
* Inhale while simultaneously contracting the anus.
* Retain the breath while also holding the contraction of the sphincter muscles.
* Exhale and release the contraction of the anus.
* Repeat for as long as is comfortable. Do not strain.

Benefits. This mudra gives one control of the sphincter muscles in the same way that a horse has control. When one performs this mudra perfectly one is able to prevent the escape of pranic energy from the body. This energy can therefore be conserved and directed upward for higher and more valuable purposes. It is an excellent preparatory exercise for Moola bandha.

Moola Bandha

The word moola means root, and bandha means to lock. This technique locks the psychic energy in the upper part of the psychic body and does not allow it to descend into the lower limbs. It also stimulates Mooladhara chakra through mental compression, which helps in the awakening of kundalini.

In the basic practice of Moola bandha the aspirant is instructed to exert muscular contraction in the area associated with Mooladhara chakra. Later, however, when the exact root point of Mooladhara has become familiar to the practitioner, the muscular contraction need not be employed and the aspirant can merely touch the correct point lightly with his awareness. If mastered completely, this subtle technique is far more powerful than the physical contraction. Aspirants, however, should resort to the muscular contraction in the initial stages of practice.

* Sit in a meditative pose with the knees firmly on the ground.
* The best asanas are Siddhasana and Siddha-yoni asana, as the pressure exerted by the lower heel in these poses improves the bandha. Place the hands on your knees in Gyana or Chin mudra.
* Close your eyes and relax the whole body.
* Concentrate on the trigger point of Mooladhara chakra.
* Try to touch this point with your awareness, and then contract it.
* Hold this contraction for as long as possible.
* Then slowly release it.
* Relax for a few seconds, and then practise it again.

Moola bandha is usually practised along with Jalandhara bandha with the breath retained either inside or outside.

Precautions. Moola bandha must be perfected gradually and with great care. Do not strain while attempting it.

Benefits. In this bandha the region of Mooladhara, located between the urinary and excretory organs, is contracted and pulled upward. This forces the Apana vayu (vital energy in the lower parts of the body below the navel) to flow upward and thereby unite with the Prana vayu (vital energy in the region between the larynx and the heart), thus generating vitality.

Ashwini-Vajroli Moola Alternation

Aspirants often do not learn to sense the subtle difference between Ashwini mudra, Vajroli mudra and Moola bandha in the early states of practice, and they simply tense all of the muscles in the pelvic region no matter which technique they are attempting. This can destroy the efficacy of the three techniques when used as parts of the advanced kriyas of kundalini yoga. The practice of Ashwini-Vajroli moola alternation assists the aspirant to distinguish between the three techniques.

Stage 1

* Sit in a meditative pose, preferably Siddhasana or Siddha-yoni asana.
* Practise Gyana or Chin mudra.
* Now perform Vajroli mudra, the simple form.
* Hold it for a slow count of ten.
* Release Vajroli.
* Then perform Moola bandha, and hold it for a count of ten.
* Release Moola bandha.
* Continue in this way for as long as possible.
* On subsequent days you can increase the count from ten to fifteen or more.

Stage 2

* Practise Vajroli mudra.
* Add Moola bandha to Vajroli.
* Now also practise Ashwini.
* Hold all three for a few seconds, then release Ashwini, Moola and Vajroli, respectively.

Notes

* This practice should be attempted only when you have learned the three basic techniques by themselves.
* Your concentration when practising should be on distinguishing the three separate areas of contraction.
* This practice has no relation with the breath.
* Practise it daily until you can distinguish the three clearly from each other.

Jalandhara Bandha

Jalandhara bandha (''chin lock'') is an important technique which compresses the pranic force in the trunk region of the body, which is useful in stimulating the kundalini energy. It has a Raja Yoga form and a Kundalini Yoga form.

Raja Yoga form

* Sit in any of the meditative poses which allow the knees to firmly touch the floor. (Sukhasana is not suitable.) Persons who cannot sit in Padmasana, Siddhasana, etc. can do Jalandhara bandha while standing.
* Place the palms on the knees.

* Relax the whole body and close the eyes.
* Inhale deeply, retain the breath, bend the head forward and press the chin tightly against the chest at the sternum. Straighten the arms and lock them in a fixed position. Simultaneously hunch the shoulders upward and forward; this will ensure the arms remain locked.
* The palms should remain on the knees.
* This is the final pose. Stay in the final pose for as long as you are comfortably able to retain the breath.
* Then relax the shoulders, bend the arms, slowly release the lock and raise the head.
* Slowly exhale.
* Repeat when the respiration returns to normal.

Kundalini Yoga form

This is the same as the Raja Yoga form, except it is practised very subtly and without any tensing of the shoulders or arms. The head is simply dropped forward till the chin touches the sternum. In this form, however, the aspirant must be mentally aware of the compression of *prana* taking place in the trunk region.

Notes. (1) The whole practice can also be performed with the breath retained outside. (2) This bandha closes the windpipe and compresses various organs in the throat by imposing a chin lock.

Precautions. Never inhale or exhale, as the case may be, until the chin lock has been released and the head is upright.

Limitations. Persons with high blood or intra-cranial pressure or heart ailments should not practise without expert advice.

Benefits. (1) This is a good practice for reducing and removing stress, anxiety and anger. It brings about relaxation of the whole body and mind. It relaxes the heart by slowing down the heartbeat. Relaxation is achieved on a physical level by the compression of the sinus receptors which are located in the throat region. These receptors are sensitive to the blood pressure in the jugular vein which supplies blood to the brain. If the pressure is high the receptors send messages to the brain and heart, which are slowed down; if the pressure is low the heart is speeded up. The receptors are pressure-sensitive and so the compression they receive during Jalandhara bandha slows down the heart and brings tranquillity to the mind. (2) The thyroid and parathyroid gland are massaged and their functioning improved. These glands, especially the thyroid, have wide influences on the human organism, growth, sexual functions and so on. The whole body consequently benefits from their enhanced efficiency.

ASANAS

Surya Namaskara (Salutation to the Sun)

This dynamic exercise, though not traditionally regarded as a part of yoga practices, is excellent for loosening up all the joints and muscles, as well as massaging all the internal organs. It is a stimulating exercise to do in the morning after a bath and before doing any other yogic exercise. If one feels tired at any time of the day, this exercise will restore vitality, both physically and mentally.

Surya namaskara comprises twelve positions, which corresponds to the twelve signs of the zodiac. One complete round of Surya namaskara consists of these twelve positions performed in succession twice. Associated with each position is a mantra, which for optimum benefits should be repeated verbally or mentally.

Position 1. Pranamasana ("Prayer Position")

* Stand erect with the feet together. Place the palms together in front of the chest. Relax the whole body.
* Breath should be normal.
* Concentrate on Anahat chakra.
* *Mantra*: Om Mitraya Namah (Salutation to the Friend of All).

Pranamasana establishes concentration and calmness needed for the ensing exercises.

Position 2. Hasta Uttanasana ("Raised Arms Pose")

* Raise both arms above the head. Keep them separated by one shoulder's width. Bend the head and upper trunk slightly backward.
* Inhale while raising the arms.
* Concentrate on Vishuddhi chakra.
* *Mantra*: Om Ravasye Namaha (Salutation to the Shining One).

Hasta uttanasana stretches the abdominal viscera, removing excess fat and improving digestion. It also exercises the arm and shoulder muscles, tones the spinal nerves and opens all the lung compartments.

Position 3. Padahastasana ("Hand-to-Foot Pose")

* Bend forward until the fingers or hands touch the ground on either side or in front of the feet. Try to touch the knees with the forehead. Do not strain but keep the legs straight.
* Exhale as you bend forward. Try to contract the abdomen in the final position to expel the maximum amount of air.
* Concentrate on Swadhisthana chakra.
* *Mantra*: Om Suryaya Namaha (Salutation to Him Who Induces Activity).

This asana is useful in eliminating and preventing stomach or abdominal ailments. It reduces surplus fat in the abdominal region, improves digestion and helps to remove constipation. It improves blood circulation, makes the spine supple and tones the spinal nerves.

Position 4. Ashwa Sanchalanasana ("Equestrian Pose")

* Stretch the right leg back as far as possible. At the same time bend the left leg but keep the left foot in the same position. The arms should remain straight and in the same position. In the final position the weight of the body should be supported on the two hands, the left foot, the right knee and the toes of the right foot. The head should be tilted backward, the back arched and the gaze directed upward.
* Inhale while stretching the right leg backward.
* Concentrate on Ajna chakra.
* *Mantra*: Om Bhanave Namah (Salutation to Him Who Illumines).

Ashwa sanchalanasana massages the abdominal organs and improves their functioning. The muscles of the legs are straightened and nervous balance is attained.

Position 5. Parvatasana ("Mountain Pose")

* Straighten the left leg and place the left foot beside the right foot. Raise the buttocks in the air and lower the head so that it lies between the two arms. The body should form two sides of a triangle. The legs and arms should be straight in the final position. Try to keep the heels in contact with the ground in this pose.
* Exhale as you straighten the left leg and bend the trunk.
* Concentrate on Vishuddhi chakra.
* *Mantra*: Om Khagaya Namaha (Salutation to Him Who Rushes in the Sky).

Parvatasana straightens the nerves and muscles in the arms and legs. It bends the spine in the opposite direction to the previous pose and so further helps to make it supple. It tones the spinal nerves and supplies them with a fresh flow in blood.

Position 6. Ashtanga Namaskara ("Salutation with Eight Limbs")

* Lower the body to the ground so that in the final position only the toes of both feet, the two knees, the chest, the hands and the chin touch the ground. The hips and abdomen should be raised slightly off the ground.
* The breath should be held outside. No respiration.
* Concentrate on Manipura chakra.
* *Mantra*: Om Pushne Namaha (Salutation to the Giver of Strength).

Ashtanga namaskara strengthens the leg and arm muscles and develops the chest.

Position 7. Bhujangasana ("Serpent Pose")

* Raise the body from the waist by straightening the arms and bend the head backward. This stage is the same as the final position of bhujangasana.
* Inhale while raising the body and arching the back.
* Concentrate on Swadhisthana chakra.
* *Mantra*: Om Hiranya Garbhaya Namah (Salutation to the Golden Cosmic Self).

In this pose, the abdomen is compressed, helping to squeeze stagnant blood form the abdominal organs and encouraging a flow of fresh blood. This pose is useful for all stomach ailments, including indigestion and constipation. Arching the back exercises the spine, making the muscles supple and revitalizing the most important spinal nerves.

Position 8. Parvatasana ("Mountain Pose")

This is a repeat of position 5.

* From the stretched back position, assume the mountain pose as described in position 5.
* Exhale as you raise the buttocks.
* Concentrate on Vishuddhi chakra.
* *Mantra*: Om Marichaye Namaha (Salutation to the Lord of Dawn).

Position 9. Ashwa Sanchalanasana ("Equestrian Pose")

This stage is a repeat of position 4.

* Bend the left leg and bring the left foot forward so that it lies near the hands. Simultaneously lower the right knee so that it touches the floor.
* Inhale while assuming the pose.
* Concentrate on Ajna chakra.
* *Mantra*: Om Adityaya Namaha (Salutation to the Son of the Infinite Cosmic Mother).

Position 10. Padahastasana ("Hand-to-Foot Pose")

This position is a repeat of position 3.

* Place the right foot next to the left foot.
* Straighten both legs and try to bring the forehead as close to the knees as possible. Do not strain if you are unable to touch the knees but do not bend the legs.
* Exhale while performing the movement.
* Concentrate on Swadhisthana chakra.
* *Mantra*: Om Savitre Namaha (Salutation to the Benevolent Mother).

Position 11. Hasta Uttanasana ("Raised Arms Pose")

This stage is a repeat of position 2.

* Straighten the whole body and raise both arms above the head. Keep the arms separated by a shoulder's width. Bend the head and arms backward slightly.
* Inhale as you straighten the body.
* Concentrate on Vishuddhi chakra.
* *Mantra*: Om Arkaya Namaha (Salutation to Him Who Is Worthy of Praise).

Position 12. Pranamasana ("Prayer Pose")

This final pose is a repeat of position 1.

* Bring the hands in front of the chest and place the palms together. Relax the whole body.
* Exhale as you assume the final pose.
* Concentrate on Anahata chakra.
* *Mantra*: Om Bhaskaraya namaha (Salutation to Him Who Leads to Enlightenment).

Note

Positions 1 to 12 constitute half a round of Surya Namaskara. For the second half, positions 1 to 12 are repeated but with a few minor changes:

(a) In position 4, instead of the right foot, stretch the left foot back.

(b) In position 9, bend the right leg and bring the right foot near the hands.

Bija Mantras

As an alternative to the twelve names of the sun, there is a series of bija mantras or seed syllables. Bija mantras do not have any literal meaning, but set up powerful vibrations of energy within the mind and body. There are six bija mantras, repeated consecutively in the following order, four times during a complete round of surya namaskara:

Om Hram--Om Hrim--Om Haroom--Om Hrain--Om Harum--Om Hrah

When Surya Namaskara is practised too fast to repeat the sun mantra, the bija mantras are sufficient.

Duration

For spiritual benefits slowly do three to twelve rounds. For physical benefits the same number of rounds are advised. Start with two or three rounds, increasing by a round on each successive day. Advanced students can practise more rounds if they wish.

Sequence

Surya namaskara is ideally practised before the other asanas. This loosens the whole body and removes sleepiness. After completing Suryaya Namaskara, the practitioner is advised to do Shavasana for a few minutes.

This will allow the heartbeat and respiration to return to normal, and relax all the muscles.

Precautions

The practice of Surya Namaskara should be immediately discontinued if a fever develops due to excess toxins in the body. These toxins should be eliminated over a period of time by practising other asanas. Surya Namaskara may be resumed thereafter. The practitioner should not do more rounds than he can comfortably preform without excessive physical fatigue.

Limitations

There is no age limit for the practice of Surya Namaskara. Women, however, should refrain from it during the menstrual cycle or after the fourth month of pregnancy.

General Benefits

1. Surya namaskara has a powerful influence on all body systems, endocrinal, circulatory, respiratory, digestive, etc. and helps bring them into balance with each other. Many diseases are caused when one or more of these systems are out of balance. Surya Namaskara puts them in equilibrium, and thus helps to remedy many ailments.
2. All the major muscles get complete exercise. Daily practice keeps the whole body healthy and removes excess fat. It revitalizes the body and mind and sharpens the thinking power.
3. All abdominal organs are alternately stretched and compressed. This ensures that the organs function correctly and efficiently.
4. Synchronization of the breath with the physical movement during Surya Namaskara ensures that the practitioner, at least for a few minutes daily, breathes deeply and rhythmically as he should. This removes stagnant, germ-filled air from the lungs and replaces it with health-giving, oxygen-rich air. Increased mental clarity is brought about by the influx of fresh, oxidized blood to the brain.
5. Surya namaskara induces perspiration, which is a vital bodily mechanism for eliminating impurities. The beneficial effect is easily seen in those plagued with boils and pimples. Surya namaskara gives them a radiant complexion
6. There is no better way to remove nervous tension, stress and anxiety than regular practice of Surya Namaskara. The movements gently massage the nervous connections throughout the whole body, allowing them to relax and become revitalized.

To summarize, surya namaskara is the ideal exercise to bestow good health.

Naukasan (Boat Pose)

* Lie flat on the back, arms at the sides, palms facing down. Inhale and raise the legs, arms, head and trunk. The head and feet should not be raised more than one foot off the ground. The arms should be held at the same level and in line with the toes. Hold the raised position for a comfortable length of time, then exhale and slowly return to the starting position. Relax the whole body. Repeat this exercise five times.
* Repeat the same process, but this time clench the fists and tense the whole body in the raised position as much as possible. While exhaling, return to the floor quickly, without causing any injury. Immediately relax the entire body.
* Inhale while raising the body. Exhale while lowering the body. Internal Kumbhaka (retention of the breath inside the lungs) while in the elevated position.
* Elevated position should be maintained until the abdominal muscles start to vibrate.

Benefits. This is a very good asana for relaxing the muscles and joints. It should be done soon after waking up in the morning. It is useful for nervous, tense persons as it brings immediate relaxation. It helps to remove stomach or intestinal worms, and improves the digestive process by stimulating intestinal peristalsis.

Paschimotanasana (Back Stretching Pose)

Sit on the floor with the legs straight in front, the lower arms on the thighs. Relax the whole body, especially the back muscles. Slowly bend the body forward, sliding the hands along the top of the legs. Try to grasp the big toes with the fingers and the thumbs. If this is impossible hold the heels, the ankles or the legs as near as possible to the feet. Again, consciously relax the muscles at the back of the legs. Keeping the legs straight and without using the back muscles, only using the arms pull the trunk a little lower toward the legs. This should be a gentle process without any sudden movement or excessive strain anywhere in the body. If possible, touch the knees with the forehead. Remain in the final position for a comfortable length of time, trying to further relax the whole body, and then slowly return to the starting position. Beginners should only bend forward as far as they can without strain.

Do not bend the legs at the knees, even though you cannot bend the body further forward. It is part of the aim of the asana to stretch the muscles at the back of the legs. Do not force them. They will elongate in time. After some weeks or months of regular practice you will be able to touch the knee with the forehead or perhaps even the chin.

Breathe normally in the sitting position. Exhale slowly while bending forward. Inhale while holding the body motionless. Exhale as you pull the trunk further forward with the arms. Breathe slowly and deeply in the final pose. Inhale while returning to the starting position. If the final pose is not held for a long time the breath may be retained outside.

Adepts can maintain the final pose for up to five minutes provided they are comfortable in it. Beginners should perform the asana a few times, staying in the final pose for only a short length of time. Spiritual aspirants should aim to stay in the final position with complete relaxation for extended lengths of time.

* Spiritual concentration should be on Swadhisthana chakra.
* Physical and mental concentration should be on the abdomen, relaxation of the back muscles or the slow breathing process.
* Use this asana as a counterpose to backward bending asanas.

Precaution. People who have slipped discs, sciatica, chronic arthritis and nerve infections should not attempt this asana.

Benefits. This asana stretches the hamstring muscles and loosens the hip joint. It effectively removes excess fat in the abdominal region and tones all the abdominal organs and removes diseases of this area, such as diabetes. It also activates the kidneys, liver, pancreas and adrenal glands. It tones the pelvic organs and is therefore especially useful for eliminating female sexual maladies. It encourages a good flow of fresh blood to the spinal nerves and muscles, thereby rendering them more healthy. This is also a powerful asana for spiritual awakening and is highly regarded in ancient yoga texts.

Bhujangasana (Cobra Pose)

Lie on the stomach with the legs straight and the feet extended. Place the palms flat on the floor under the shoulders. Rest the forehead on the ground and relax the body. Slowly raise the head and shoulders off the ground, bending the head as far back as it will go. Try to raise the shoulders without using the arms, only using the back muscles. Now bring the arms into action and slowly bend the back as much as possible without strain until the arms are straight. Keep the navel as near to the ground as possible. Hold as long as comfortable.

Practise up to five times.

Inhale while raising the body from the ground. Breathe normally in the final pose. If the final pose is held for a short time, retain the breath inside.

Precaution. People with peptic ulcers, hernia, intestinal tuberculosis or hyperthyroidism should not attempt this asana.

Benefits. This asana helps to remove female sexual disorders such as leucorrhea, dysmenorrhea and amenorrhea. It tones the ovaries and uterus, stimulates the appetite and eliminates constipation. It is beneficial for all abdominal organs, especially the liver and kidneys. It relocates slipped discs, removes backache and keeps the spine supple and healthy.

Sarvangasana (Shoulder-stand Pose)

Lie flat on the back with the feet together, the arms by the sides and palms flat on the ground. Using the arms as levers raise the legs and back to a vertical position. Bend the elbows and use the arms as props to steady the back by pressing it with the palms. The trunk and legs should extend straight upward, forming a right angle with the neck, the chest pressing against the chin.

Retain the breath inside while assuming and returning from this asana. Practise normal breathing when steadied in the raised position.

* Spiritual concentration should be on Vishuddhi chakra.
* Physical concentration should be on thyroid gland or respiration.

Advanced practitioners can practise up to fifteen minutes. Beginners should practise for a few seconds and increase by a few seconds daily. For general health benefits, three to five minutes is adequate.

Precaution. Not advised for suffers of enlarged

thyroid, liver or spleen, high blood pressure or heart ailments.

Benefits. This asana stimulates the thyroid gland and thereby improves the balance of the circulatory, digestive, reproductive, nervous and glandular systems. It adjusts improper body growth and clears psychological disturbances by bringing a rich supply of blood to the brain. It relieves asthma, bronchitis and elephantasis. It releases the normal gravitational pressure from anal muscles, relieving piles. It tones the legs, abdomen, the female reproductive organs, spine and neck. It inhibits hydrocele and eliminates waistline fat. Leucorrhea and diabetes can be remedied. Mastery of this asana gives conscious control over body temperature.

Halasana (Plough Pose)

Lie flat on the back with the arms straight and beside the body, palms facing downward. Keeping the legs straight, slowly raise them to the vertical position above the body. Only use the stomach muscles to raise the legs; do not use the arms. Simultaneously bend the trunk upward, hips first. Slowly lower the legs over the head and touch the floor with the toes of both feet. Keep the legs straight, bend the arms and place the hands on the back. Relax the body. Remain in the final pose for a comfortable period of time and then return to the starting position.

Retain breath inside while assuming and returning from this pose. Breathe slowly and deeply in the final pose.

* Spiritual concentration should be on Vishuddhi or Manipura chakra.
* Physical and mental concentration should be on the abdomen, relaxation of the back muscles, respiration or the thyroid gland.
* Adepts can hold the final pose of Halasana for more than ten minutes. Beginners should hold for fifteen seconds and increase by a few seconds daily.

Precaution. This asana is not advised for old and infirm people, sufferers of sciatica and other back ailments, or high blood pressure.

Benefits. This asana adjusts the functioning of the abdominal organs, especially the kidneys, liver and the pancreas. It activates digestion, relieves constipation and removes fat from the waist. Beneficially influences all the visceral organs and regulates the activities of the thyroid, thereby balancing all the body's metabolic rates. It helps to remedy diabetes, eliminate piles, loosen the vertebrae and tone the spinal nerves, thereby encouraging optimum health.

Shalbhasana (Locust Pose)

Lie on the stomach with the hands under the thighs, palms facing down. Stretch the legs and tense the arms. Raise the legs and abdomen as high as possible without bending the legs.

Practice up to five times.

Inhale deeply in the prone position. Retain the breath inside while raising the legs and abdomen. Exhale while returning to the starting position.

* Spiritual concentration should be on Vishuddhi chakra.
* Physical concentration should be on the abdomen, lower back or heart.

Precaution. This asana is not to be practised by sufferers of peptic ulcer, hernia, intestinal tuberculosis or weak heart.

Benefits. This asana tones and adjusts the liver and other abdominal organs, especially the intestines, pancreas, and kidneys. It is useful for relieving and eliminating diseases of the stomach and bowels, and it stimulates the appetite. It strengthens the lower spine and heart, and tones the sciatic nerves.

Chakrasana (Wheel Pose)

Lie on the back with the knees bent and the heels touching the buttocks. The feet should be about one foot apart. Place the palms on the ground beside the temples, with fingers pointing toward the shoulders. Slowly raise the trunk. Let the head rotate slightly and allow the crown to support the weight of the upper body. The legs will form right angles at the knees. Straighten the arms and legs, lift the head off the ground and raise the body to its fully arched height. You can straighten the knees almost completely by moving the trunk upward. Slowly lower yourself back to the ground and then return to the supine position.

Initially practise Chakrasana with the breath retained inside. After some regular practice, Chakrasana may be maintained for long periods by breathing normally in the fully raised position.

Practise Chakrasana once for as long as you con comfortably maintain it.

* Spiritual concentration should be on Manipura chakra.
* Physical concentration should be on the back, abdomen or respiration.

Precaution. Chakrasana should not be practised by sufferers of high blood pressure, coronary ailments, stomach ulcer, toxic intestines, partial deafness, dilated eye capillaries, or by anyone who has recently fractured bones or undergone abdominal operations. It is not to be attempted until the practitioner is able to do the more preliminary backward bending poses.

Benefits. This asana is beneficial for the entire nervous and glandular systems. It influences all hormonal secretions and relieves varied ailments of the female reproductive system. It fully stretches the back and abdominal muscles, making them supple. It powerfully compresses and massages the abdominal organs.

Dhanurasana (Bow Pose)

Lie flat on the stomach and inhale fully. Bend the knees and hold and ankles with the hands. Tense the leg muscles and arch the back. Simultaneously raise the head, chest and thighs as high as possible. Keep the arms straight. Hold for as long as is comfortable.

Practise up to five times.

One may rock back and forth in the final position. Do not repeat until the breath returns to normal.

The breath may be retained inside in the final pose or slow, deep breathing may be practised.

* Spiritual concentration should be on Vishuddhi chakra.
* Physical concentration should be on the abdominal region or back.

Precaution. This asana should not be practised by people with hernia, peptic ulcers, intestinal tuberculosis or by people with a crooked spine.

Benefits. This asana powerfully massages the abdominal organs and muscles, removes gastro-intestinal disorders, dyspepsia, chronic constipation and sluggishness of the liver. It quickly reduces excess fat in the abdominal area.

Vajrasana (Thunderbolt Pose)

Stand on the knees with the feet stretched backward and big toes crossed. The knees should be together, heels apart. Lower the buttocks on to the insides of the feet, the heels at the sides of the hips. Place the hands on the knees, palms downward.

Practice Vajrasana as much as possible, especially right after meals for at least five minutes to enhance the digestive functions.

Concentrate on the normal breathing process. This will bring tranquillity to the mind if practised with the eyes closed.

Benefits. Vajrasana alters the flow of blood and nervous impulses in the pelvic and visceral secretions. This pose increases the efficiency of the entire digestive system and is especially useful for indigestion. It reduces the blood flow to the genitals and massages the nerve fibers which feed them. This makes it useful for men with dilated testicles. It strengthens the pelvic muscles which serve as prevention against hernia and aids women in childbirth. It is very useful in relieving stomach ailments such as peptic ulcer or hyperacidity.

Ushtrasana (Camel Pose)

Sit in Vajrasana with the knees apart. Stand on your knees and stretch the arms to the sides. Lean backward and put the hands on the heels. Stretch the neck backward and let the body weight rest on the arms. Arch as far back as possible. Return to kneeling position, then back to Vajrasana.

Inhale while assuming the knee-based position. Exhale while bending backward and while lowering to Vajrasana.

Practise a maximum of ten times as a dynamic exercise. Hold up to three minutes as a static pose.

* Spiritual concentration should be on Vishuddhi or Anahata chakra.
* Physical concentration should be on the abdomen, thyroid gland or spine.

Benefits. This asana is beneficial for the digestive, excretory and reproductive systems. It stretches the stomach and intestines, eliminating constipation. It is useful for removing backache, lumbago and rounded back.

Uttanpadasana (Raised Foot Pose)

Lie flat on the floor, face upward. Place the legs together with the arms on each side. The arms should remain passive during the whole practice. Close the eyes. Try to relax your whole body for a short period. Breathe out deeply. Then breathe in as deeply as possible. Slowly raise your legs keeping these together and straight. It is important that the arms remain as relaxed as possible. The raising of the legs should be achieved by contraction of the abdominal muscles. This is important for it ensures that the abdominal muscles are strengthened and the internal organs massaged. Do not raise the legs too high; the feet should be held so that they are between 30 to 60 cm above the ground. Hold your legs to the final raised position while simultaneously holding your breath. Do not straighten but remain in the final pose for as long as you can without experiencing any discomfort. Then slowly lower the legs as you breathe out. On reaching the floor completely relax the entire body. When your breathing rate has returned to normal the asana can be repeated.

Breathing should be normal while lying on the floor, followed by deep inhalation. Practise retention while raising and holding the legs in the final pose. Exhale while lowering the legs. Practise normal breathing while relaxing after completion of the asana.

Concentration should be on the abdomen and the breathing pattern.

Hold the final position only for as long as you comfortably can. Do not strain. Repeat the asana as many times as you wish, although three times is a reasonable number.

Benefits. Uttan Padasana is excellent for straightening the abdominal muscles, massaging the internal organs, removing wind and eliminating constipation.

Pawanmuktasana (Wind Releasing Pose)

Lie flat on the back. Relax the whole body. Bend the right leg and bring the thigh and knee as near as possible to the chest. The other leg should remain straight. Place the hands over the knee and interlock the fingers. Gently pull the knee nearer the chest. Relax the whole body keeping the straight leg, back and head on the floor. Breathe in deeply and slowly while simultaneously raising the head and shoulders. At the end of inhalation the forehead, nose, chin or neck should touch or be as close as possible to the right knee. Hold your breath for a short time in the raised position. Then exhale slowly and lower the head and shoulders to the floor to resume the starting position. Inhale while again raising the body and repeating the procedure. Do a number of rounds. Then straighten the bent leg and relax the whole body for a short time.

Now fold both legs to the chest and repeat the asana. Afterwards relax the whole body with concentration on breath.

Breath should be deep and synchronized with the movement. This asana gives the most benefits if one holds the breath while in the raised position for as long as is comfortable.

One should be aware of breath and the compression of the abdomen throughout the practice.

For general health benefits do three to five rounds.

Benefits. This asana gives an excellent massage to the abdomen. It increases the circulation of the blood and stimulates the nerves which connect the organs to the brain or nerve complexes. It is useful for removing constipation and flatulence. This asana also tones up the back muscles and spinal nerves.

Shavasana (Corpse Pose)

Lie on the back with the arms beside and in line with the body, palms facing upward. Move the feet slightly apart to a comfortable position and close the eyes. Relax the whole body. Do not move any part even if discomfort occurs. Let the breath become rhythmic and natural. Become aware of inhalation and exhalation. Count the number of respirations: 1 in, 1 out, and so on. Continue to count for a few minutes. It the mind starts to wander bring it back to the counting. If you can keep the mind on the breath for a few minutes, the mind and body will relax.

The longer the better in general. During asana practice a minute or two is sufficient.

Concentrate on the breath and counting.

Benefits. Relaxes the whole psychophysiological system. Ideally practised before sleep, before or during asana practice and particularly after dynamic exercises such as Surya Namaskara.

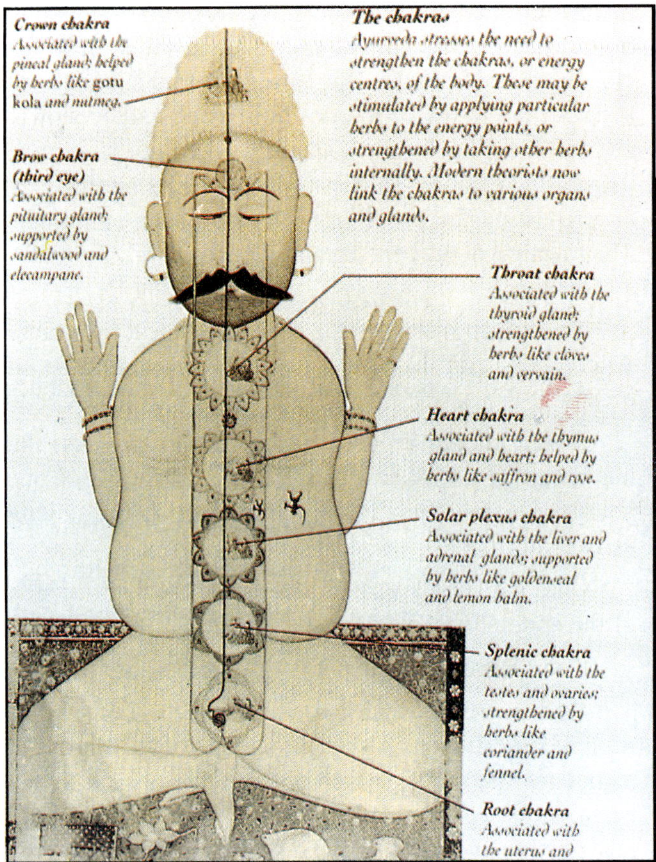

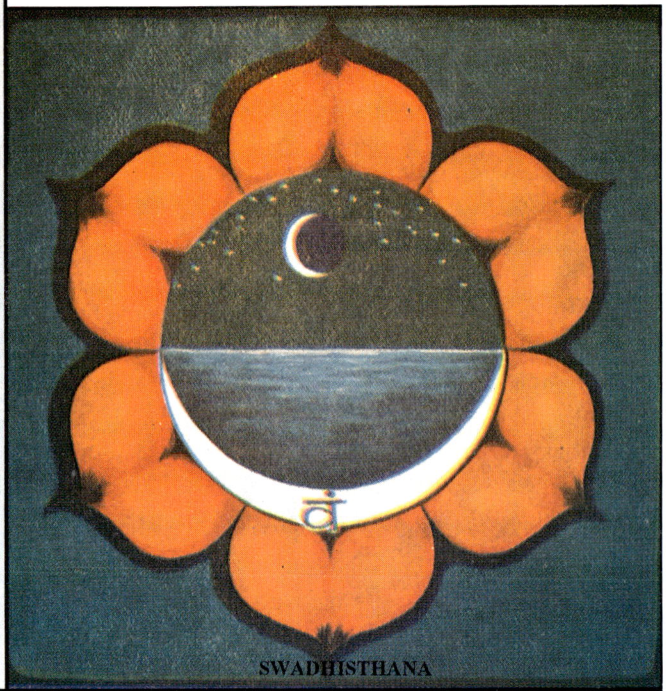
SWADHISTHANA

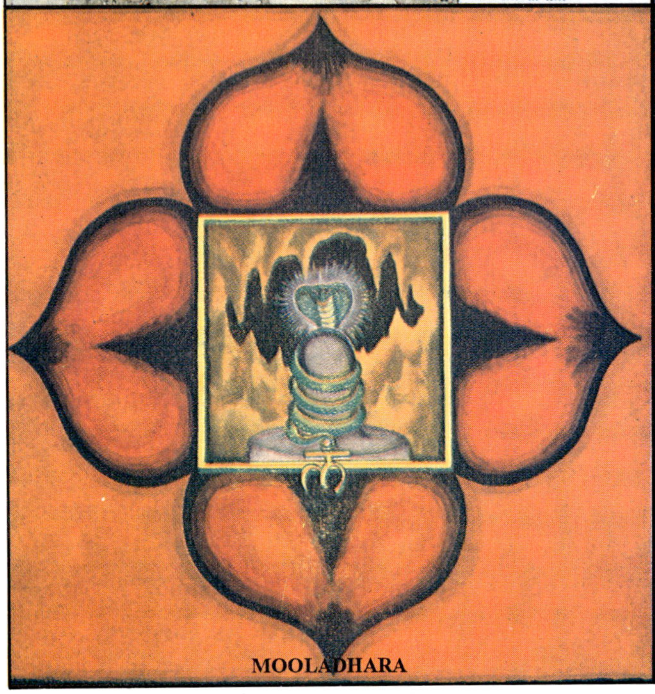
MOOLADHARA

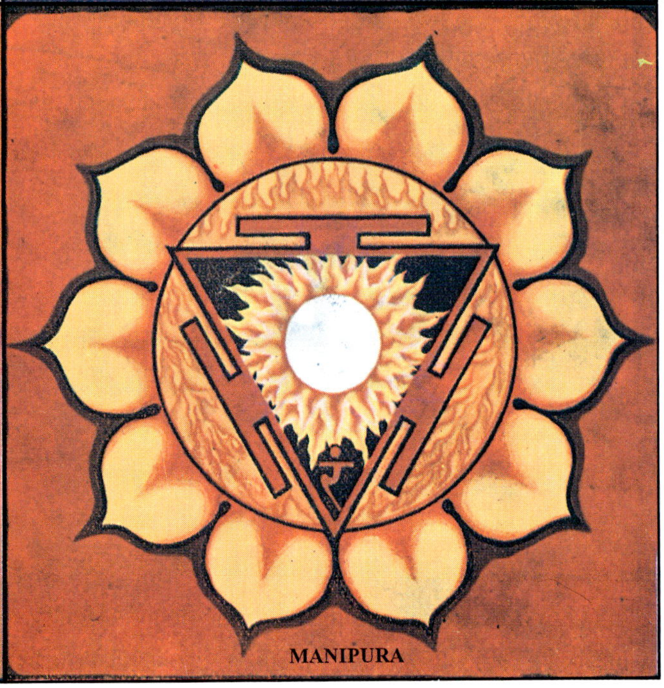
MANIPURA

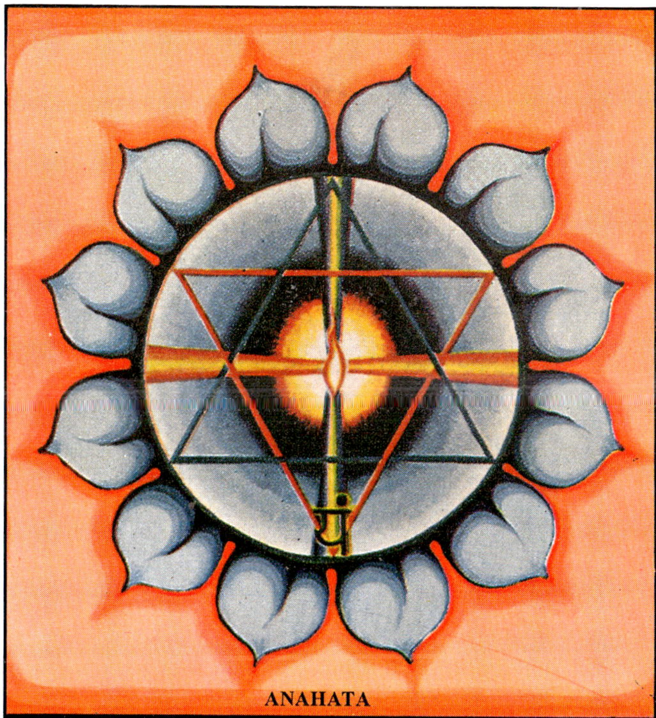

ANAHATA

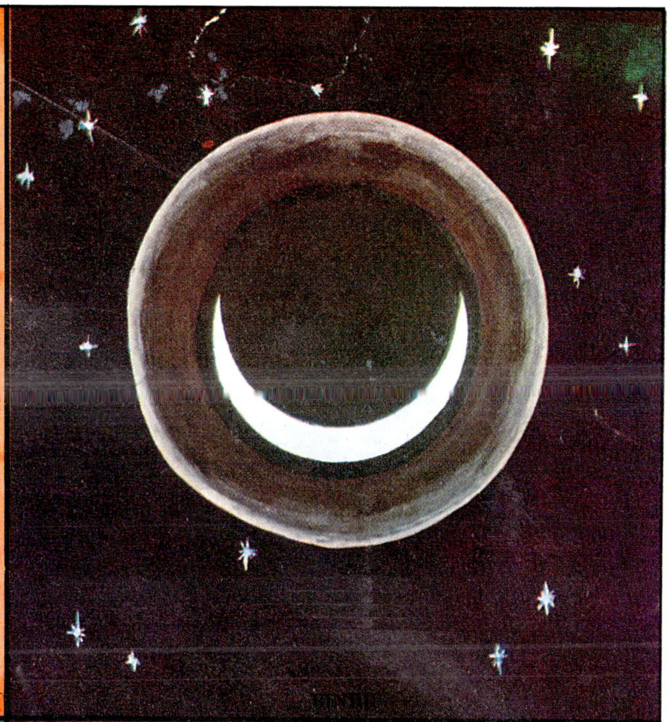

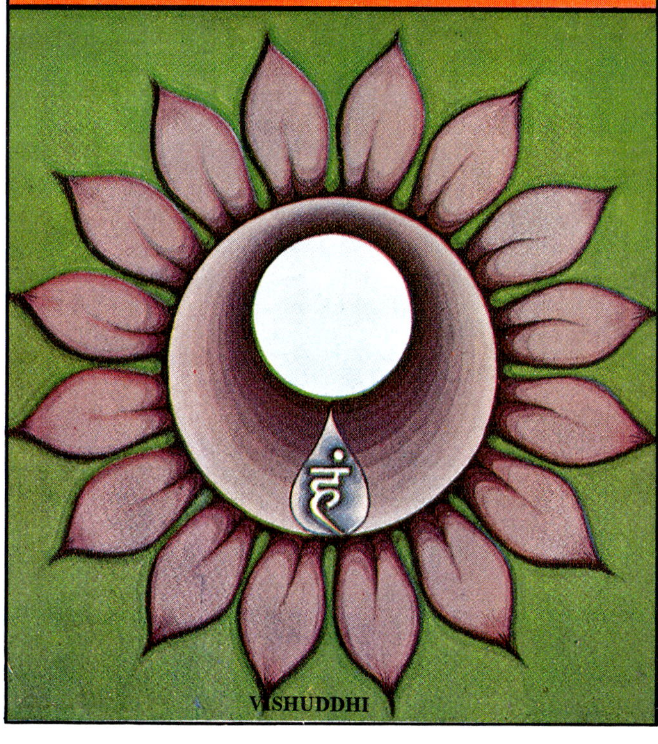

VISHUDDHI

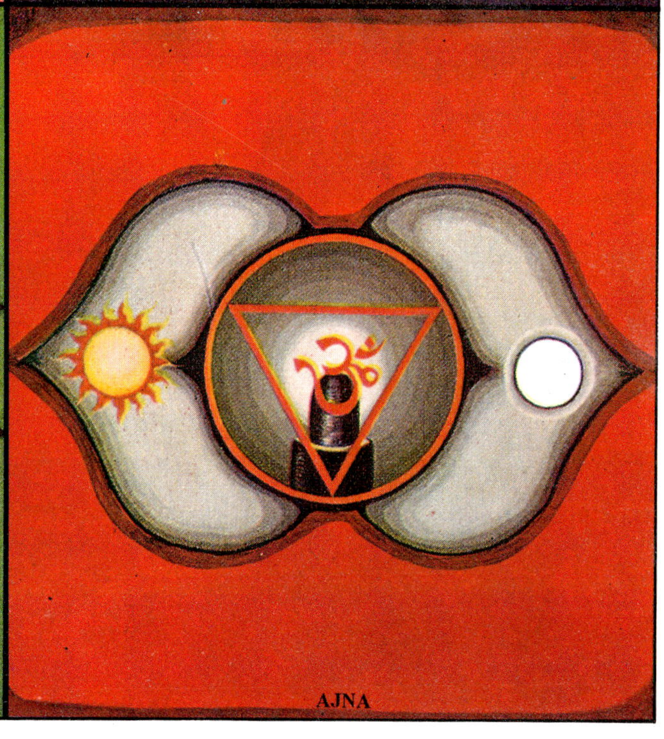

AJNA

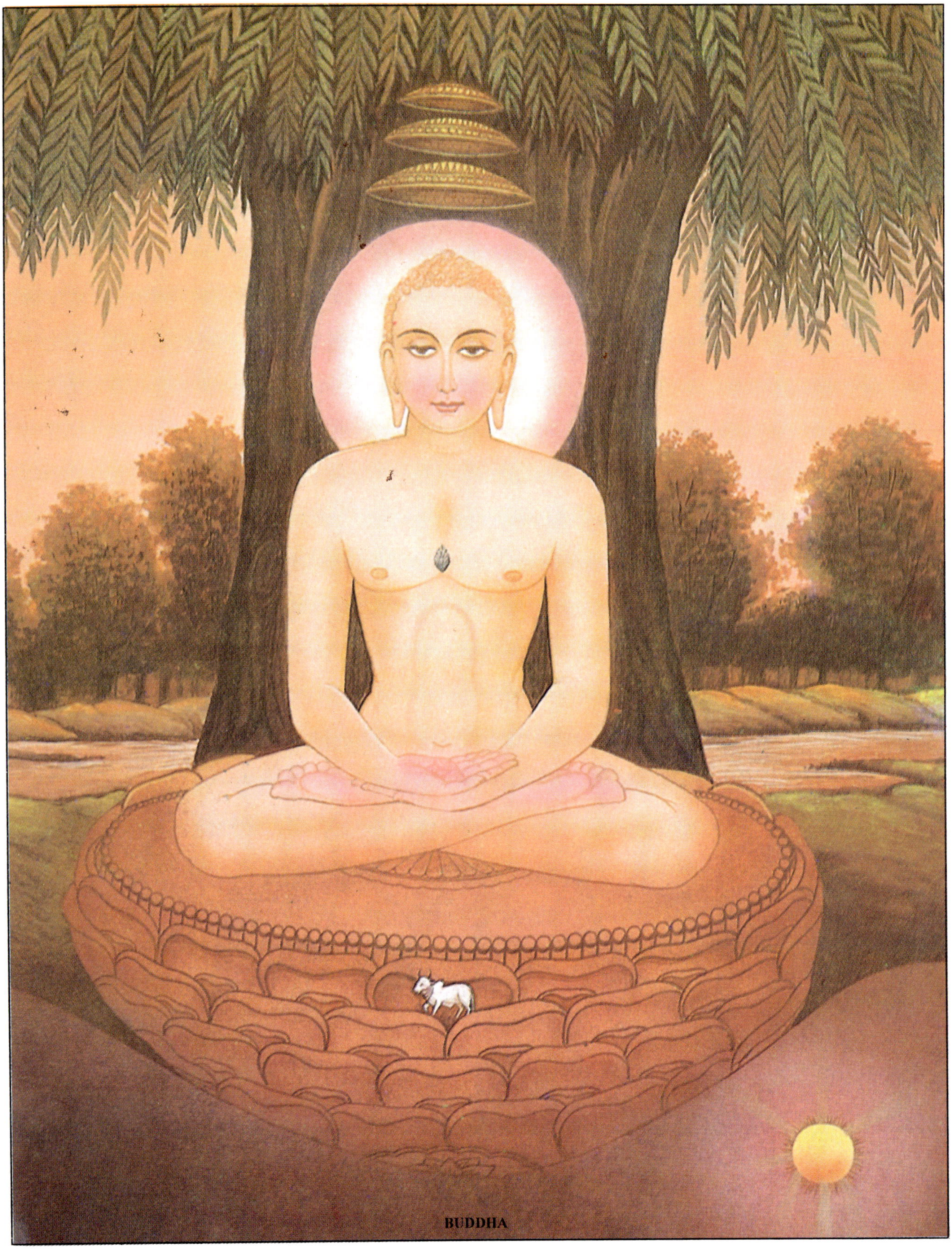

BUDDHA

MUDRAS AND BANDHAS

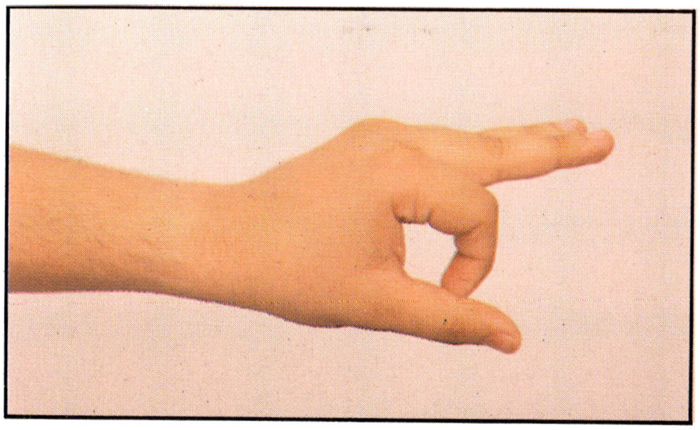

Gyana Murdra

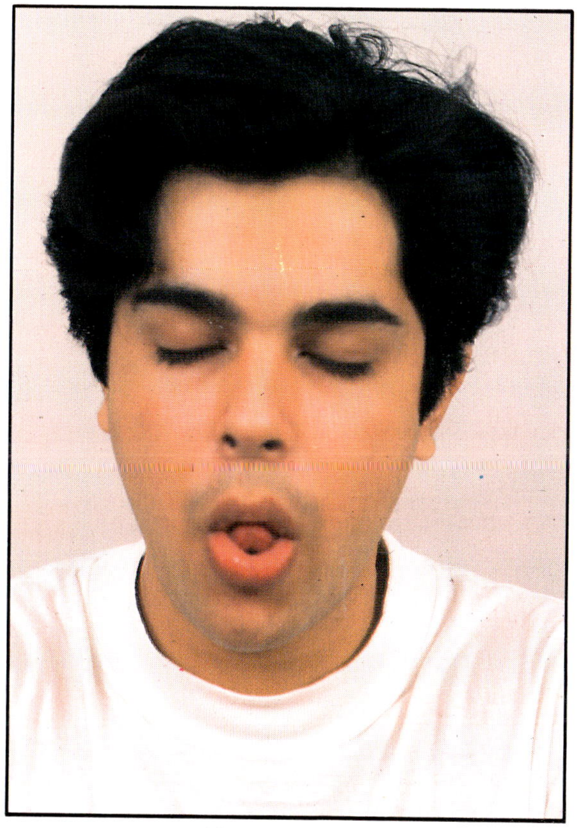

Khechari Murdra

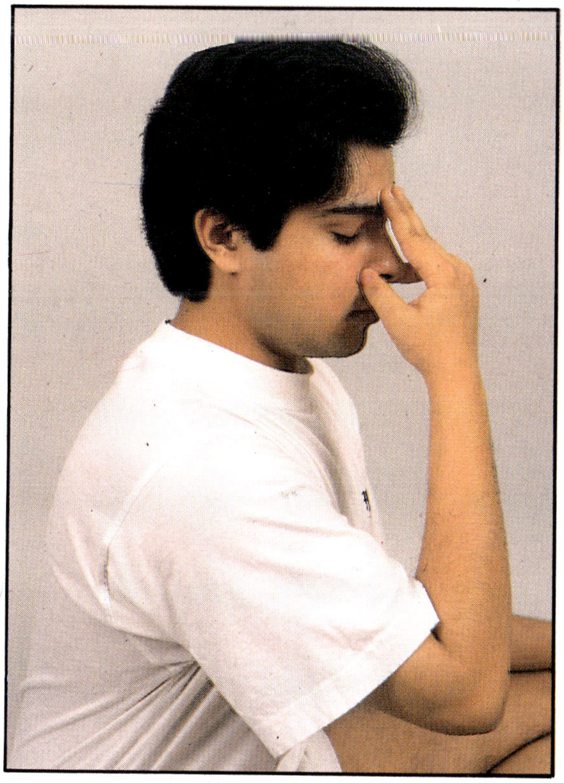

Nasagra Mudra

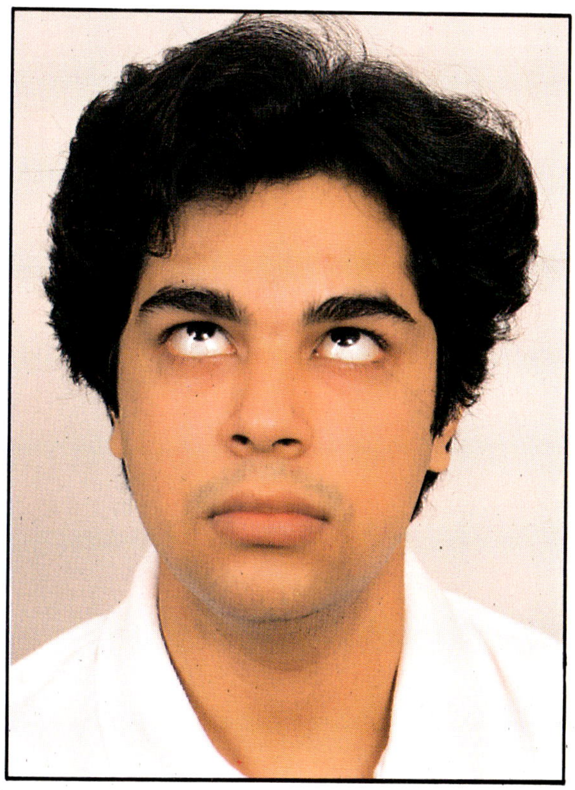

Shambhavi Mudra

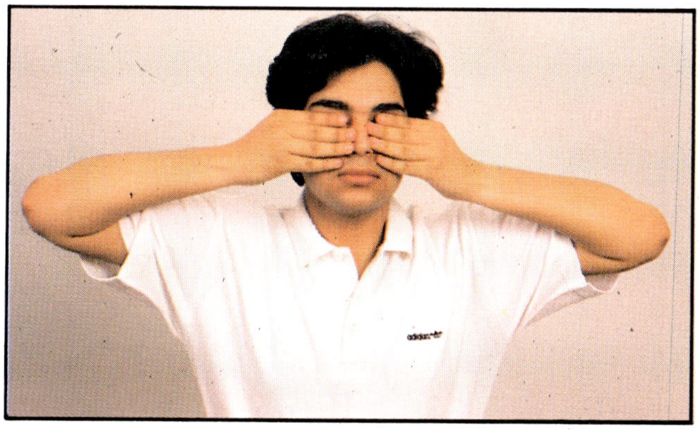

Yoni Mudra

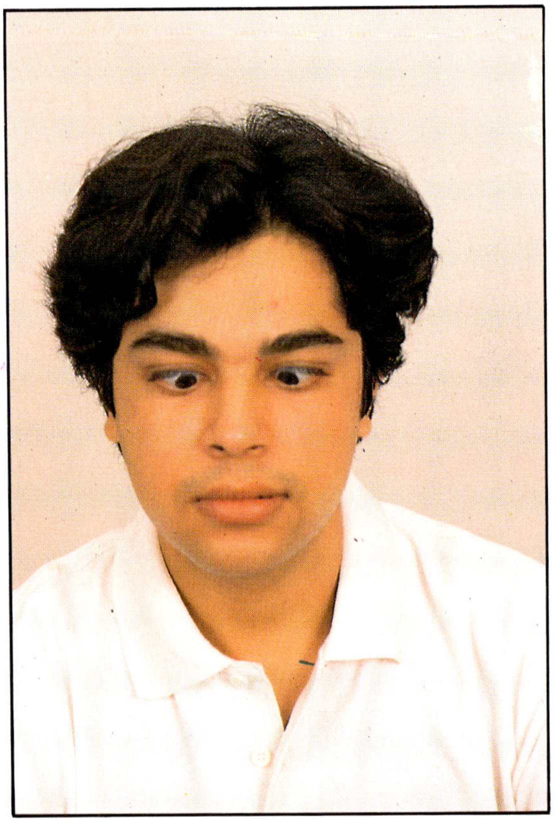

Agochari Murdra

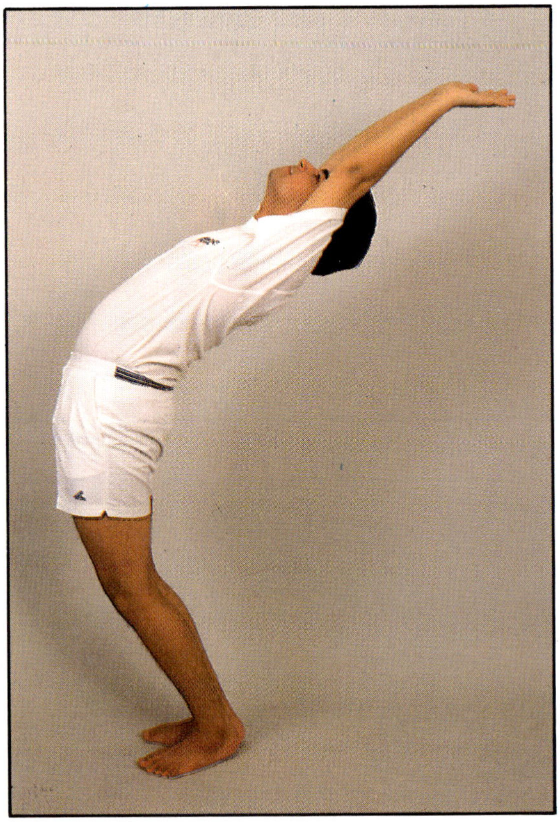

Hasta Utlanasana (Raise Arm Pose)

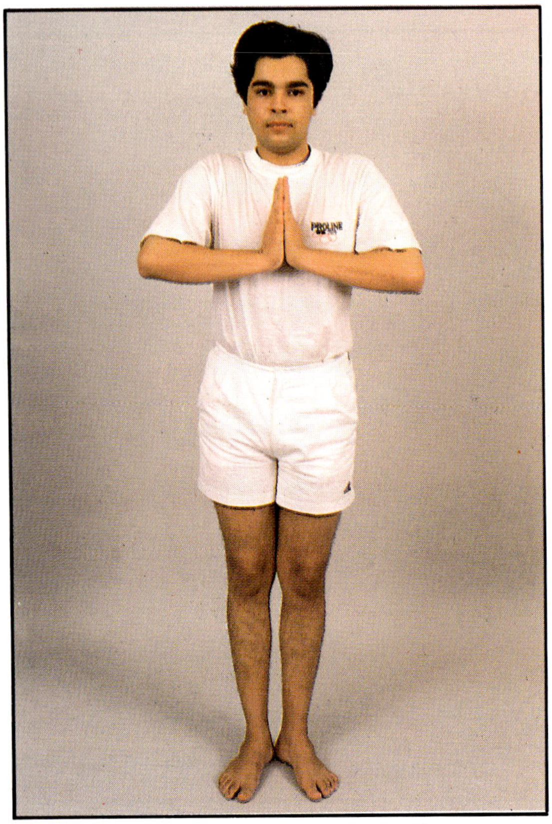

Pranamasana ("Prayer Position")

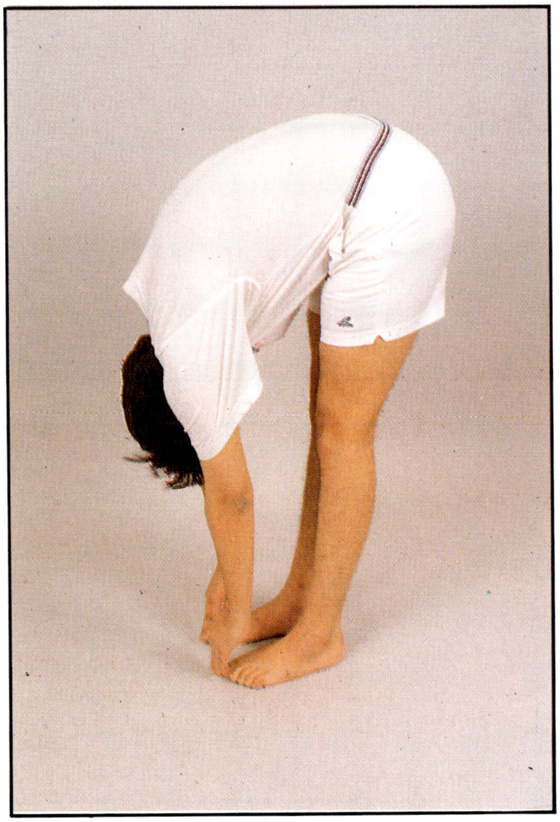

Padahastasana ("Hand – to – Foot Pose")

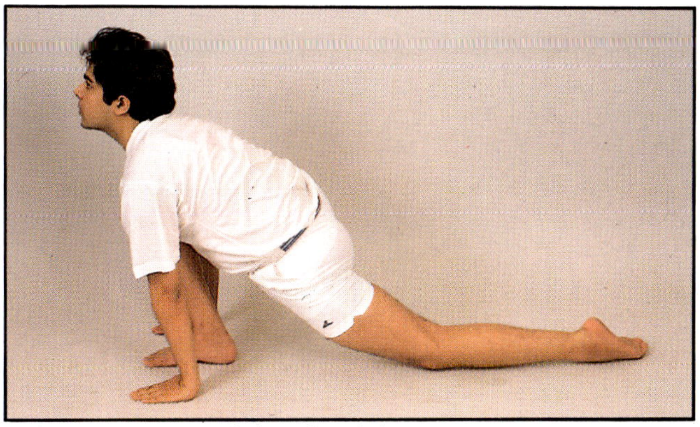

Ashwa Sanchalanasana
(The Equestrian Posey)

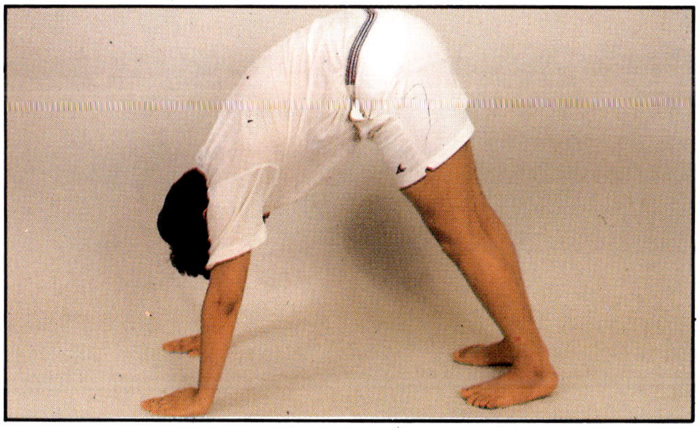

Parratasana ('Mountain Pose')

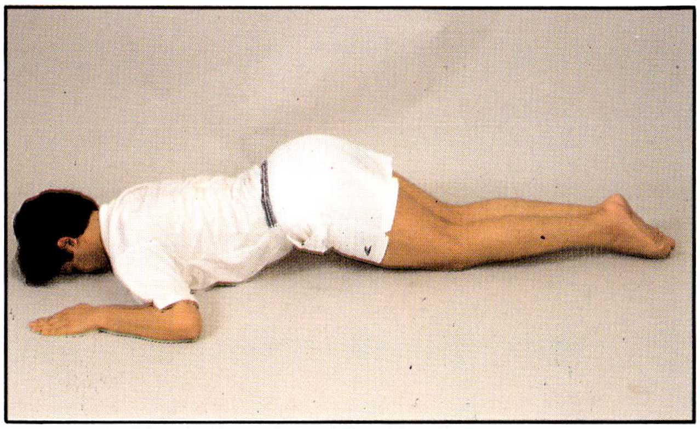

Ashtanga Namaskara Worship with Eight Points

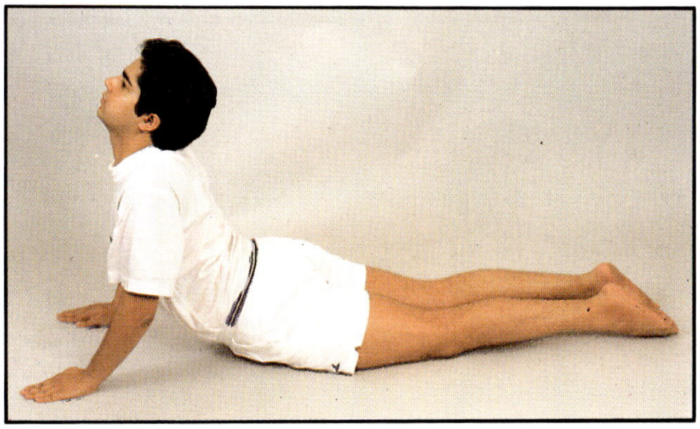

Bhujangasana ("Serpent Pose")

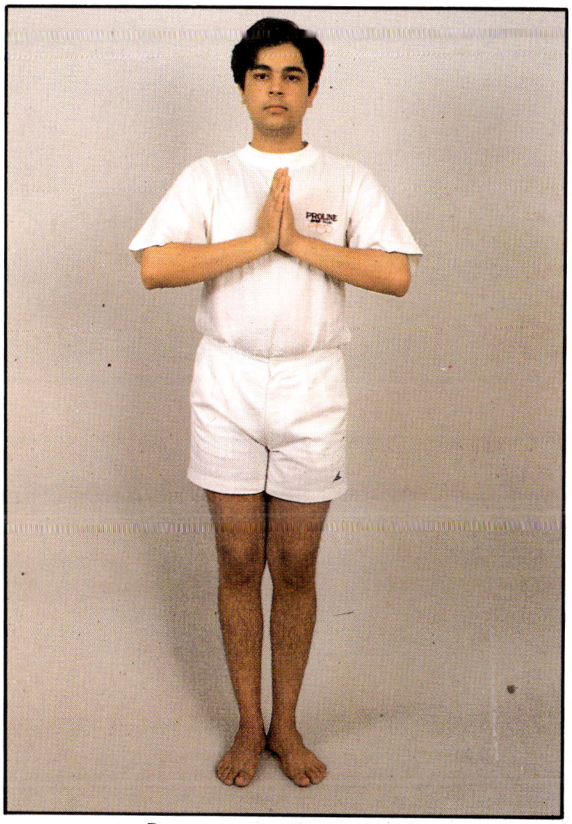

Pranamasana ('Prayer Pose')

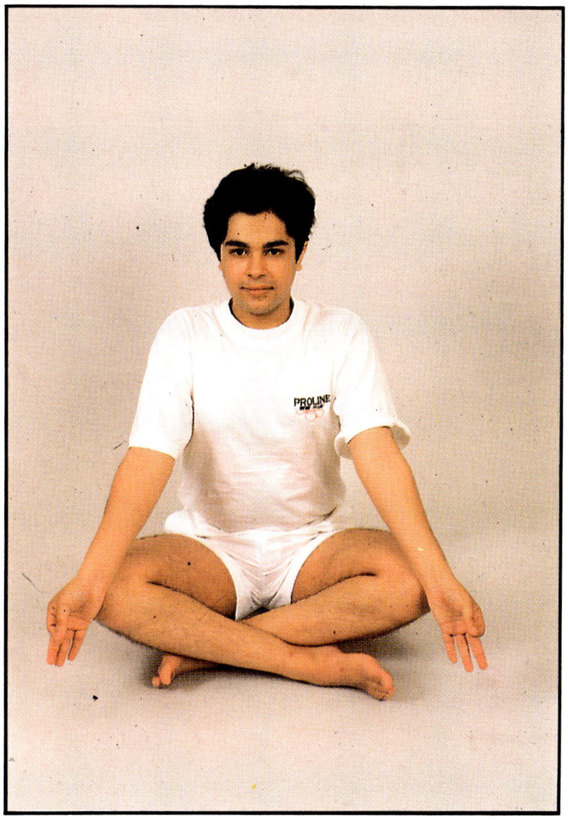

Meditation Pose

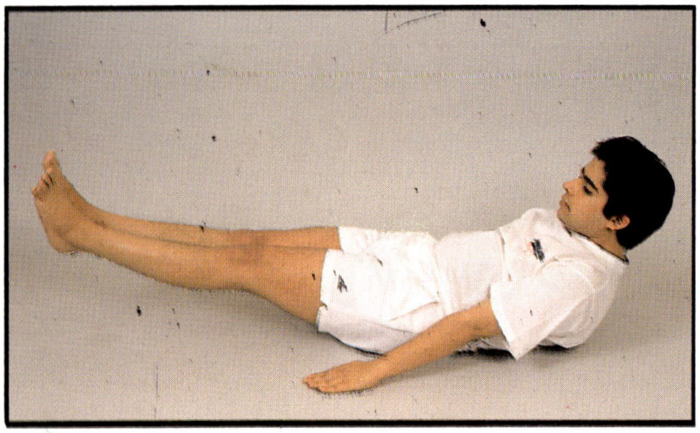

Nauka Sana ('Boat Pose')

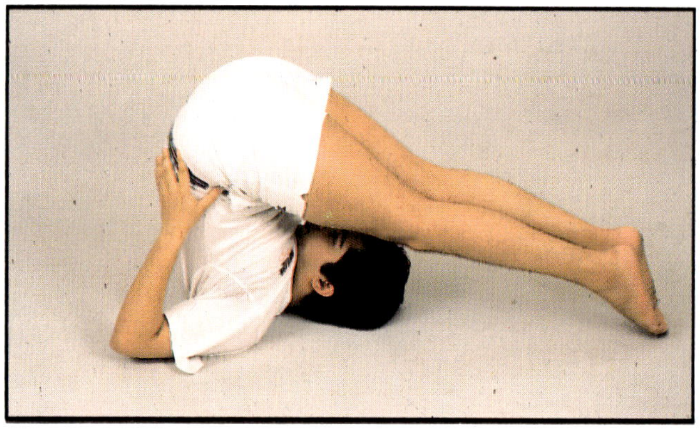

Halasana (Plough Pose)

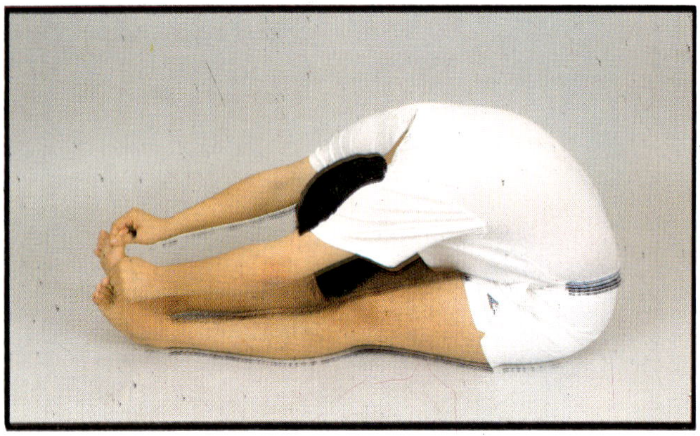

Paschimotanasana ("Black Stretching Pose"

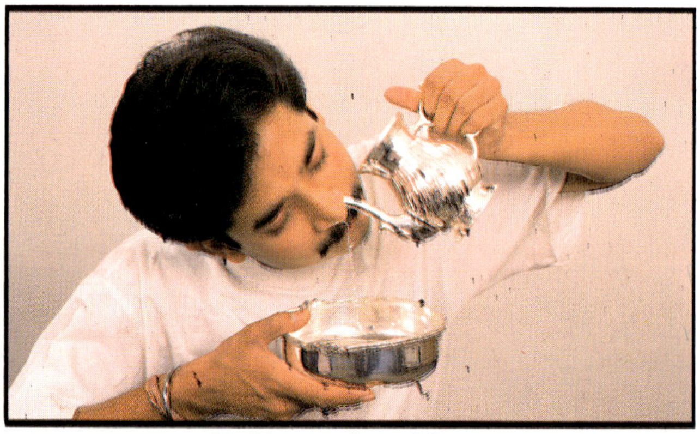

Shalbhasana (Locust Pose)

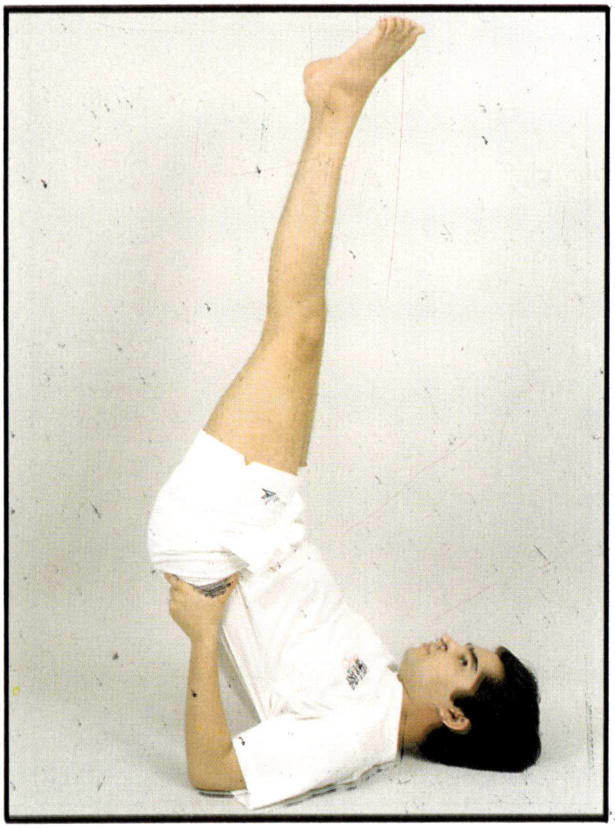

Sarrangasana (Shoulder – stand Pose)

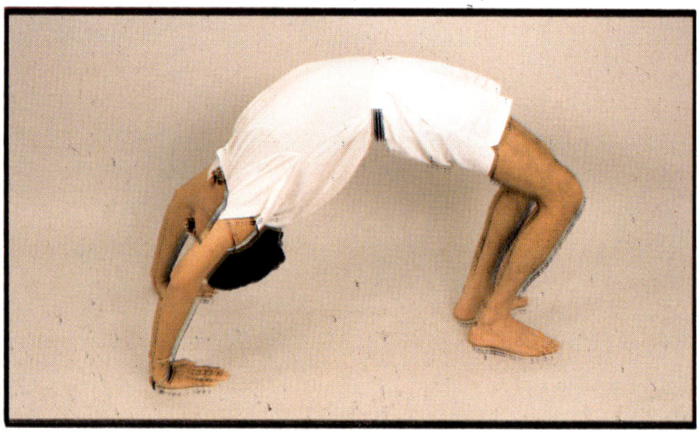

Chakrasana (Wheel Pose)

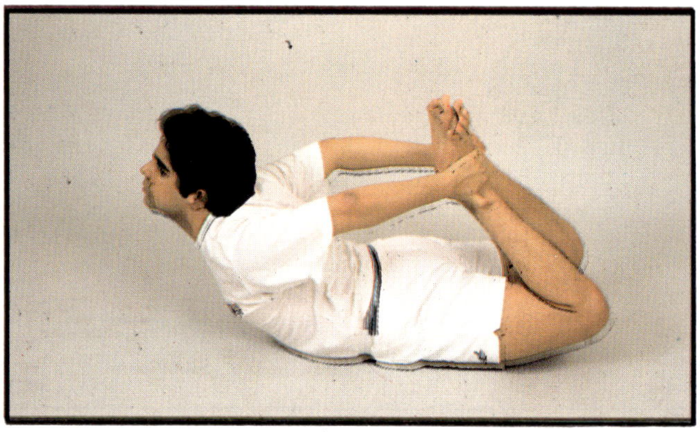

Dhanurasana (Bow Pose)

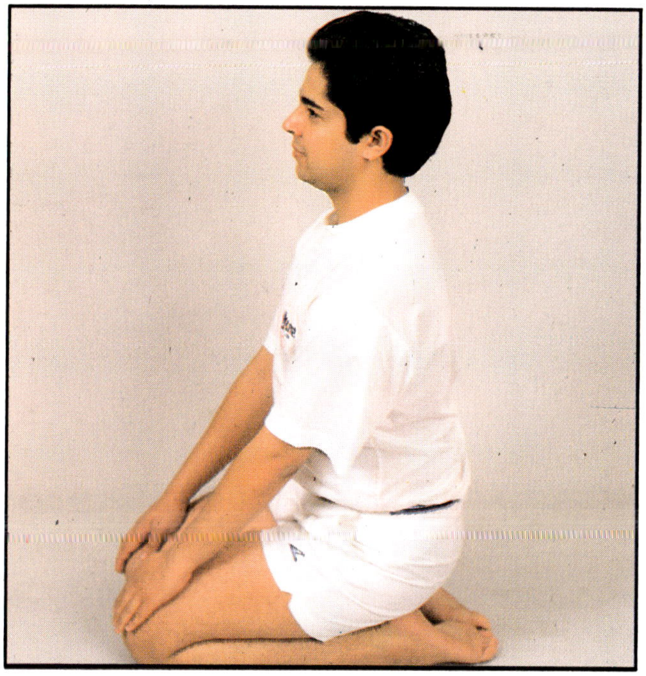

Vajrasana (Thunder Bold Pose)

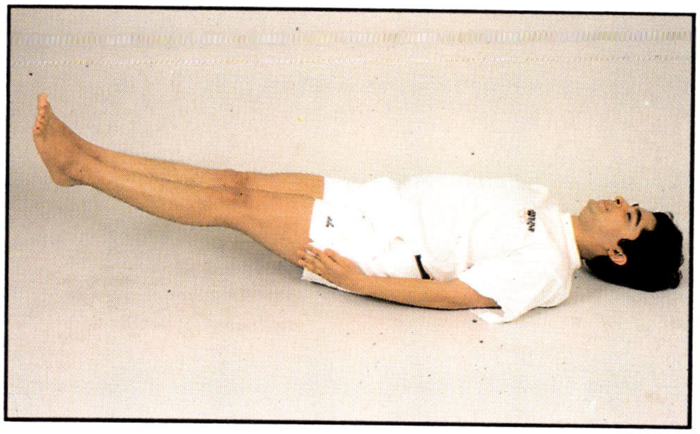

Uttan Padasana (Raised Food Pose)

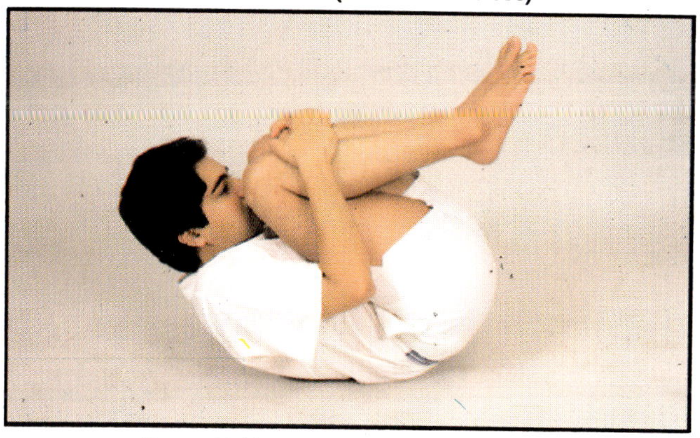

Pawan Muktasana (Wind Releasing Pose)

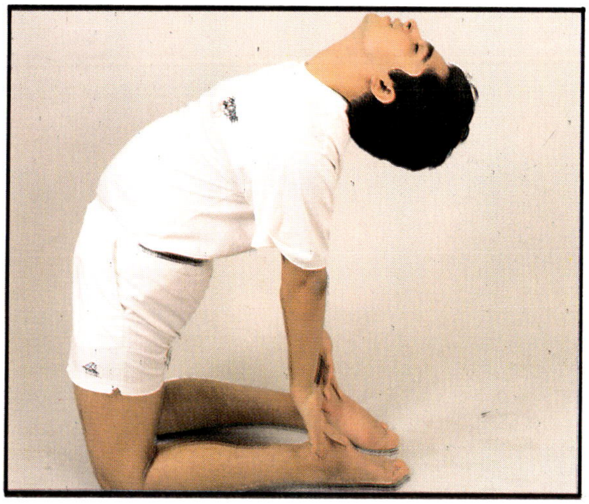

Ushtrasana (Camel Pose)

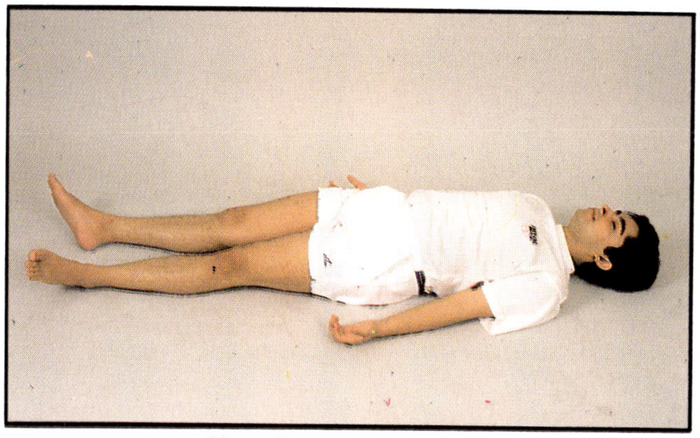

Shava Sana (Corpose Pose)

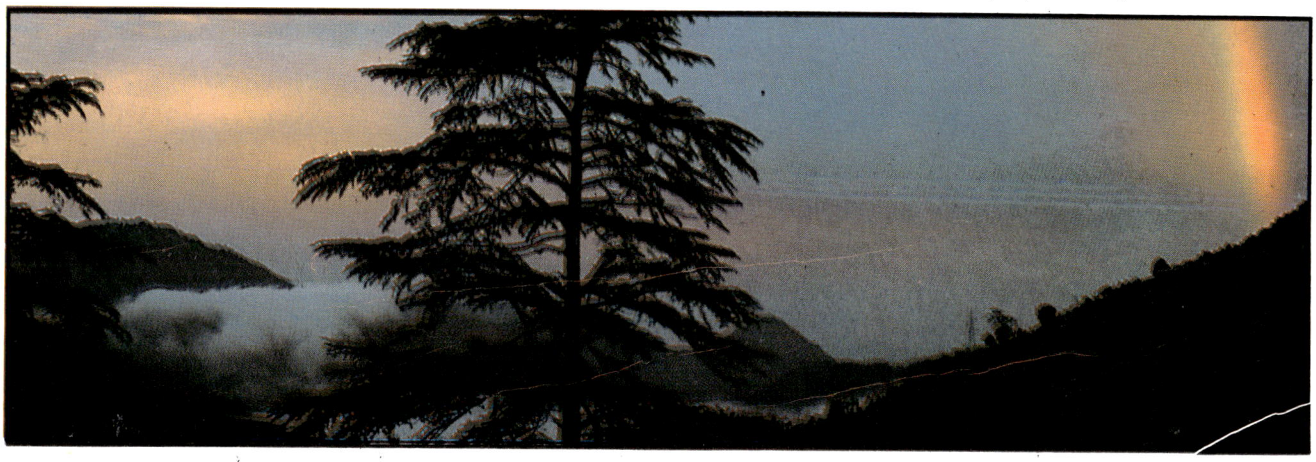

Watch Out danger Sign for

CANCER

Keep a Sharp Eye Out For any of these SYMPTOMS

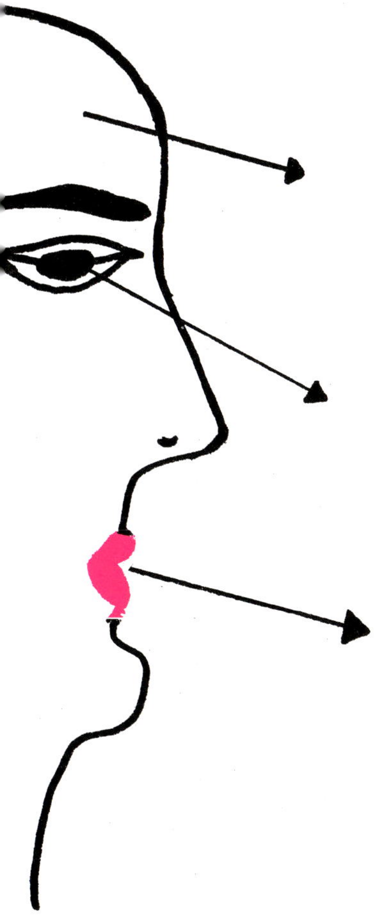

LEARN

SEE

INFORM

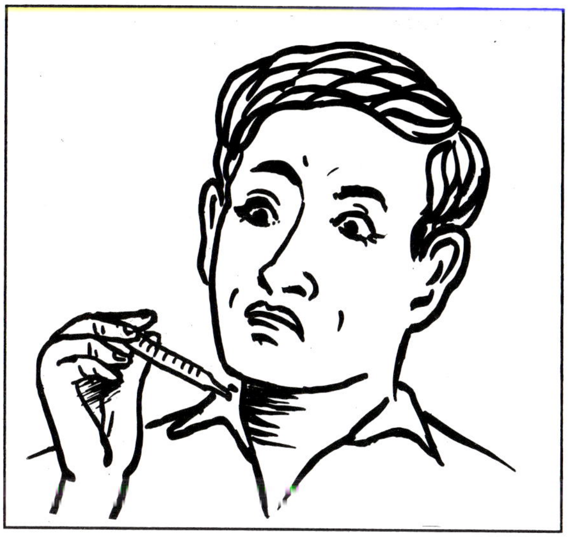

Low Grade Fever Frequent & Persistent

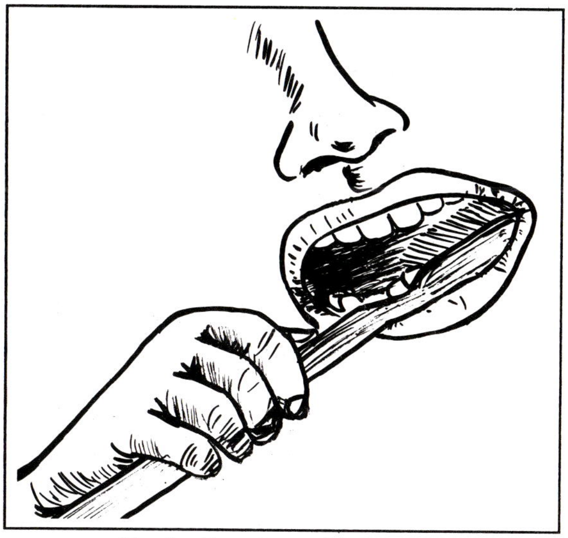

Bleeding From Gums while Brushing

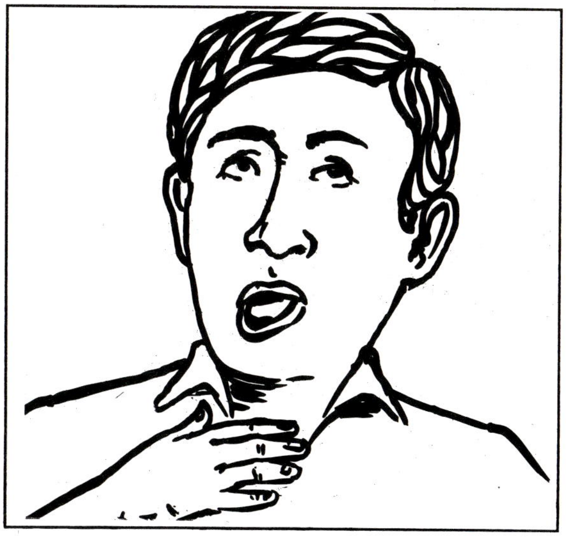

Chest Pain

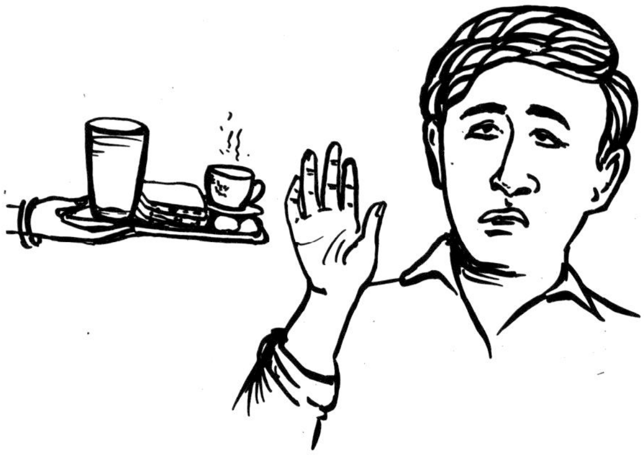

Low of Appetite

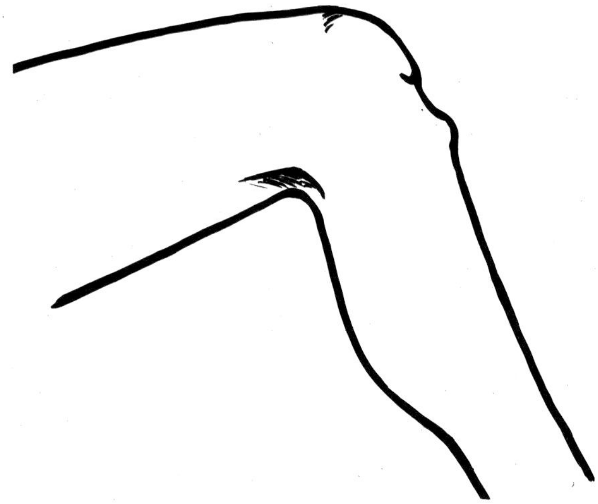

Thickening or Lump in the Brest of Else Where in the Body

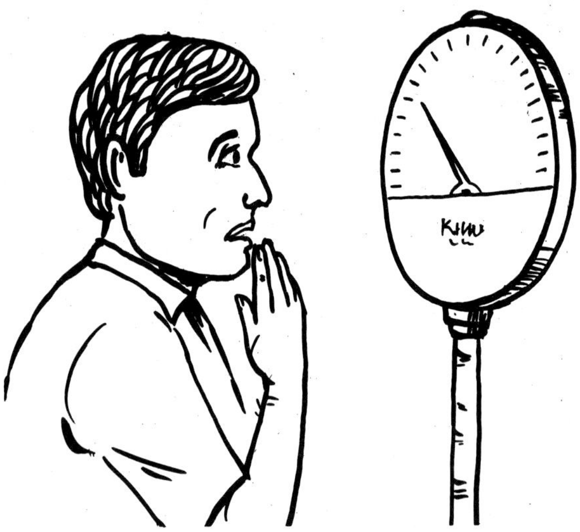

Loss of Weight

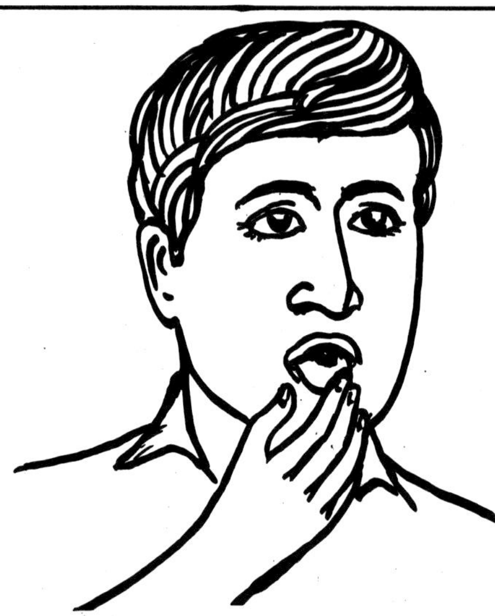

Indigestion or Difficulty in Swallowing

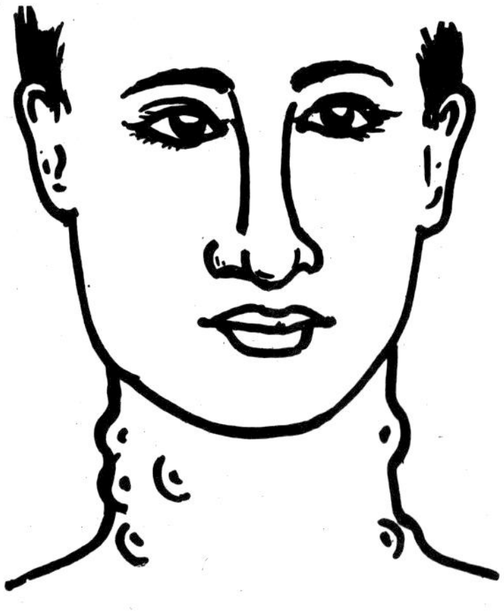

CANCER INVADE AND CROWD out Neighbouring tissues and Organs. Sometimes they From LUMPS. These lumps Press on vital Parts of the body like the Food Pipe and Brain Causing Problem.

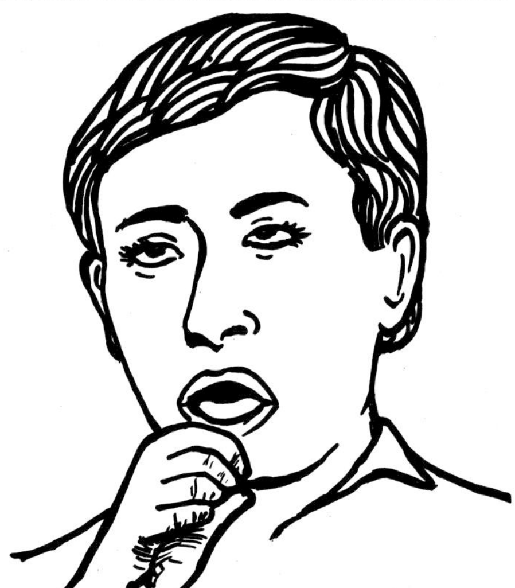

Nagging Cough or Hoarseness

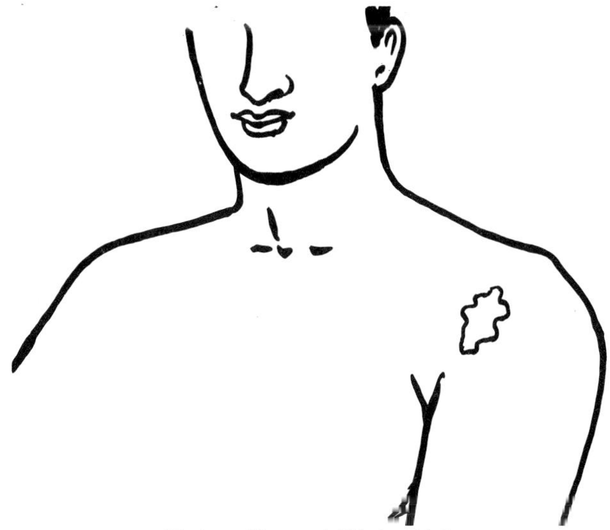

Obvious Change in Wart or Mole

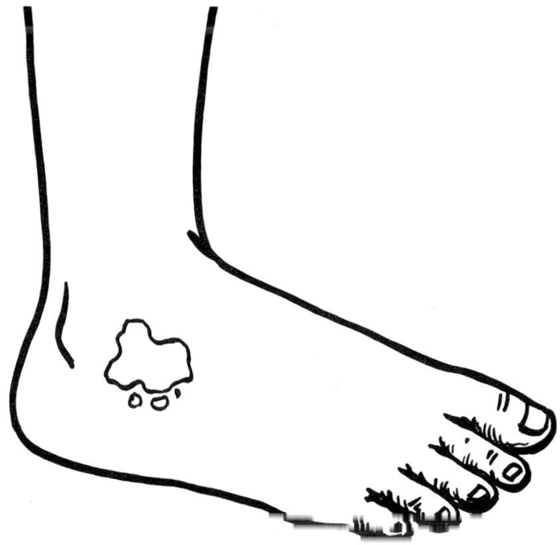

A SORE that does not Heal

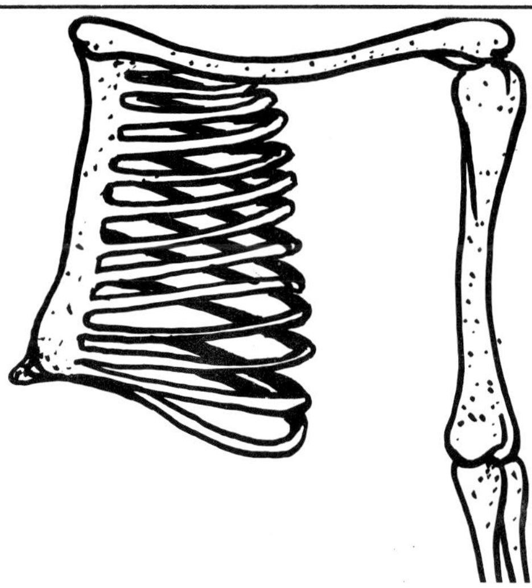

All Cancers Do not show as lumps Blood Cancer Starts in the Bone Narrow and Spread in Blood.

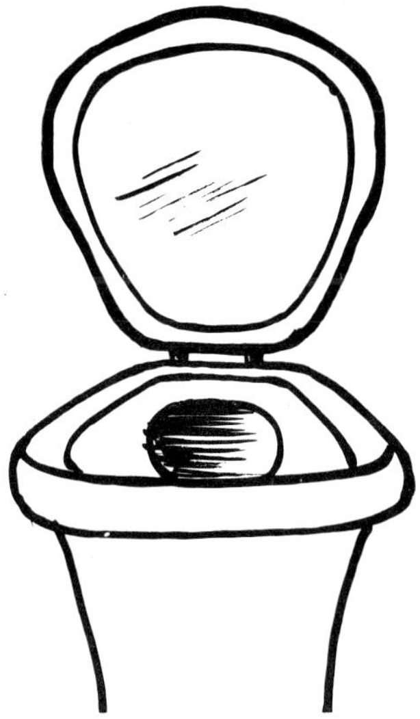

Change in Bowel or Bladder Habit

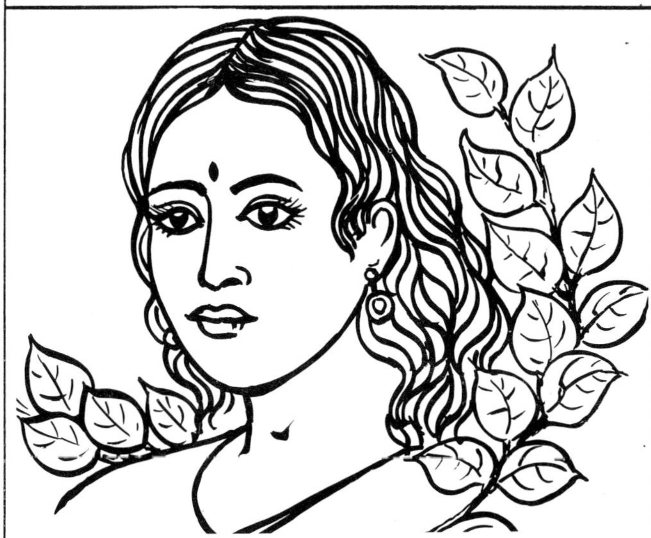

At the First Hint of the Trouble. You should see your Doctor

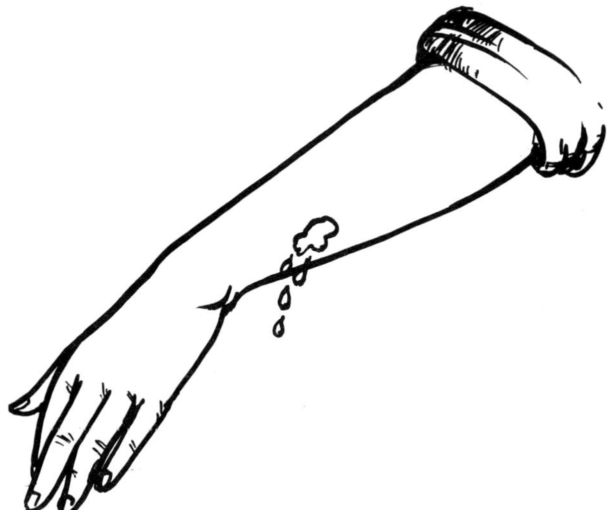

Unusual Bleeding or Discharge

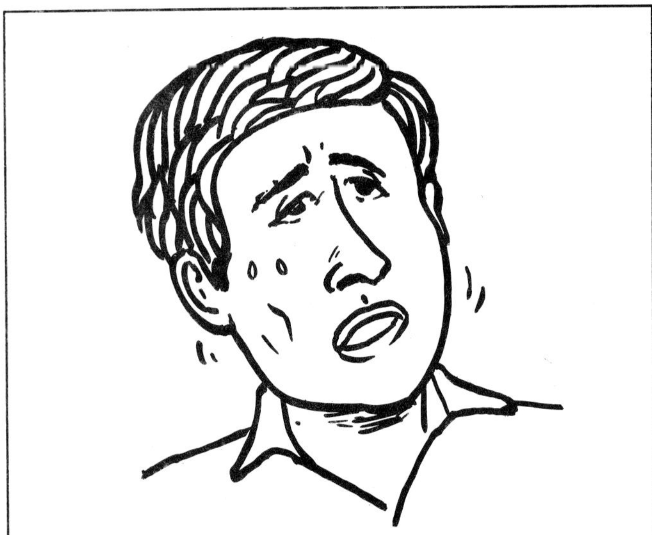

Difficulty in Breathing ?

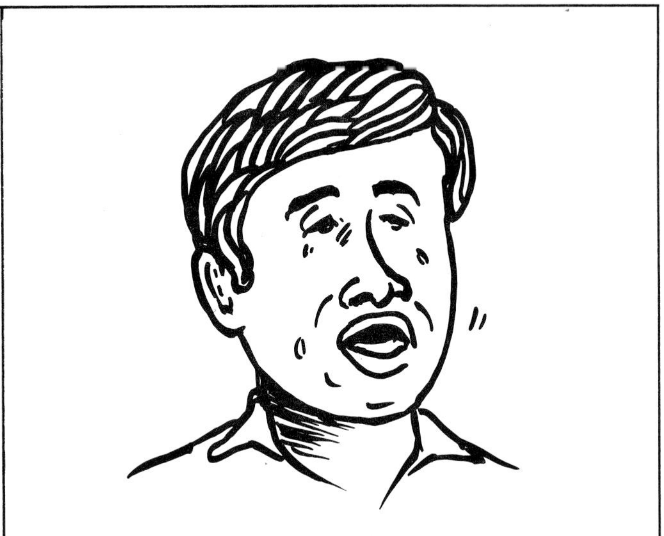

Pollor, Weakness or Frequent tiredness

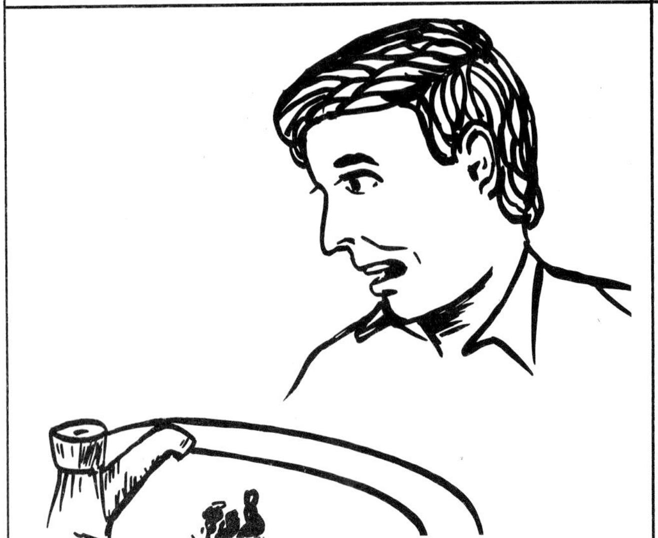

Is there Blood in Your Sputum ?

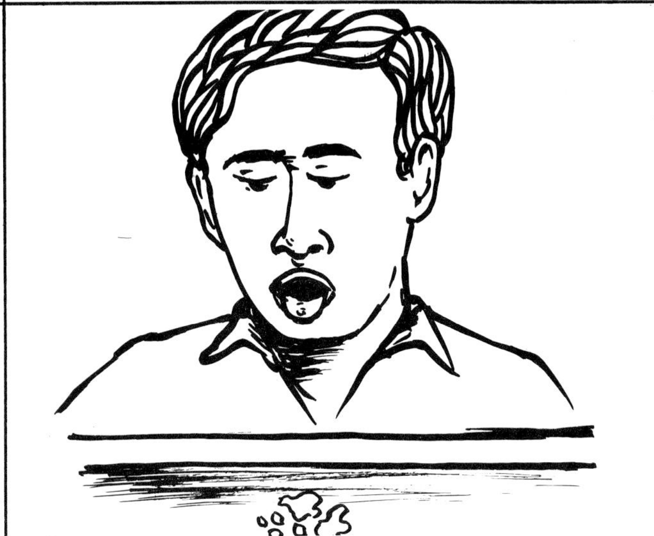

Appearance of Blood in Cough, Urine or Stool.

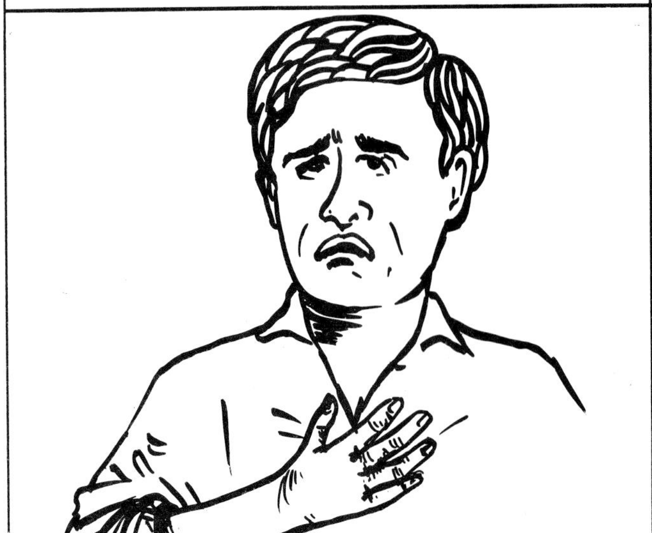

Infections – Cough, sore – throat, Boils which Apper Frequently

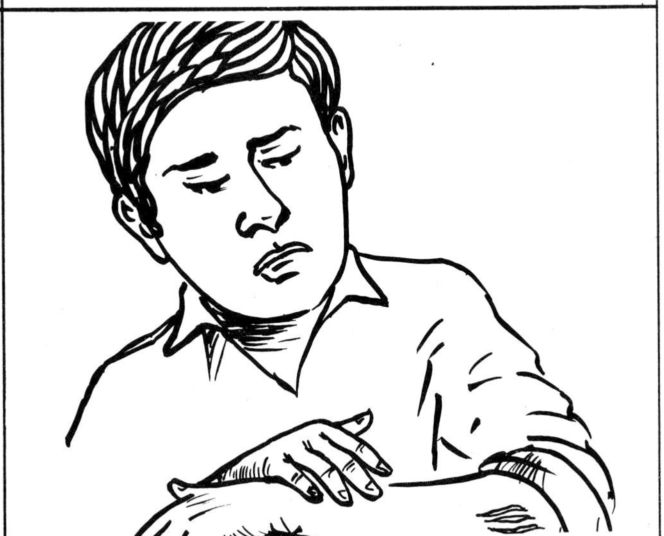

Frequent Bruising with or Without Reason

THE TECHNIQUES OF NATUROPATHY

HOW TO TAKE AN ENEMA

The following points should be kept in mind while taking an enema:

1. Lie down on a hard bed: the foot of the bet must be four inches higher than the head. Of cours, you can take the enema while lying on the floor, but in that case your buttocks should be higher than the rest of your body in order to facililate the introduction of the liquid through the rectum.
2. The vessel in order to faciliate the hot the enema should be suspended from a nail at a height of three feet from the body. The nozzle should be introduced in the rectum to allow the water to go in.
3. If you raise your knees,it would faciliate the introduction of the enema into the rectum.
4. Check that the nozzle is not blocked : in that process some of the liquid should be allowed to run off. That will also ensure that there is no air trapped in the tube which may penetrate the intestine with enema.
5. Let the water go into the rectum, retain it for two to three minutes before you visit the toilet.
6. Do not strain at stools after an enema. Straining will not help clean the bowels as they should be cleared.

An enema with warm water (from one to one-and-a-half litres) should be taken daily when you are on a diet of fruit or are fasting. If you do not take an enema, there is no derived to be derived from fasting or living on fruits alone. Such enema can help when constipation is very severe or when your are starting the naturopathic treat-ment. In the case of ordinary costiveness, a strengthening enema is advised. For that about 250 millilitres of cold water should be introduced into the intesting and retianed for five to ten minutes. Cold water enervates the intestine and gives it tone. Such an enema cab be taken daily and even twice in the day if one feels like it. But it should be taken the last thing at night before retiring.It will not harm you even if you take it for months on end.

Whether the enema water is small is quantity or not, you must let the water come out its own. Do not starian, nor be in a hurry. In the beginning you might have to spend up a half an hour in the latring after you have taken the enema.

MUD PACKS

The best way to prepare a mud pack is to take clay from about four inches below the surface of the earth. Ensure that the clay does not contain any impurities, like compost or pebbles. If there are nay pebbles, grind the clay and pass it through a sieve. Mix it with cold and see that it has a consistency like soft dough. It should stick and not be thing enough to slide down when used in the pack. If the pack is to be applied on the abdomen (from the navel to the pubes) spread the mud evently on a piece of cloth. See that it is about half an inch thick. Then place it gently with the cloth up and the mud touching the skin. Remove the cloth on the mud. You may even let the cotton remain over the mud, but cover it with a thick woolen. If that is done the patient can keep lying down without covering himself with a blanket or a sheet.

The mud pack should be used for 20 to 30 minutes. After is removed, clean the skin using a soft piece of cloth dipped in cold water.

Clay is to be found in different shades in different places, but whatever the color, it is eqally beneficial.If the mud is loamy and has a tendency to stick to the skin, some sand can be mixed with it.

HIP BATH

You must have been specially made tuds for hup baths. The tub is oval in shape and one end of it is raised so that the patient can rest his back against it. This is the ideal tub for taking a hip bath.

Fill the tub with cold water. The level of the water should be so adjusted that it touches your navel when you sit in it. Your feet will be outside the tub and you can support them by keeping a low stool in front of the tub. You can rest your back against the raised portion of the tub and remain in the half-supine position.

Take rough towel and rub your abdomen from the right to the left. Do it gently so that the skin is not scraped Do not apply too much pressure in rubbing.

A hip bath can be taken from ten to twenty minutes. Thin persons should take it for only ten minutes and the stout ones can continue for 20 minutes. During winter the duration of the hip bath should be reduced by about 25 per cent.

In the beginning, the hip bath should be taken only for a minute or two; the time should be increased gradually to ten or twenty minutes, as indicated above.

If it is too cold, rub your body with your palms for five to seven minutes before getting into the tub. A vigorous rubbing of the body will bring warmath to it and you will not experience any discomfort when you start the hip bath.

Wipe your body with a towel when you get out of the tub, dress, quickly and go for a walk or take some other exercise. Those too weak to engage in any such activity should get into bed and wrap a blanket around them and rest for half an hour to bring back warmth to their body.

You can take bath a couple of hours after the hip bath and not before.

GENITALS BATH

Keep a stool one foot long, six inches wide and six inches high in the tub. It would be all the batter if there is a circular cut in from of it. If a stool is not readily available keep four bricks, two upon two to raise the level and sit on them. The water level in the tub should be such that it is one inch above the stool. The water should be cold; during summer the water of an earthen pitcher can be used for the purpose.

Take off your clothes sit on the stool. Take a piece of cloth, dip it in water and gently rub your abdomen with if for two minutes. Then take hold of the foreskin of your penis in two fingers and rub it lightly with a soft piece of cloth dipping cold water oftger. This can be continued for ten to twenty minutes. A lean person can do it for only ten minutes,and the hefty one for as long as twenty minutes. After the rubbing of the foreskin is completed, rub the entire spine with a wet towel for two minutes. You can take hold of the wet towel in two hands and move it up and down ou your spine.

Women should rub their abdomen.They should take a piece of sof cloth, pull up the lips of the vagina and rub them slowly. And in the end they should also rub the spine as above. No hip bath or genitals bath should be taken at the time of menstruation.

You must take exercise, walk or lie down in a bed and wrap yourself in a blanket tol restore the body heat lost due to immersion in water.

If a tub is not available, this bath can be taken in the sun. In that case, spread a wet towel on the stool on which you sit. Keep a bucket full of water near the stool and take the bath as indicated above.

HOT FOOT BATH

When you have to take a foot bath, sit on a stool and lower your feet in a bucket full of hot water. The level of the water should, ideally, come up to knees. The temperature of the water should not be to much above the body temperature. As the water gets cold, go on adding more hot water. Take care to see that hot water added later does not scald the feet.

Cover yourself with a blanket. Wrap it around your body: even if the bucket is covered, it will be all right. The head should be covered with a towel wetted with cold water. As the coldness of the towel evaporates dip it in cold water, wring it lightly and again cover your head with it.

Take some hot water before your lower your feet into the bucket water. Go on sipping hot water throughout the time your feet are in the bucket.

A hot foot bath should be taken for 20 minutes. Wash your feet with cold water afterwards and wipe them with a towel. If you have perspired, wipe your body with a wet towel and dress yourself. An ordinary bath can be taken after the hot foot bath.

HOW TO TAKE A BATH

A bath is a daily ritual, but few people understand its purpose or importance. That is why most of us merely throw water over our heads and the bodies and think that we have done our duty. Throwing water over the body is beneficial, but it is not what a bath is.

The twin purposes of a bath are: cleanliness and reactivating the circulation of the blood by the tingling sensation that cold water produces as it comes into contact with the skin. The firstr purpose, i.e. cleanliness can be better served by hot watter. The skin of the body has millions of pores through which the skin breathes as we do through our lungs. It the pores are clogged, the lungs are over worked. Over work may lead to fatigue or exhaustion of the lungs. And them, closed pores do not pass any perspiration which is a must to clear the blood or morbid humours. Closed pores are a danger to the general health of human beings.

Cold water is alos a cleaning agent, but it cannot deal with the grease and dirt infestingf the pores of the skin. Hot water mixed with lemon juice is the bestg cleansing agent for the skin. Or, better still, take a lemon and loast it light over a fire, then cut in into two parts, dip a part in hot water and rub it over your skin. This will cleanse your skin as no soap can do. But a hot bath should not be taken daily. It generally brings lethargy, weakness and shows down the digestive processes. Once or twice a week is enough if your have to take a hot bath. The temperature of the water should not be more than one of two degrees above body temperature.

A hot bath retiring for the night is the best ofr your heath. It helps you to sleep better and if you cover your body after a hot bath, it will save you from the danger exposure. A bath, hot or cold, should be taken one hour before meals or three hours after it.

Really hot water for a bath has its own advantages but it sould be used sparingly. If you are suffering from a cold, take a hot bath, cove yourself with woolens and get into bed. It will drive away the cold. A really hot bath when you are tired acts as a tonic: it drives away fitigue as nothing else does.

A bath with hot water has its uses, but a daily with should be cold water. When the skin is cooled by cold water, blood rushes to warm it up. The circulation of the blood is activated and the blood is also cleansed is a prelude to old age. A cold bath is, therefore, instrumental in keeping us young.

The best way to start a bath is to rub the whole of your body with your palms or with a rough towel . Start with your scalp, forehead, face and the neck .Then go on to you wrists and then to the shoulders through the arms. Afterwards rub your chest, the arm pits and abdomen and the back. The feet should be last to receive attention. Keep your feet straight when you rub them. Start from the feet and come upto the thighs. In the beginning, rub gently but later increase the pressure.

After the vigorousd rubbing, take a cold bath. Wipe your body with a towel. Start with the head and then dry up the whole body. You will feel a peculiar kind of pleasure whey you rub your body after a bath. For weak persons a rubbing can do the job of exercise.

If this methods of taking a bath is adopted, there will not be any danger of any skin eruptons or itch. The face will be free of pimples and other blemishes which mar its beauty. The skin will acquire a healthy glow and if it is rough and leathery, it will become pink and soft. You will have the feeling as if you have been having an oil massage.

If the palms of the hand are used to dry up the body after a bath instead of a towel, it will be doubly benefical. It gives a pleasant sensation during winter.

WET PACK FOR THE WAIST

The bandage to be used as a wet pack forf the waist be seven to eight feet long and six inches broad. It should be of soft cotton cloth. Dip it in cold water, wring it lightly and wrap it around your waist. It should cover the areas from the navel to a little above the pubes and should remain in direct contect with the skin. Cover the wet bandage with a woolen cloth of equal dimensions and secure and with a safety pin or a string so that it does not lossen up.

There will be a cold sensation on the skin covered by the wet pack but after about ten minutes, warmth will return. If you still feel cold after ten minutes, that is an indication that the bandge has been wrapped lightly and has to be tightened. Or, the bandage has not been properly wrung out or it is thicker than it should be.

The wet pack for the waist can be used from half and hour to two hours at a time.

WET PACK FOR THE CHEST

The dimensions of the bandage for the chest should be same as for the waist. It should be similarly dipped in cold water, wrung out and wrapped round the chest and covered by a woolen piece of cloth. It should be wrapped in such a way that it should cover the chest, the upper part of the shoulders and the corresponding portion of the back. The woolen covering for the wet pack should be secured with a safety pin or a piece of string as in the case of the waist pack.

This pack can also be used for half an hour to two hours.

SUNBATHING

Sunbathing is an important tool of the naturopath. Even though people in the west use it for cosmetic purposes, it plays an important part in restoring health.

In Indian conditions, the ideal times for a sunbath during summer is six to six thirty in the morning and during winter from seven to seven thirty.

Take off all your clothes and sit in a secluded corner away from interruptions. The whole of your body should be exposed to the health-giving rays of the sun.

In the beginning take a sun bath for only two to three minutes but increase the timing gradually to fifteen to twenty minutes.

When the sunlight is very hot, cover your head with a towel. If you cannot find a secluded place to take the sun bath, cover yourself with a light cotton sheet.

SUNBATHING FOR INDUCING PERSPIRATION :

Sweat can be induced through a sun bath. For this purpose the sun is hot enough at ten to eleven in the morning in summer and two in three in the afternnon in winter. Take hot water and lie down naked on a mattress or spread on the floor. If the wind is strong, Choose a place in the lee of the wind.

You will start sweating in about ten to fifteen minutes after you have lied down. After fifeen to twenty minutes the sweat will start running down your body. The sun bath can be continued for fifteen to twenty minutes. Whether you sweat or not, you must take a cold bath just after it.

Some people may not perspire in the beginning but after repeating the sun bath for three or four days, their sweat glands will be activated and they will perspire.

You must cover your head with a your head with a wet towel while taking a sun bath, but at the same time go on sipping warm water to aid the body to produce the sweat.

SPONGING THE BODY :

When you are running a temperature, a sponge bath is more advisable than a bath. The patient shoudlbe covered with a sheet or blanket and his body should be wiped with a wet towel. Wipe his feet first, one after the other, rub them with them wet towel for four to five minutes and then wipe them witha dry towel. But even when the feet have been dried rub them with the palms of the hands so that some heat it generated in the body. In the case of fever, such rubbing is not advised.

After the feet been attended to, go to the calves and the rest of the legs, the abdomen, the chest, the back, the face and the neck. The hands should be rubbed for five or six minutes and the abdomen, chest and the back a little longer.

The total time taken for a sponge bath is on an average half an hour. The ideal time for a sponge bath is mid day.

FASTING :

Nothing but water should be taken when you are fasting. The intake of water must be two to two and a half litres. One feels fresh if one counties drinking water and the intake of water also help the expulsion of morbid matter from the body.

In the evening of the first day of the fast and the morning after, an enema of hot water should be taken to clean the bowls.

One day's fasting should be followed by a food intake 25% less than one normally takes. A two days' fast should be followed by ingestion of fruits only the next day; normal food should follow the next day. A three days' fast should be followed the next day by fruit juices and soup of vegetables (the soup must be clear, without addition of any thickening agents or condiments). On the fifth day eat fruits only and on the sixth breakfast on fruits, lunch on bread and boiled vegetables and repeat a fruit diet for your dinner. It is only afterwards that you should resume your normal diet.

FRUITS, FRUITJUICES AND MILK DIETS:

When you have been advised to live on fruit juices or juices or soups of vegetables, you should take about 250 millions of fruit juice or juice or clear soup of a vegetable three or four times in the day. The best juices are those of oranges, pineapple, rose apple, raspberry and tomatoes. If the juice is too thick, mix it with plain water in the porportion of 1: ¾th.

Juice of gourd, tomatoes and carrot can be taken in its natural form. If you do not have a juicer (a machine to extract the juice of fruits) grate the fruits or vegetables and squeeze them though fine muslin or other finemeshed cloth.

Other vegetables have to be half a kilogram and should be boiled in 250 millilitres of water and the juice drunk.

When you are living on fruit, take them thrice daily. But take one kind of fruit at one meal. For example, you can take the same fruit at all meal times, it would be still better.

The whole intake of fruits in the day should be more than one to one and a half kilograms.

When a diet of fruit and milk is indicated, take 250 to 300 millilitres of milk with the fruits. If your appetite improves, as it should, the quantity of the milk can be increased to half a litre at one time. Unboiled milk should be taken in the morning and even during lunch time milk boiled in the morning can be ingested. Sip the milk as you munch the fruit. It will be more beneficial then eating the fruit and drinking the milk.

Even when you are on a diet of fruit juices, do not forget to drink one to two litres of water in the day. If your bowels do not move automatically during the fruit and diet, take recourse to an enema. But the bowels must be evacuated properly and no morbid humors or substances should be allowed to accumulate in the body.

WATER AND FOOD INTAKE OF WATER :

One must drink one to one a half litre of water in 24 hours. The best time for taking water is the first thing in the morning, one hour before meals and two hours after. If you must drink water during the meals, see that the quantity does not exceed 200 to 250 millilitres. If you have taken water one hour before the meal, you will not feel the need to take it during eating. But still, water may be taken during the meal according to need and inclination.

TIME OF MEALS :

The interval between two meals should be five hours or more. The last meal of the day must be eaten two or three hours before you get bed. Breakfast between seven to eight in the morning, lunch between 12 noon and one in the afternoon and dine between six and seven in the evening.

WHOLEMEAL BREAD :

The best wheat flour is when you have cleaned and dried the wheat and ground it through a hand mill (chakki). Do not pass the flour through a sieve so that the bran is not separated. Bran is the substance which provides roughage needed to avoid constipation and it also contains the necessary vitamins. The dough should be kneaded two to three hours before it is used for chapatis.

The chapati should be thick, but it needs patience to cook it properly. A thin chapati is, of course,the best since most people are likely to count the number of chapatis they take without regard to their size or thickness.

Do not eat the chapati with the vegetables since you may not chew it properly. Eat them separately or alternate mouthfuls of chapatis and vegetables.

PORRIDGE :

Good qualty, properly cleaned wheat should be used for being ground into porridgo. Each wheat grain should be broken into eight to ten pieces. Flour and larger should be separated at the porridge should be toasted over a hot plate lightly till it turns brown. It should not be too thick or too thin.

It should be cooked over a slow fir till it is properly done. It should not be mixed with salt or milk, even though people are in the habit of adding these substances to porridge.

The best sweetening agent for the porridge would be raisins added to it while it is being boiled.

RICE :

Unmilled rice is the best. The necessary vitamins which are found in this cereal are lost in the process of milling and polishing. The paddy should be treated at home with the help of a pestle which only separates the husk and leaves other elements intact.

Add only enough water to cook the rice. If too much water is added, it would have to be either dried up/by heat or passed through a sieve, destroying its starch and also some other vital elements.

VEGETABLES :

Vegetables which can be eaten with their rind on, should be eaten unpealed. If the outer covering is hard, scarp it with a sharp knife. Wash the vegetables before the cutting them into smaller pieces.

Add a little ghee or sesame, coconut or groundnut oil and add a few cumminseeds and let vegetables contain natural moisture and water does not have to be added to them for cooking. The most that you can do is to cover them with a lid and put a little water over it so that some moisture is added to the pen in which the vegetables is cooking. Try to see that the natural moisture of the vegetable is not burnt by excessive heat since many vital elem are thus lost.

Salt, turmeric, cumminseed may be added as seasoning. The less salt you take the better it is. If you feel like taking ghee, add it after the vegetable has been cooked and not before.

SALADS :

A salad is prepared out of raw vegetables. All vegetables which can be eaten raw can form part of the salad. For example, you can eat cucumber, carrot, radish, onions, tamatoes, spinach, green cofriander and cabbage for salad. Take any three of these vegetables and cut them into small pieces, season them with salt if you must, but the would be to eat them as they are. The normal amount of salad per head (adult) should not be more than 250 grams.

You can add a little curd also to the salad if you like.

A salad can be made out of fruits also. The best time to take the salad is before is meal.

WALKING, DEEP BREATHING AND SLEEP

During a walk, you most move briskly. Your back should be straight and the arms moving.

The normal speed of walking should be about four miles per hour. Take a different route for a walk every day as that would be more enjoyable instead of taking the same route every day.

Five to six miles walk in the morning and two t three miles in the evening is the best. Those who are starting to take a walk should not overstrain themselves but increase the distance gradually.

DEEP BREATHING :

Deep breaths should be taken during a walk. Inhalation should become a natural become a rhythm with you. Inhalation and exhalation should both be done slowly.

SLEEP :

Sleep should be sufficient to give a sense of relief from exhaustion. But do not oversleep, nor laze about in bed when your are not sleeping.The ideal time for sleep is form nine O' Clock in the night to five in the morning. Those who feel sleepy all the time return to normal sleeping hours after some days.

During summer, a siesta for an hour or so will refresh you. If you cannot sleep, relax for an hour after lunch.

How to sprout:

For sprouting moisture and warmth are needed. The procedure for sprouting is very simple and easy, As explained below:

1. Clean the seeds throughtly and weed out the defective ones as also tiny pieces of hard substances.
2. Wash the seeds with water several times to ensure that no dirt remains.
3. Soak these washed seeds in water, preferably in an earthern pot The water should be 5 to 7 centimeters (two to three inches) above the seeds.
4. The sees should remain soaked in water for six to ten hours. Some harder Seeds, such as soybeans, will require more time, while other will require less time. Ten hours is the maximum time because after that they will to rot. By soaking, the seeds absorbed sufficient moisture necessary for bringing them into life. This purpose is fully served in six to ten hours. The best course is to soak before going to bed and take them out in the morning.
5. After taking out trhe soaked seeds from the water, wash them several times with fresh water.
6. Take a thick piece of cloth of a size according to the quantity of the sprouts to made. Soaked and washed seeds should be put into this piece of cloth and loosely tied. This small bundle may be hung on a peg or kept some where. It may be useful to expose this bundle to the morning sun for an hour or so.
7. After 10 to 14 hours, the seeds will germinate. Tiny sprouts will poke their way out and began to grow. The time will very according to season. In hot season the germination takes less than in cold season.
8. During the period the seeds are kept tried in the cloth, it should be ensured that this bundle does not go dry. water is to be sprinkled over it several times during the day especially in hot season to kept it always wet. Twice or thrice during the day the seeds are to flushed with water several times to remove the shine that generally accumulates on them.
9. Soybean or similar other seeds require more time for sprouting. They require more warmth also. Seeds, after being tied in cloth, should be fully covered with some woolen piece all around and kept some where, with heavy weight placed on them. Let remain there for ten or fifteen hours and they will sprout. The time required will be more or less, according to season.
10. After the seeds sprout, they are ready for use. If the sprouting is allowed to continue longer, the nutritonal value increases tremendously.

11. If the sprouts are exposed to indirect sunlight for the last two hours before consumption, they will became green and affractive.

12. After sprouting and before consumption, remove all the defective and hard seeds which have not sprouted. This picking has to be necessarily done in the case of soybean, pulses like moth and moong otherwise while eating if any hard seed comes under your teeth, the whole taste is spoiled. A little time spent in weeding out defective seeds will make you relish the sprouts more.

13. It is the best to wash and rinse the sprouts before eating. Afterwards they should be placed in a thick dry cloth and tied tightly to remove excess moisture. You will relish more if the sprouts have less moisture.

14. After the seeds have sprouted, they can be placed in a covered container and kept in the refrigerator. They can last of several days without spoiling. Please remember to keep them covered. They will not spoil even when kept outside thed refrigerator also but must be washed and then their extra moisture removed as explained earlier.

15. Each sprouted seed can be eaten by itself without the addition of salt of any other condiments. They have their own delicious taste. why spoil it with any additions? However, to create variety and taste, mix several sprouts such as moong, moth (Kidney bean) gram and alveoli. In the beginning take sprouts in a small quantity and after pounding or grinding them in a blender or otherwise. When they are easily digested, increase their proportion in your diet.

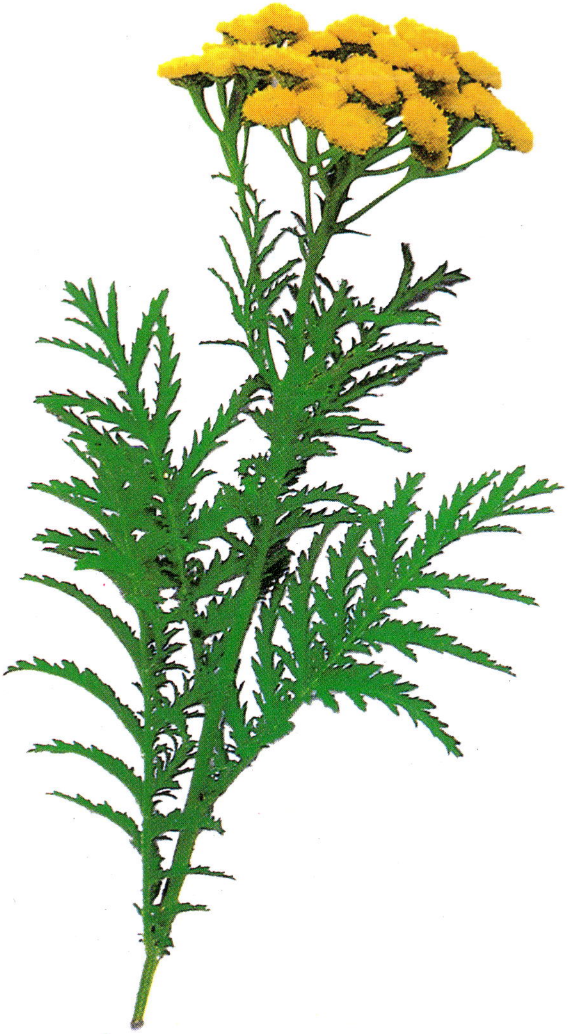

Bibliography

1. Bailey & Love's short Practice of Surgery: Mann, Russell, ELBS.
2. Robins, Pathologic Basis of Disease, WB Sannders Company.
3. Swami Satyanand Saraswati, A System Course in the Ancient Tantrik Techniques of Yoga and Kriya.
4. Alan W. Watts, Nature Man and Woman.
5. Zachgry F. Landsdowne Ph.D., The Chakras & Esoteric Healing.
6. BKS Iyengar, Light on Yoga Sutras of Patanjali.
7. Cancer Research, Official Journal of the American Association for Cancer Research (Vol. 51 No. 11)
8. Cell DF, Review of the article by Meyerowitz BE, Heinrich RL, Coscarelli Schag CA, Helping patients cope with cancer.
9. Swinehart 1968, quoted from Johnson JD, Meishcke H: Differences in evaluations of communication channels for cancer related information.
10. Floravanti M., Di Cesare F, Ramellil et al.: Pre-surgery information and psychological adjustments to enterrostomy.
11. Brown P., Ames N., Mettger W et al.: Closing the comprehension gap: Low literacy and the cancer information service.
12. Michielutte R., Dignan MB, Wells Hb, Development of a community cancer education program: The Forsyth Country, NC cervical cancer prevention project.
13. Waitzkin H: Information giving a medical care.
14. Reid AAL, 1977, quoted from Freimuth VASANT VIHAR, Stein JA., Kean TJ: Searching for health information: The Cancer information services model.
15. Marcus AC, bettinghous EXPORT MANAGER, Mazan KD et al.: The cancer information servicer: A 15 year history of service and research-introduction.
16. Humphrey GB, Littlewood JL, Kamps WA: Physician/patients communication model considering the interaction of physicians' therapeutic strategy and patients coping style.
17. Meyerowitz BE, Heinrich RL, Coscarelli Schag CA: Helping patients cope with cancer.
18. Astrological Magazine, India

INDEX